Essential Burn Care
for Non-Burn Specialists

Jong O. Lee
Editor

Essential Burn Care
for Non-Burn Specialists

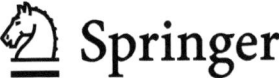 Springer

Editor
Jong O. Lee
Department of Surgery
University of Texas Medical Branch
Galveston, TX, USA

ISBN 978-3-031-28897-5   ISBN 978-3-031-28898-2   (eBook)
https://doi.org/10.1007/978-3-031-28898-2

This Springer imprint is published by the registered company Springer
Nature Switzerland AG
The registered company address is: Gewerbestrasse 11, 6330 Cham, Switzerland

To my mom and dad, Kwang and Ik.

To my sister, Amanda, and nephews, Trent and Andrew.

For their love and support.

To my mentors Drs. Richard Moore and David Herndon.

For their encouragement.

Contents

1 **Epidemiology** 1
   Barclay T. Stewart

2 **Pathophysiology and Hypermetabolic
   Response to Burn** 29
   Roohi Vinaik, Dalia Barayan,
   and Marc G. Jeschke

3 **Initial Assessment of Burn Patient** 85
   Matthew A. DePamphilis and Robert L. Sheridan

4 **Initial Management and Resuscitation** 113
   Leopoldo C. Cancio and Jill M. Cancio

5 **Inhalation Injury** 145
   Axel Rodriguez and Alexis McQuitty

6 **Burn Wound Management** 167
   Paige J. South, Deepak K. Ozhathil,
   Amina El Ayadi, and Steven E. Wolf

7 **Treatment of Facial Burns** 181
   Alen Palackic, Robert P. Duggan, Rahul Shah,
   Jong O. Lee, and Ludwik K. Branski

8 **Treatment of Hand Burns** 197
   Tina L. Palmieri

9 **Burn Wound Infection** 213
   Joseph E. Marcus, Kevin K. Chung,
   and Dana M. Blyth

10 Pediatric Burns 233
Eric S. Ruff, Nikhil R. Shah,
Ramon L. Zapata-Sirvent, and Jong O. Lee

11 Elderly Burns 255
Robyn Richmond and Sharmila Dissanaike

12 Electrical Injuries 267
Manrique Guerrero, Casey Kohler,
and Brett Arnoldo

13 Chemical Burns 285
Henry B. Huson and Herb A. Phelan

14 ICU Care of Burn Patients 301
Molly Hunter and David T. Harrington

15 Pain Management in Burn Patients 315
Jordan B. Starr, Paul I. Bhalla, and Sam R. Sharar

16 Outpatient Burn Care 335
Barclay T. Stewart and Nicole S. Gibran

17 Telemedicine 365
Lauren B. Nosanov and Amalia Cochran

18 Burn Disasters 383
Wendy Y. Rockne, Victor C. Joe,
and James C. Jeng

**19 Exfoliative Skin Diseases: Stevens-Johnson
Syndrome and Toxic Epidermal Necrolysis** 405
Felicia N. Williams and Jong O. Lee

20 Burn Scar and Contracture Management 415
Jorge Leon-Villapalos, David Zergaran,
and Tom Calderbank

21 Burn Rehabilitation 433
Lynne Benavides, Betsey Ferreira,
Oscar E. Suman, and Jeffrey C. Schneider

22 Anesthesia for Burn Patients .449
Jamie L. Sparling and J. A. Jeevendra Martyn

Index 479

Chapter 1
Epidemiology

Barclay T. Stewart

Burden of Disease

In the absence of systematic injury data collection and minimal burn injury surveillance activities, much of the data available to estimate the burden of burn injuries or temporal trends has been gathered through hospital registries, police and fire service reports, mortuary reports, and isolated representative, community-based surveys. Each of these modalities for data collection has specific strengths and limitations regarding ability to detect injuries and fatalities, bias related to differential abilities to access care, and infrastructure requirements. As a result, the patchwork of data available makes it difficult to accurately, comprehensively, and longitudinally describe the burden of burn injuries globally. Several key definitions and concepts provided in Table 1.1 might be useful prior to reading this chapter and considering how you might use epidemiological information to reduce the burden of burn injuries in your region.

B. T. Stewart (✉)
Division of Trauma, Burn and Critical Care Surgery, UW Medicine Regional Burn Center, University of Washington, Harborview Medical Center, Seattle, WA, USA
e-mail: barclays@uw.edu

© The Author(s), under exclusive license to Springer Nature Switzerland AG 2023
J. O. Lee (ed.), *Essential Burn Care for Non-Burn Specialists*,
https://doi.org/10.1007/978-3-031-28898-2_1

TABLE I.I Key definitions and concepts to promote understanding and use of epidemiological data to reduce the burden of burn injuries locally and regionally

Term	Definition or concept
Incidence	Rate of occurrence of a condition or injury (e.g., new cases) measured as number per number-at-risk per unit time (e.g., 10 burns per 1,000 children per year).
Prevalence	Proportion of a population who have a specific characteristic in a given time period.
Active surveillance	A system that tasks staff members to regularly contact emergency care systems, health care providers, or populations to seek information about burns. Active surveillance provides more accurate and timely information, but it is also expensive and resource intensive.
Passive surveillance	A system by which a health jurisdiction receives reports submitted from emergency care services, hospitals, clinics, public health units, mortuaries, or other sources. Passive surveillance is a relatively inexpensive strategy to cover large areas, and it provides critical information for monitoring a community's health. However, because passive surveillance depends on people in different institutions to provide data, data quality and timeliness are difficult to control. Additionally, the data are skewed toward populations with fewer barriers to care.
Integrated surveillance	A combination of active and passive systems that use a single infrastructure to gather information about multiple conditions, injuries, or behaviors.

(continued)

TABLE 1.1 (continued)

Term	Definition or concept
Syndromic surveillance	An active and/or passive system that uses case definitions that are based entirely on clinical features without any clinical or laboratory diagnosis (e.g., burn injuries rather than flame, scald, electrical). Because syndromic surveillance is inexpensive and simple, it is often the first kind of surveillance begun in a low-resource setting.
Community-based survey	Representative sampling of a population, typically through household surveys, in order to gain information about risk factors, conditions, and deaths within a preceding time period. Community-based surveys are the most accurate method for determining injury epidemiology and mitigate some of the selection bias associated with barriers to care in passive surveillance systems but are also the most costly and time consuming.

Incidence

It is estimated that there are between 7 and 12 million people who sustain burn injuries that require medical care, cause prolonged absence from work or school, or result in death each year [1]. As a result, burns from fire, heat, and hot substances are the fourth most common etiology of injury globally behind road traffic incidents, falls, and violence. For comparison, the incidence of burn injuries is greater than that of HIV/AIDS and tuberculosis combined and approaches the incidence of all malignant neoplasms [2].

Using highly modeled data from varied sources (e.g., passive surveillance systems, burn center registries, mortuaries, fire services) and with some rare exceptions, there is evidence that the age-standardized incidence rate has not changed significantly for most countries except the most wealthy, where it has likely decreased by about 10% [1]. These declines in incidence in high-income countries are the result of increasing socioeconomic status of specific population groups, improved working conditions, national safety policies, and awareness campaigns [3]. In addition to national income, the incidence of burn injuries and deaths varies markedly by age, gender, socioeconomic status, national income, region, and several other factors.

Injuries Managed at Hospitals and Burn Centers

The incidence of people who seek care are admitted or die from burn injuries represents the minority of injuries that occur (Fig. 1.1). However, people with burn injuries evaluated at hospitals represent an opportunity to decrease preventable morbidity and mortality with timely and effective service delivery. Therefore, understanding the epidemiology of this injury group can be used to guide optimal resource allocation and reduce disability.

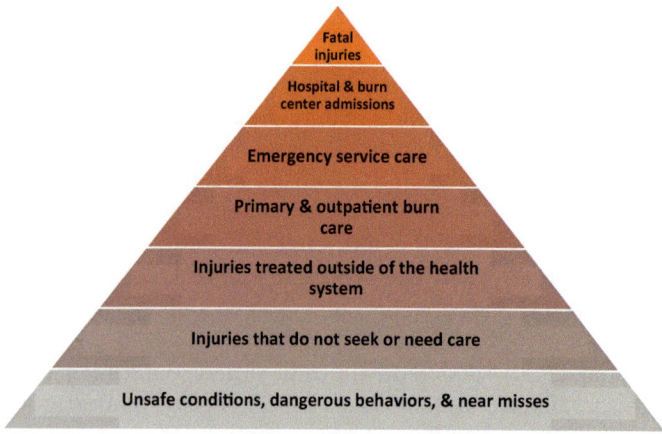

FIGURE 1.1 Epidemiological pyramid of burn hazards and injuries

The incidence of burns managed in emergency departments and outpatient clinics globally that require inpatient care for their injuries is between 5 and 26 patients per 100,000 population [4]. This represents the minority of people with burn injuries who require care and are admitted to a hospital, particularly in regions where outpatient services are well-established. As example, a study from the United States reported that 8% of burn-injured patients evaluated in an emergency department were admitted or transferred to a regional burn center [5]. However, the incidence of burns that require hospital-based care are markedly higher in many low- and middle-income countries due to both higher incidence and less ability to provide outpatient burn care (e.g., 8.0 per 10,000 children in Ethiopia, 6.3 per 10,000 children in Ghana) [4, 6].

Emergency departments and outpatient clinics in high-income and some regions within lower income countries (e.g., United States, United Kingdom) have witnessed a decrease in the number of burn injury-related encounters for more than two decades [7]. It is hypothesized that this is due to a decreasing incidence and severity of injury due to systematic prevention and control initiatives, as well as an increasing availability of burn first aid and outpatient care resources [8].

The majority of people who have sustained a burn injury and seek care can safely be managed as outpatients. In a European review of 76 reports that involved 186,500 patients, the annual incidence for burn injuries requiring admission to a multidisciplinary burn center was 0.2 to 2.9 per 10,000 people [9]. In the Netherlands, the incidence approached 1 per 100,000 person years for burns ≥20% total body surface area (TBSA). Other studies from high-income countries including Australia, Singapore, and United States have reported that burns ≥20% TBSA comprise less than 20% of burn injuries requiring inpatient care [10, 11].

Mortality

Between 100,000 and 350,000 people die each year from burn injuries [1, 4, 12]. The overwhelming majority of burn injuries and deaths occur in low- and middle-income countries, which are frequently ill-equipped to success-fully prevent and care for burns and where data are sparse. As example, mortality to incidence ratios of low- and middle-income countries are multiple times higher than those in high-income countries due to advances in burn prevention (e.g., building codes, fire and smoke alarms, safer cooking arrangements) and mature emergency and burn care systems [1]. Although data sources are sparse, there may be a general decline in burn injury-related mortality globally.

The University of Washington (UW) Institute of Health Metrics and Evaluation (IHME) Global Burden of Disease Study (GBD) modeled the burden of fire, heat, and hot substances in 2017 by updating key fatal and non-fatal data, leveraging covariables to improve estimation in data-sparse regions, and utilizing state-of-the-art spatiotemporal statistical modeling techniques [1, 3]. IHME models suggested that the global age-standardized mortality rate was 1.6 per 100,000 injuries (95% UI 1.3 to 1.7), which equated to 120,632 deaths (95% UI 101,630 to 129,383) in 2017. Based on these estimates, the world might have witnessed a 46.6% (95% UI −49.7 to −38.8) decrease in age-standardized mortality from 1990 to 2017. The greatest declines in mortality were witnessed by high-income countries and the lowest by sub-Saharan Africa, South and Central Asia, and Eastern Europe.

Although these estimates are encouraging, numerous experts in burn prevention and control have suggested that these reductions do not seem consistent with injury-related mortality broadly, cluster-randomized community-based surveys of burn injury, and gains in burn prevention and care capacity in low- and middle-income countries specifically. Some of the limitations of these data include:

1. Relative absence of data from low- and middle-income countries where incidence of injury, prevalence of disability, and death are the highest
2. Patchwork of data from active and integrated surveillance systems, hospital registries, fire service records, mortuary data, and community-based surveys
3. Differences in criteria for and behavior in seeking burn center-level care have changed over time, making longitudinal comparison challenging
4. Classification schemes of cause codes and injuries (e.g., burns, amputation, bodily harm) vary in operationalization in registries across hospitals and countries

Global and Local Inequities

As differences in the incidence, hospital admissions, and mortality provided above demonstrate that the burden of burn injuries are not equitably distributed globally. The health, social, and financial burdens are unfairly carried predominantly by people living in low- and middle-income countries where prevention and control programs are uncommon, and access to organized emergency, trauma, and burn care systems is limited [13]. Burn injuries are a dramatic example of the inequity of injury globally and even across socioeconomic divides within countries.

As examples, about 90% of deaths from burn injuries occur in low- and lower middle-income countries compared to 7% in upper middle-income and 3% in high-income countries [1]. The rate of child injury death from fire and flames is more than 10 times higher in low-income countries than in high-income countries [4, 6, 14]. In high-income countries, the child mortality rate from fire and flames is 3% of the rate of death from unintentional injuries of all types; in low-income countries, the child mortality rate is over 10% [15].

Burn injuries occur disproportionately to racial and ethnic minorities and minoritized people in high-income countries. In the United States, the proportion of Black infants who require hospitalization for burn injury is double the proportion of Black infants in the general population [16–18]. In Canada, the age-standardized mortality rate for fire-related mortality among First Nations people was 4.3 times that of other races combined [19]. This disparity has also been reported in the United States, Greenland, and Australia [20–24].

The very low incidence of non-fatal burn injuries among Hispanic people, in comparison to other people with other ethnicities, treated in the United States suggests that many Hispanic people living with burn injuries are being treated in their homes, potentially in manners that are below standard-of-care [4]. Even in countries with mature health systems and surveillance programs, representative community-based surveys can play important roles. As example, community-based surveys are needed in the United States to establish the degree to which minoritized and undocumented patients utilize the healthcare system for treatment of burn injuries. Only with an accurate appreciation of the burden and distribution of burn injuries within a population can effective interventions and advocacy initiatives be created.

Risk Factors for Fires and Burn Injuries

Major fire and burn injury risk factors include age, gender, socioeconomic status, race and ethnicity, and comorbidities. These risk factors often co-exist within people and populations and act synergistically and exponentially exacerbating the problem. Conversely, when risk factors and hazards co-exist, they can be addressed simultaneously with targeted prevention and control initiatives with minimal additional resources.

Age

Age is consistently and strongly associated with the etiology, incidence, and mortality of burn injuries regardless of national income. With markedly changing local and global population structures, the epidemiology of burn injuries will too change. Prevention professionals, policymakers, burn centers, and health systems will need to anticipate these changes and adapt their interventions and service delivery capabilities to meet future demands.

Children

Infants and children aged <5 years are at high risk of injury. Infants commonly sustain scald injuries related to hot bottles, being near mothers and older siblings who are cooking, and spills. Toddler-aged children are newly mobile and curious and have little inhibitions or prior knowledge and experience with flame, scald, and electrical hazards. Beginning at six months of age, children start reaching for objects and crawling and are fully mobile by 18 months. This escalation in motor skills and activity increases the chances that children will encounter hot liquids and solids, electrical cords, candles, fireplaces, microwaves, treadmills, curling irons, ovens, cookstoves, chemicals, and other harmful agents. As example, the majority of scald burns in the United States are children between the ages of six and 36 months from hot foods and liquids (e.g., soup, tea, coffee) spilled in the kitchen or eating area [25–28]. A major risk factor for toddler-aged burn injuries is lack of supervision [29–31]. The ability to supervise infants is complex and related to maternal and child ages, socioeconomic status, education level, social support, cooking arrangement, home design, availability of older children, household and societal norms, school availability, health promotion and awareness campaigns, and other reasons. Interventions that aim to support child supervision and introduce protective barriers when supervision may be difficult (e.g., home visits and education, distribution of playpens, creation of community creches) reduce incidence and severity of multiple injury types, including burn injuries [30, 31]. Numerous other factors are associated with child burn injury and death, including use of working smoke alarms, residential fire sprinklers, fire-retardant chemicals in fabrics and upholstery, and healthcare systems that prioritize pediatric care education and resources [4, 32]. Fire-related mortality rates increase again after age 15 years, presumably related to greater exposure to and severity of hazards, experimentation with high-risk behaviors, and new employment. Fires and burns are the third most common cause of unintentional injury and death in children.

The majority of burns sustained by children are non-fatal. The United States National Center for Injury Prevention and Control reported that 90% of children who sustain burn injury in the United States and evaluated in emergency departments are not admitted to the hospital. Further, two-thirds of children admitted to the hospital for burn injuries were reported to have sustained burns <10% total body surface area (TBSA) [33]. Regardless, in countries with limited burn care capacity or among populations with limited access to care, even small injuries can result in significant disabilities [34]. As example, a community-based survey of burn injuries in four low- and middle-income countries found that 17% of children with burn injuries experienced disability that lasted >6 weeks, and 8% were anticipated to experience lifelong disability due to their injury [35].

Elderly

Older people (i.e., age ≥60 years) are also at high risk of burn injury. Their susceptibility is related to deterioration in dexterity, coordination, balance, judgment, and cognition secondary to aging, medications, and comorbidities. Along with infants, the elderly are at the highest risk of dying in structure fires and being burned by hot baths and showers [4, 36, 37]. Unlike children, the elderly poorly tolerate even small and shallow burn injuries, signaling the negative impacts of the pathophysiological cascades that stem from injury and healthcare interventions, as well as burns being a symptom of frailty and poor physiological reserve [38–40]. As a result, the elderly have the highest mortality to incidence ratio of any age-group. Age, alongside burn size and inhalation injury, is one of the three factors most associated with in-hospital mortality after burn injury. Whereas the percentage of TBSA burned at which 50% of patients will die (LA_{50}) in high-income settings is over 90% in children aged <5 years, the LA_{50} for patients aged 70–79 is <40% TBSA, and for those aged ≥80 years the LA_{50} is <20% TBSA. Data from the United States National Burn Repository suggests that in-hospital mortality is 9% for elderly in the seventh decade of life, 16% for those in the eighth decade of life, and 25% for those ≥80 years. These mortality rates are particularly striking when compared to those of adults aged 18–49 years (3%) and children (<1%). A large proportion of the elderly who lived at home prior to their injuries are discharged to skilled nursing facilities or long-term acute care facilities following hospitalization for burn care [41].

Several behaviors increase the inherent risks faced by elderly. For instance, older individuals who smoke are more likely to die of fire, smoke inhalation, and burns than younger people who smoke [4]. Many elderly people also live in households that do not have smoke detectors or may be unable to maintain them (e.g., leave the home to purchase batteries, climb on a step ladder to reach the detector, deploy the dexterity to change the batteries) [42]. Similarly, many elderly also suffer from energy poverty and may be exposed to unsafe heating hazards, which have been documented to be the most common reason for elderly residential fires in the United States.

Gender

Burns, like other injuries, have significant gender-related differences that appear soon after infancy. Boys are more likely to be injured and about 25 to 70% more likely to die from an injury than girls [4, 43]. Several explanations for these differences have been proposed and validated in some populations: boys are less likely to be supervised and allowed to roam further from home with fewer limits; boys socialize differently and engage in higher risk behaviors more frequently; and boys have higher activity levels and behave more impulsively than do girls. Gender differences are also observed in adults. Burn injury rates among people who seek healthcare in the United States have been reported to be about 50% greater among men than women (270 vs. 180 per 100,000, respectively) [44].

After infancy, differences in exposures to hazards like unsafe cookstoves and cooking arrangements, household work, and clothing between high- and low-income countries are, in large part, responsible for women and girls experiencing a higher incidence and mortality rate from burn injuries than men and boys. Clothing ignition is a common cause of burn injuries, particularly in countries where the predominant attire worn by women is loose fitting and flammable, like saris, chadarees, paranjas, and burqas (e.g., South Asia, Central Asia, Middle East and North Africa, sub-Saharan Africa). As a result and in contrast to the epidemiology in high-income countries, the mortality rate among females is more than twice that of males in many low- and middle-income countries, particularly in sub-Saharan Africa, Eastern Mediterranean, South Asia, and Southeast Asia [1, 45, 46].

Cooking and Cookstoves

About 90% of burn injuries occur in and around the home—most of which are related to cooking [47]. In areas without electrification, use of open flames and rudimentary cooking arrangements (e.g., 3-stone fires, clay pots) are common [6, 48]. Further, cooking arrangements are often inside of the home and on the ground, which is accessible to even small children. Common fuels for such cookstoves include biomass (e.g., wood, charcoal, leaves, dung), kerosene, and paraffin. The risk of injury related to cookstoves is increased by a lack of enclosure for open fires, cookstove instability, nearby storage of flammable fuels, flammable and loose-fitting clothing, combustible household materials, insufficient smoke alarm mechanisms, and lack of multiple exits.

Nearly half of the world's population is exposed to harmful levels of indoor air pollution and unnecessary fire and burn injury risks from rudimentary cooking arrangements. More than 4 million children and adults die prematurely each year from consequences of exposures to these cooking arrangements, with upwards of 300,000 deaths per year from cooking-related burns [49]. Transitioning households to improved or liquid propane gas (LPG) cookstoves can save lives, prevent disability, mitigate deforestation during the collection of solid biomass fuels, and promote social and gender equity related to more efficient cooking arrangements. However, as more households in resource-limited settings move away from biomass and kerosene as a fuel source for domestic stoves and heaters, there has been a subsequent increase in the number of injuries sustained from the use of natural gas and propane cookstoves [48]. While much research and program development have gone into the design of energy-efficient cookstoves and implementation of improved and LPG cookstoves, little has been done to document and improve key safety features in real-world settings (e.g., tip ability, projection of flame, radiant heat, contact points) [50]. Developing safer cookstoves with policies and regulations that facilitate their use is critically needed.

Occupation

Occupational exposure to hazards and work-specific behaviors also exert differential burn injury risk within populations. About 10–20% of burn injuries that present to United States emergency departments are work related [44]. However, this is likely skewed upward due to pressure from employers and workers' compensation plans to present for evaluations in burns that would otherwise be managed with emergency care. Workers in the construction, welding, utilities, concrete, transportation, mining, agriculture, and firefighting fields are particularly at high risk of injury and being unable to return to work after injury with dedicated vocational rehabilitation [51,

52]. Additionally, homemakers and informal workers (e.g., undocumented migrant laborers, lawn maintenance workers, jacks-of-all-trades) are likely at high risk given their exposures to hazards and lack of formal protections, but data around injuries in these contexts are sparse.

Climate and Seasonality

Colder and high-altitude climates are variably associated with increased risk of burn injury. Residential fires that occur in winter months that are not associated with smoking or electrical faults in the United States are most often caused by heating appliances or cooking-related fires. Energy poverty necessitates the use of hazardous fuels, such as kerosene or open biomass (e.g., wood) fires to maintain warmth. As example, Nepal has an annual burn injury epidemic in the winter months, particularly among populations who live in mountainous and rural areas [46, 53]. In Nepal, like in many cold-climate countries, older children and women are often responsible for lighting and tending to fires, managing cookstoves and lamps, and maintaining warmth. These practices significantly increase their risk of burn injury and burn-related death.

Conversely, the colder northeastern region of the United States has a generally lower fire and burn-related mortality rate (0.97 per 100,000) than the more temperate southeastern region (1.49 per 100,000) [4]. Further, the fire and burn mortality rate of some of the coldest states in the United States are lower than the average national rate (1.23 per 100,000). As example, the fire and burn mortality rate in New Hampshire and Vermont was 0.5 per 100,000 population compared to Minnesota where it was 0.7 per 100,000. Nonetheless, Alaska had the highest fire and burn mortality rate in the United States (2.72 per 100,000). Although temperate climates are not protective, warmer climates in the United States do seem to have lower fire and burn death rates, as reported in Arizona (0.87 per 100,000) and Florida (0.84 per 100,000).

In locations with significant seasonal variations of temperature, burns occur more frequently in the colder winter months. In some countries and during holidays (e.g., the Fourth of July in the United States, Diwali in India and Nepal, Greek Orthodox Easter in Greece, Hari Raya in Malaysia, and New Year's celebrations globally), firework-related injuries become common, particularly among older male children [54]. Firework injuries often affect the hands, neck, face, and eyes and are not lethal. As a result, they exact a disproportionate morbidity for their incidence.

Comorbidities

Comorbidities that have been associated with a higher risk of burn injury include epilepsy, peripheral neuropathy, and other physical and cognitive disabilities. In low- and middle-income countries where access to medications for epilepsy and diabetes is often limited, these comorbidities are a common predisposing factor for burn injury. Epilepsy in particular is a common cause of fires, severe burns, and burn-related fatalities as those suffering from the condition may fall into an open fire, onto a cookstove, or disrupt an ignition source [55]. The risk and severity of injury are further exacerbated by stigma and traditional beliefs about epilepsy. As example, in some communities the concerns about epilepsy being contagious prevent people from helping to put out the fire or lending first aid. Epilepsy among people who practice religious fasting, which in some communities include medications, also are at high risk and must be counseled about avoiding proximity to flames, chemicals, and hot substances while they are not on a seizure medication. As example, a prospective study of burns among people living with epilepsy in Saudi Arabia reported that 40% of injured patients sustained burns while fasting, in part, because they did not take their medications [56].

Burn injuries among people living with peripheral sensory neuropathy (e.g., from diabetes, leprosy, spinal cord injury) are common regardless of national income. Practices like soaking feet in "warm" water, warming feet in front of fires, and touching hot objects and substances without the sensation that generates a withdrawal response often cause severe burns in tissues with poor perfusion, which lead to infection, need for reconstruction and/or amputations in many cases.

Other physical and cognitive disabilities have been associated with burn injuries, particularly those resulting from residential fires and scald and contact injuries. With a growing aging population, including people without access to cardiovascular disease management in much of the world, cognitive disabilities from stroke, vascular dementia, Alzheimer's disease, and age-related cognitive dysfunction are a major cause of burn injuries [57]. Further, elderly patients with dementia tend to have poorer outcomes despite smaller injuries, and rehabilitation is typically limited [36, 41].

Interpersonal and Collective Violence

The vast majority of burns in the world are unintentional. However, self-immolation and assault-by-burning occur worldwide although are more common in some regions and among specific populations [43]. In the United States, assault (including child abuse) is responsible for about 2% of injuries admitted to burn centers, and less than 1% of admissions are from self-immolation or attempted suicide [58]. Similar proportions have been reported from Europe and Taiwan [59].

Chemical assault—the use of acid or another caustic or corrosive substance by one person against another with the intent to injure or disfigure—has been perpetrated for centuries and is increasing in a number of communities [60, 61]. Recent high-profile attacks and advocacy campaigns have brought chemical assault to public attention and survivors are seeking systematic change to the way chemical assault is viewed and controlled through legislation [61–63]. Although such attacks are thought to be more common in the low- and middle-income countries, their incidence is on the rise in higher income countries too [61, 64]. However, little is known about the incidence and distribution of these events globally or the ways in which health systems and governments are addressing chemical assault [60].

In many cases, chemical assaults occur as a manifestation of gender-based (GBV) or intimate partner violence (IPV). These motives in particular have inspired local, national, and global campaigns to address chemical assaults and empower women and girls in communities with pervasive gender inequity [65, 66]. Reports from several countries have described local efforts to limit access to corrosive substances, facilitate the prosecution of assailants, and increase support for victims [60, 61, 63, 67]. A recent systematic review of legislation around chemical assault collated policies and regulations to propose a comprehensive legislative framework to prevent chemical assaults and mitigate their effects on victims, and included five legislative priorities: (i) apply a public health approach; (ii) adopt legal definitions specific to chemical assault; (iii) control chemical supply, sales, and procurement; (iv) facilitate justice; and (v) support survivors [68].

The United Kingdom has a remarkably high incidence of chemical assault and acid violence that is predominantly perpetrated by men and boys against men and boys [69]. Unlike in other regions with high rates of chemical assault, the risk factors in the United Kingdom tend to be related to organized crime. Acid Survivors Trust International, a United Kingdom-based, international, non-profit organization, is an exemplar in their use of epidemiological data to drive targeted interventions in different regions and populations, support advocacy initiatives, and generate evidence-based policy to prevent and control chemical assault.

Collective violence and the complex humanitarian emergency that ensues are another form of violence that generate burn injuries at rates far greater than those in safe societies. Most wartime burn injuries are related to explosive devices (e.g., land mines, unexploded ordnances), breakdown of infrastructure (e.g., electricity, formal housing), and poor fire prevention practices. A representative, cluster-randomized, community-based survey of civilians in post-invasion Baghdad (2003–2014) determined that burn injuries occurred in 117 per 100,000 persons, which is three times greater than the rate of burn injuries pre-invasion (39 per 100,000 population) [70]. Further, burn injuries represented 10% of all injuries in Baghdad during the decade post-invasion. In the wake of turmoil, the lack of organized burn care led to a high mortality rate (16%). Additionally, 40% of burn-injured people were left with major disabilities and about half experienced catastrophic health expenditure and/or food insecurity because of their injury. A report from Médecins Sans Frontières Operations Center Brussels described surgical care from projects in 15 countries over seven years [71]. Eleven percent of all operations were for burn injuries, including those for general surgical, obstetric, gynecologic, pediatric, and other conditions. People receiving surgical care at conflict relief projects had nearly twice the odds of having a burn operation compared to people requiring surgery in communities affected by natural disaster.

Data for Burn Injury Prevention and Control

Given the enormous and intolerable burden of burn injuries globally, prevention and control initiatives should be priorities of community organizations, burn centers, health systems, professional societies, and governments. Better data can inform burn injury prevention and control efforts, particularly data from community-based surveys, surveillance systems, and national and multi-national registries.

The approach to injury prevention and control is comprised of four core functions (i.e., surveillance, analysis, intervention, evaluation). Injury prevention and control practitioners undertake a spectrum of activities to understand the problem, address hazards systematically and holistically, and reduce the burden of injury:

- Surveillance and data collection
- Strengthening individual knowledge and skills

- Educating healthcare professionals
- Changing practices of institutions and agencies
- Fostering coalitions and networks
- Mobilizing neighborhoods and communities
- Influencing policy and legislation

A precise understanding of the problem and factors that contribute to it is the basis for planning effective interventions. In much of the world, data regarding hazard distribution and burn injuries are scarce, inaccurate, or both. A lack of sufficient and high-quality data limits the development, implementation, and evaluation of potentially lifesaving and morbidity reducing interventions. The Haddon Matrix is a tool to conceptualize host-agent-environment factors that must be considered when collecting data for planning prevention and control interventions (Table 1.2). A third dimension has been added to the matrix that includes common causes of intervention success and failure (e.g., equity, stigma, preferences, feasibility, cost) (Fig. 1.2). These issues can facilitate priority setting and decision-making, but only have value in light of the epidemiological characteristics associated with burn injury in specific populations and communities.

There are exemplars of comprehensive national burn registries (e.g., Australia and New Zealand, Taiwan) and a nascent, global, hospital-based burn registry supported and promulgated by the World Health Organization [48, 72]. These registries currently and will continue to inform key burn injury prevention and control strategies. However, where these databases do not yet exist or are not utilized, active surveillance programs and representative community-based surveys are required to ensure that key risk factors and vulnerable populations that hide in the shadows of health systems are understood. Data and patterns from these surveys from Ghana, Bangladesh, Ethiopia, Iran, Nepal, Uganda, and Rwanda have taught us that hazards are not equally distributed within communities, countries of similar national incomes, or regions [6, 14, 73, 74]. No one set of prevention and control interventions will be effective or cost-effective without such granular data.

TABLE 1.2 Haddon Matrix applied to childhood burn injury from residential fires caused by cookstoves

	Host	Agent	Physical environment	Social environment
Pre-event	• Teach children about risk of fires • Provide barriers • Create community creches	• Childproof matchboxes • Safer cookstoves • Safer fuel storage	• Lower flammability of structures • Separate living and cooking spaces when able	• Support transition to safe cookstoves • Use community groups to disseminate safe cooking best practices
Event	• Teach stop, drop and roll • Plan and practice fire escape plan	• Keep fire blanket near cookstove • Regulate flammable fabrics and upholstery	• Install smoke and CO detectors • Distribute fire extinguishers	• Pass subsidies for smoke detectors • Fund fire response programs
Post-event	• Provide first aid education to lay people • Ensure rapid first response	• Install auto-shutoff regulators on LPG stoves	• Ensure access to telephone to call emergency response	• Increase availability of burn stabilization points and care centers

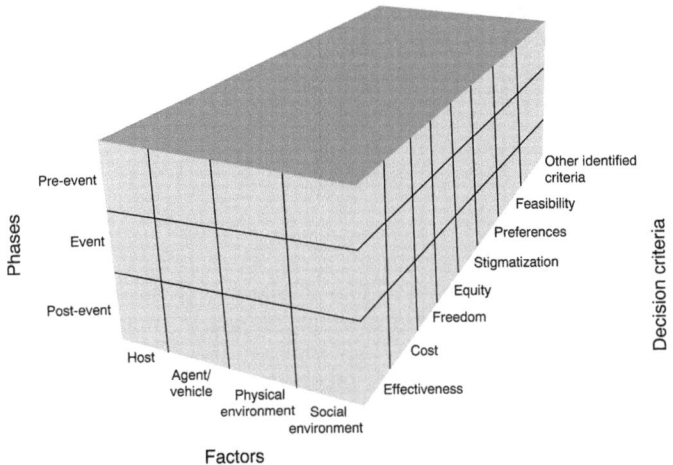

FIGURE 1.2 Haddon Matrix with a third dimension that incorporates high-value domains for decision-making [75]

Conclusion

The vast majority of burns can be prevented with targeted, context-specific interventions that are responsive to the diversity of people, ways-of-life, home and work environments, and competing interests that exist locally and globally. There are major inequities in incidence of burn injury between and within populations and the prevalence of disabilities from un- or under-treated burns globally. Mitigating exposure to known hazards and changing behaviors are key to reducing the burden of burn injuries and promoting restorative health justice among disadvantaged populations. The first step is to generate epidemiological data to describe the problem, identify opportunities to prevent injuries and improve service delivery, and benchmark interventions. Every stakeholder in the burn community has a role in supporting high-quality data collection and utilization, including those who focus on epidemiology and injury prevention, but also those in fire services, emergency departments, burn centers, health systems, and patient advocacy groups. Together, we can reduce preventable death and disability from burn-related hazards and eliminate one of the greatest health inequities on our planet.

References

1. James SL, Lucchesi LR, Bisignano C, et al. Epidemiology of injuries from fire, heat and hot substances: global, regional and national morbidity and mortality estimates from the Global Burden of Disease 2017 study. Inj Prev. 2020;26:i36–45.
2. Diseases GBD, Injuries C. Global burden of 369 diseases and injuries in 204 countries and territories, 1990-2019: a systematic analysis for the Global Burden of Disease Study 2019. Lancet. 2020;396:1204–22.
3. Crowe CS, Massenburg BB, Morrison SD, Naghavi M, Pham TN, Gibran NS. Trends of Burn Injury in the United States: 1990 to 2016. Ann Surg. 2019;270:944–53.
4. Peck MD. Epidemiology of burns throughout the world. Part I: Distribution and risk factors. Burns. 2011;37:1087–100.
5. DeKoning EP, Hakenewerth A, Platts-Mills TF, Tintinalli JE. Epidemiology of burn injuries presenting to North Carolina emergency departments in 2006-2007. Burns. 2009;35:776–82.
6. Mehta K, Gyedu A, Otupiri E, Donkor P, Mock C, Stewart B. Incidence of childhood burn injuries and modifiable household risk factors in rural Ghana: A cluster-randomized, population-based, household survey. Burns. 2021;47:944–51.
7. Correction: a review of the international burn Injury Database (iBID) for England and Wales: descriptive analysis of burn injuries 2003-2011. BMJ Open 2019;9:e006184corr1.
8. O'Brien SP, Billmire DA. Prevention and management of outpatient pediatric burns. J Craniofac Surg. 2008;19:1034–9.
9. Brusselaers N, Monstrey S, Vogelaers D, Hoste E, Blot S. Severe burn injury in Europe: a systematic review of the incidence, etiology, morbidity, and mortality. Crit Care. 2010;14:R188.
10. Gabbe BJ, Cleland H, Watterson DM, et al. Long term outcomes data for the Burns Registry of Australia and New Zealand: Is it feasible? Burns. 2015;41:1732–40.
11. Song C, Chua A. Epidemiology of burn injuries in Singapore from 1997 to 2003. Burns. 2005;31(Suppl 1):S18–26.

12. Peck M, Pressman MA. The correlation between burn mortality rates from fire and flame and economic status of countries. Burns. 2013;39:1054–9.
13. Reynolds TA, Stewart B, Drewett I, et al. The impact of trauma care systems in low- and middle-income countries. Annu Rev Public Health. 2017;
14. Gyedu A, Stewart B, Mock C, et al. Prevalence of preventable household risk factors for childhood burn injury in semi-urban Ghana: a population-based survey. Burns. 2016;42:633–8.
15. Sleet DA. The global challenge of child injury prevention. Int J Environ Res Public Health. 2018;15:1921.
16. Kahn SA, Bernal N, Mosier MJ. Pearls from the national burn repository. J Burn Care Res. 2018;39:626–7.
17. Soleimani T, Evans TA, Sood R, Hartman BC, Hadad I, Tholpady SS. Pediatric burns: kids' inpatient database vs the national burn repository. J Surg Res. 2016;201:455–63.
18. Latenser BA, Miller SF, Bessey PQ, et al. National Burn Repository 2006: a ten-year review. J Burn Care Res. 2007;28:635–58.
19. Friesen B. Haddon's strategy for prevention: application to native house fires. Circumpolar Health. 2003;84:105–9.
20. Bjerregaard P. Fatal non-intentional injuries in Greenland. Arctic Med Res. 1992;51(Suppl 7):22–6.
21. Fraser S, Grant J, Mackean T, et al. Burn injury models of care: a review of quality and cultural safety for care of Indigenous children. Burns. 2018;44:665–77.
22. Moller H, Falster K, Ivers R, Clapham K, Harvey L, Jorm L. High rates of hospitalised burn injury in Indigenous children living in remote areas: a population data linkage study. Aust N Z J Public Health. 2018;42:108–9.
23. Moller H, Harvey L, Falster K, Ivers R, Clapham KF, Jorm L. Indigenous and non-Indigenous Australian children hospitalised for burn injuries: a population data linkage study. Med J Aust. 2017;206:392–7.
24. Kimble RM, Griffin BR. Reducing the incidence of burn injuries to Indigenous Australian children. Med J Aust. 2017;206:389–90.
25. Allen CE, Figueroa J, Agarwal M, Little WK. Pediatric scald injuries sustained from instant soup and noodle products. Clin Pediatr (Phila). 2021;60:16–9.
26. Bentivegna K, McCollum S, Wu R, Hunter AA. A state-wide analysis of pediatric scald burns by tap water, 2016-2018. Burns. 2020;46:1805–12.

27. Baggott K, Rabbitts A, Leahy NE, Bourke P, Yurt RW. Pediatric sink-bathing: a risk for scald burns. J Burn Care Res. 2013;34:639–43.
28. Palmieri TL, Alderson TS, Ison D, et al. Pediatric soup scald burn injury: etiology and prevention. J Burn Care Res. 2008;29:114–8.
29. Tyler MD, Richards DB, Reske-Nielsen C, et al. The epidemiology of drowning in low- and middle-income countries: a systematic review. BMC Public Health. 2017;17:413.
30. Ablewhite J, McDaid L, Hawkins A, et al. Approaches used by parents to keep their children safe at home: a qualitative study to explore the perspectives of parents with children aged under five years. BMC Public Health. 2015;15:983.
31. Mashreky SR, Rahman A, Svanstrom L, Linnan MJ, Shafinaz S, Rahman F. Experience from community based childhood burn prevention programme in Bangladesh: implication for low resource setting. Burns. 2011;37:770–5.
32. Peck M, Molnar J, Swart D. A global plan for burn prevention and care. Bull World Health Organ. 2009;87:802–3.
33. Shields BJ, Comstock RD, Fernandez SA, Xiang H, Smith GA. Healthcare resource utilization and epidemiology of pediatric burn-associated hospitalizations, United States, 2000. J Burn Care Res. 2010;31:506–7.
34. Potokar T, Bendell R, Chamania S, Falder S, Nnabuko R, Price PE. A comprehensive, integrated approach to quality improvement and capacity building in burn care and prevention in low and middle-income countries: an overview. Burns. 2020;46:1756–67.
35. Hyder AA, Sugerman DE, Puvanachandra P, et al. Global childhood unintentional injury surveillance in four cities in developing countries: a pilot study. Bull World Health Organ. 2009;87:345–52.
36. Pham TN, Kramer CB, Wang J, et al. Epidemiology and outcomes of older adults with burn injury: an analysis of the National Burn Repository. J Burn Care Res. 2009;30:30–6.
37. Marshall SW, Runyan CW, Bangdiwala SI, Linzer MA, Sacks JJ, Butts JD. Fatal residential fires: who dies and who survives? JAMA. 1998;279:1633–7.
38. Romanowski K, Curtis E, Barsun A, Palmieri T, Greenhalgh D, Sen S. The frailty tipping point: Determining which patients are targets for intervention in a burn population. Burns. 2019;45:1051–6.

39. Maxwell D, Rhee P, Drake M, Hodge J, Ingram W, Williams R. Development of the Burn Frailty Index: a prognostication index for elderly patients sustaining burn injuries. Am J Surg. 2019;218:87–94.

40. Romanowski KS, Barsun A, Pamlieri TL, Greenhalgh DG, Sen S. Frailty score on admission predicts outcomes in elderly burn injury. J Burn Care Res. 2015;36:1–6.

41. Pham TN, Carrougher GJ, Martinez E, et al. Predictors of discharge disposition in older adults with burns: a study of the burn model systems. J Burn Care Res. 2015;36:607–12.

42. McGwin G Jr, Chapman V, Rousculp M, Robison J, Fine P. The epidemiology of fire-related deaths in Alabama, 1992-1997. J Burn Care Rehabil. 2000;21:75–3; discussion 4.

43. Peck MD. Epidemiology of burns throughout the World. Part II: intentional burns in adults. Burns. 2012;38:630–7.

44. Fagenholz PJ, Sheridan RL, Harris NS, Pelletier AJ, Camargo CA Jr. National study of Emergency Department visits for burn injuries, 1993 to 2004. J Burn Care Res. 2007;28:681–90.

45. Sengoelge M, El-Khatib Z, Laflamme L. The global burden of child burn injuries in light of country level economic development and income inequality. Prev Med Rep. 2017;6:115–20.

46. Gupta S, Mahmood U, Gurung S, et al. Burns in Nepal: a population based national assessment. Burns. 2015;41:1126–32.

47. Peden M, Oyegbite K, Ozanne-Smith J, et al. World report on child injury prevention. Geneva, Switzerland: World Health Organization; 2008.

48. Mehta K, Thrikutam N, Nakarmi KK, Hoyte-Williams PE, Peck M, Stewart BT. Epidemiology and outcomes of cooking and cookstove-related burn injuries: a World Health Organization (WHO) Global Burn Registry (GBR) report. J Burn Care Res. 2021;42:51–2.

49. Rosenthal J, Quinn A, Grieshop AP, Pillarisetti A, Glass RI. Clean cooking and the SDGs: Integrated analytical approaches to guide energy interventions for health and environment goals. Energy Sustain Dev. 2018;42:152–9.

50. Gallagher M, Beard M, Clifford MJ, Craig M, Watson. An evaluation of a biomass stove safety protocol used for testing household cookstoves, in low and middle-income countries. Energy Sustain Dev. 2016;33:14–25.

51. Carrougher GJ, Bamer AM, Mandell SP, et al. Factors affecting employment after burn injury in the united states: a burn model

system national database investigation. Arch Phys Med Rehabil. 2020;101:S71–85.

52. Carrougher GJ, Brych SB, Pham TN, Mandell SP, Gibran NS. An intervention bundle to facilitate return to work for burn-injured workers: report from a burn model system investigation. J Burn Care Res. 2017;38:e70–e8.

53. Gupta S, Groen TA, Stewart BT, et al. The spatial distribution of injuries in need of surgical intervention in Nepal. Geospat Health. 2016;11:359.

54. Sandvall BK, Jacobson L, Miller EA, et al. Fireworks type, injury pattern, and permanent impairment following severe fireworks-related injuries. Am J Emerg Med. 2017;35:1469–73.

55. Boschini LP, Tyson AF, Samuel JC, et al. The role of seizure disorders in burn injury and outcome in Sub-Saharan Africa. J Burn Care Res. 2014;35:e406–12.

56. Al-Qattan MM, Al-Zahrani K. A review of burns related to traditions, social habits, religious activities, festivals and traditional medical practices. Burns. 2009;35:476–81.

57. Livingston G, Huntley J, Sommerlad A, et al. Dementia prevention, intervention, and care: 2020 report of the Lancet Commission. Lancet. 2020;396:413–46.

58. Forjuoh SN. The mechanisms, intensity of treatment, and outcomes of hospitalized burns: issues for prevention. J Burn Care Rehabil. 1998;19:456–60.

59. Tung KY, Chen ML, Wang HJ, et al. A seven-year epidemiology study of 12,381 admitted burn patients in Taiwan—using the Internet registration system of the Childhood Burn Foundation. Burns. 2005;31(Suppl 1):S12–7.

60. Mannan A, Ghani S, Clarke A, Butler PE. Cases of chemical assault worldwide: a literature review. Burns. 2007;33:149–54.

61. Ahmed F, Maroof H, Ahmed N, Sheridan R. Acid attacks: a new public health pandemic in the west? Int J Surg. 2017;48:32–3.

62. Bagcchi S. Private hospitals are told to treat acid attack victims free of charge. BMJ. 2015;350:h2224.

63. Kay M. Indian court restricts the sale of acid to try to curb attacks on women. BMJ. 2013;347:f4762.

64. Sugrue R, Reilly F, Kelly J, Clover J. The discordant relationship between acid attack incidence and advances in management. Burns. 2018;44:236–7.

65. Justice? What Justice?: tackling acid violence and ensuring justice for survivors. J. Sagar Associates, India: Acid Survivors Trust International and TrustLaw; 2017.

66. Alishahi Tabriz A, Dabbagh H, Koenig HG. Medical ethics in qisas (eye-for-an-eye) punishment: an islamic view; an examination of acid throwing. J Relig Health. 2016;55:1426–32.
67. Bagcchi S. Acid attack victims should have same rights as disabled people, Indian Supreme Court rules. BMJ. 2015;351:h6787.
68. Kazerooni Y, Mishra B, Gibran N, et al. A systematic review and comprehensive legislative framework to address chemical assault globally. Health Policy Plan. 2020;35:1188–207.
69. Nagarajan M, Mohamed S, Asmar O, Stubbington Y, George S, Shokrollahi K. Data from national media reports of 'Acid attacks' in England: a new piece in the Jigsaw. Burns. 2020;46:949–58.
70. Stewart BT, Lafta R, Esa Al Shatari SA, Cherewick M, Burnham G, Hagopian A, Galway LP, Kushner AL. Burns in Baghdad from 2003 to 2014: Results of a randomized household cluster survey. Burns. 2016;42(1):48–55. https://doi.org/10.1016/j.burns.2015.10.002. Epub 2015 Oct 31.
71. Stewart BT, Trelles M, Dominguez L, et al. Surgical burn care by Medecins Sans Frontieres-Operations Center Brussels: 2008 to 2014. J Burn Care Res. 2016;37:e519–e24.
72. Peck M, Falk H, Meddings D, Sugerman D, Mehta S, Sage M. The design and evaluation of a system for improved surveillance and prevention programmes in resource-limited settings using a hospital-based burn injury questionnaire. Inj Prev. 2016;22(Suppl 1):i56–62.
73. Mashreky SR, Rahman A, Chowdhury SM, et al. Consequences of childhood burn: findings from the largest community-based injury survey in Bangladesh. Burns. 2008;34:912–8.
74. Dave DR, Nagarjan N, Canner JK, Kushner AL, Stewart BT, Group SR. Rethinking burns for low & middle-income countries: differing patterns of burn epidemiology, care seeking behavior, and outcomes across four countries. Burns. 2018;44:1228–34.
75. Runyan CW. Using the Haddon matrix: introducing the third dimension. Inj Prev. 1998;4:302–7.

Chapter 2
Pathophysiology and Hypermetabolic Response to Burn

Roohi Vinaik, Dalia Barayan, and Marc G. Jeschke

Introduction

Burn injuries represent one of the most severe forms of trauma affecting more than two million people in North America each year [1]. According to the World Health Organization, there are an estimated 300,000 deaths per year worldwide related to thermal injury [2]. In Canada, there are approximately 43,000 emergency visits and over 2000 hospitalization per annum due to burn injuries [3].

R. Vinaik · D. Barayan
Sunnybrook Research Institute, Toronto, Canada
e-mail: roohi.vinaik@mail.utoronto.ca;
dalia.barayan@sri.utoronto.ca

M. G. Jeschke (✉)
Hamilton Health Sciences, Hamilton, ON, Canada

McMaster University Hamilton, ON, Canada
e-mail: marc.jeschke@hhsc.ca

© The Author(s), under exclusive license to Springer Nature Switzerland AG 2023
J. O. Lee (ed.), *Essential Burn Care for Non-Burn Specialists*,
https://doi.org/10.1007/978-3-031-28898-2_2

Outcomes have improved over the years due to establishment of specialized burn centers and improvements in resuscitation, dedicated burn-specific protocols, improved wound coverage and infection control, and improved management of inhalation injury [4]. However, burn patients still experience unacceptably high rates of morbidity and mortality despite improved clinical care.

Poor outcomes in severe burns, or burns encompassing more that 20% of the total body surface area (TBSA), are attributable in part to the debilitating hypermetabolic stress response, which is unrivaled in terms of its magnitude and persistence [5]. Post-burn hypermetabolism is associated with negative sequelae, including sepsis and multi-organ failure — leading causes of death in burn patients [4]. Essentially, metabolic dysfunction in burns is characterized by two distinct phases, an initial "ebb phase" during which metabolism and tissue perfusion are decreased, and a following "flow phase" defined by elevated resting energy expenditure (REE) >110% of predicted REE [6]. The flow phase is accompanied by pronounced muscle catabolism and lipolysis, loss of total and lean body mass, and stress-induced diabetes, which eventually lead to physiologic exhaustion. However, although the phenomenon of hypermetabolism has been well documented, the mechanisms underlying this response are still not completely elucidated. An improved understanding of post-burn hypermetabolism, accompanying changes, and management are necessary to optimize patient care.

In this chapter, we define the hypermetabolic response after burns, highlighting the key metabolic consequences. In particular, we focus on glucose, lipid, and protein metabolism. Then, we discuss the various organ systems affected by post-burn hypermetabolism including the cardiac, renal, gastrointestinal, and immune systems. We conclude with a discussion of management of hypermetabolism in the clinical setting, namely focusing on how to calculate energy expenditure, conservative measures such as nutritional supplementation and early mobilization, and pertinent pharmacological intervention.

What Is Hypermetabolism?

Several reports demonstrated that post-burn metabolic changes occur in a biphasic fashion. Two distinct patterns of metabolic regulation can be observed following injury [7]. The first phase is early shock hypometabolism (ebb phase), which usually occurs within 48 h post-burn. This response is characterized by decreased cardiac output, oxygen consumption, and metabolic rate as well as impaired glucose tolerance associated with the hyperglycemic state [8]. Within the first five days post-injury, however, these metabolic variables gradually increase to a plateau phase. This second hypermetabolic phase (flow phase) is characterized by a hyperdynamic circulation and increased metabolic rate with resulting increases in body temperature, oxygen and glucose consumption, CO_2 production, and futile substrate cycling [8]. Typically, patients are considered hypermetabolic when their REE is increased 10% or more above normal [5]. This hypermetabolic stress response is initiated to provide sufficient energy for maintaining organ function and whole-body homeostasis under demanding trauma conditions [4, 7–9].

While initially ubiquitous and essential, prolonged post-burn hypermetabolism has negative consequences that are a byproduct of pronounced metabolic derangements. For example, elevated circulating levels of catecholamines, glucagon, and cortisol after injury stimulate excess release of free fatty acids (FFAs) and glycerol from fat (450% increase in triglyceride-fatty acid cycling), eventually resulting in organ alterations associated with organ damage and dysfunction. Increased lipolysis is further accompanied by increased glucose production by the liver (250% increase in glycolytic-gluconeogenic cycling) and insulin release that is twice that of controls in response to glucose load, indicative of profound insulin resistance [10–14]. Stress hormones induce proteolysis to increase availability of amino acids leading to cachexia (all summarized in Fig. 2.1). The extent and duration of this altered metabolic demand (discussed below) are directly

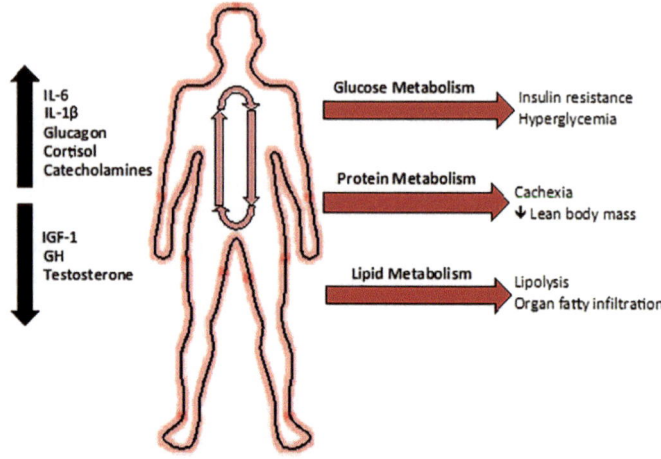

FIGURE 2.1 Schematic depicting key post-burn hypermetabolic alterations

related to the degree of burn injury quantified based on total body surface area (TBSA) with partial- and full-thickness burns [15–17].

Magnitude and Duration

A recent comparison of genomic alterations in white blood cells (WBCs) following acute lipopolysaccharide (LPS) exposure, blunt trauma, and severe burns demonstrated that gene expression returns to normal within 24 h of LPS exposure [18] and one month after blunt trauma [19]. However, the WBC genome of burn patients uniquely remains altered for up to one-year post-injury—the furthest time point studied. The duration of the genomic response to burn trauma parallels that of the metabolic perturbations induced by the injury [1, 20, 21]. Within the first few months after burn, metabolic rate increases ~40–80% above normal and remains elevated for up to one-year post-injury [22]. Although both poly-trauma [23] and sepsis [24] also trigger a similar metabolic response, the degree of this hypermetabolic state is less than that of burns and resolves more promptly. For patients with >40% TBSA full-thickness burns, resting metabolic rate at thermal neutral temperature (30°C) has been shown to surpass 140% of normal at admission and is reduced to 130% once wounds are fully healed, to 120% at 6 months, and then to 110% at 12 months post-injury [25]. While this hypermetabolic response decays significantly in the first 6 months after burn, more recent studies have revealed that severely burned patients can remain hypermetabolic for up to 3 years post-injury [22, 26, 27].

The magnitude and persistence of this stress response depend not only on burn size, age, and body composition but also the patient's preprogrammed genetic response to an insult. Inhalation injury or another insult such as an infection can further accentuate and prolong the increased metabolic rate after injury [15]. Unfortunately, persistent hypermetabolism after burn trauma is a major concern as it is associated with a profound catabolic state in almost every organ system of the body [22, 28] (Fig. 2.1). To date the cellular and molecular mechanisms underlying burn-induced hypermetabolism have not been fully identified and despite improved clinical care, the detrimental sequelae of this complex response are major contributor to post-burn morbidity and mortality.

Biomarkers and Mediators

As discussed above, marked and sustained increases in catecholamine, glucocorticoid, glucagon, and dopamine secretion are involved in initiating the acute hypermetabolic response and its ensuing catabolic state after injury [1, 29–37] The rise in these catabolic hormones is accompanied by a decrease in the normal endogenous activity of anabolic agents, primarily human growth hormone and testosterone, which together combine to result in a large net protein loss [38, 39]. Cytokines such as interleukin 6 (IL-6) and tumor necrosis factor (TNF), endotoxin, neutrophil-adherence complexes, reactive oxygen

species, nitric oxide, and coagulation as well as complement cascades have also been implicated in mediating and
maintaining the post-burn hypermetabolic state [28]. Once
these cascades of events are initiated, their mediators and by-
products further drive the persistent and increased metabolic
rate accompanied by alterations in glucose, lipid, and amino
acid metabolism [40]. This self-perpetuating process is specu-
lated to drive an entire spectrum of metabolic abnormalities
that are observed after severe burn injury. Thus, management
of burn-induced hypermetabolism remains a clinical priority.
If left untreated, this protective stress response becomes auto
destructive, ultimately causing vast cachexia, multi-organ failure, and even death [1–11, 13, 14]. In the ensuing section, we
will discuss some of the key metabolic sequelae after burns
in detail, along with the specific organ systems targeted in
thermal injuries.

Metabolic Consequences: Glucose, Lipids, Amino Acids

Glucose Metabolism

Glucose homeostasis in healthy subjects is tightly regulated.
Under normal circumstances, post-prandial elevations in circulating glucose levels stimulate pancreatic β-cells to release
insulin—a potent anabolic hormone. Insulin release promotes peripheral glucose uptake into skeletal muscle and
adipose tissue and suppresses glucose production (i.e., gluconeogenesis) in the liver, thereby restoring blood glucose concentrations [41, 42]. However, post-burn metabolic alterations
cause significant shifts in energy substrate metabolism in
order to provide glucose—a major fuel source to vital organs.
In order to satisfy the high energy demands of the post-burn
hypermetabolic state, glucose levels are markedly increased
by (1) releasing the above-mentioned stress mediators, primarily glucagon and cortisol, to oppose the anabolic actions
of insulin, (2) activating hepatic gluconeogenesis to increase

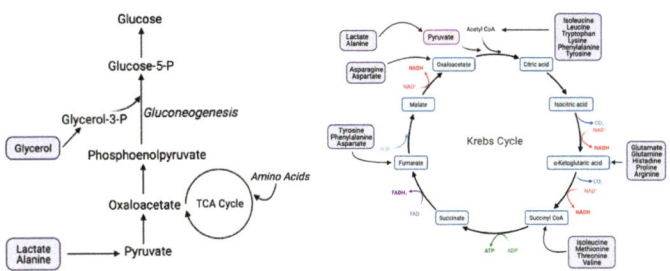

FIGURE 2.2 Lipolytic and proteolytic byproducts as gluconeogenic and glycolytic/TCA substrates

production, and (3) enhancing adipose lipolysis and muscle proteolysis to provide gluconeogenic and glycolysis/TCA substrates like glycerol, alanine, and lactate (Fig. 2.2).

In burn patients, the rate of glucose production in the liver is around twofold greater than in healthy controls [14, 43]. This increased glucose production is excessive for tissue use and leads to the "diabetes of stress." [14, 44] Moreover, unlike in healthy individuals, exogenous glucose infusion does not fully attenuate hepatic gluconeogenesis in burn patients (only about 50%) [43]. While the exact cause is not entirely defined, it appears that burn patients undergo a "double hit" where both central and peripheral insulin sensitivity are impaired after injury, resulting in poor glucose control. More specifically, insulin exerts a diminished ability to suppress hepatic glucose output (central insulin resistance) and/or a diminished ability to stimulate glucose disposal into skeletal muscle (peripheral insulin resistance) [44]. Therefore, although glucose remains a preferred substitute for tissue energy post-burn, there is a well-defined limit to its use given the insulin resistance. The result of this metabolic abnormality is (1) hyperglycemia; (2) profound catabolism; (3) increased ectopic fat deposition; and (4) wasted energy.

Of major importance is recent evidence suggesting that impaired glucose metabolism post-burn is detrimental and contributes to adverse clinical outcomes after injury. Studies have shown that hyperglycemia not only leads to profound wasting and cachexia in severely burned patients but is also linked to increased incidence of infection, pneumonia, sepsis, and even death [10–14, 21, 45, 46]. These findings were further supported by a prospective randomized trial, which demonstrated that glycemic control is beneficial for post-burn organ function and morbidity outcomes. Retrospective cohort studies also confirmed the survival benefits of glycemic control in severely burned patients [12, 46]. Together, these studies clearly highlight the significant clinical challenges associated with post-burn insulin resistance and hyperglycemia and the importance of treatment after injury.

Lipid Metabolism

Lipid metabolism is another key metabolic pathway that is significantly altered during the post-burn hypermetabolic period. As with other forms of trauma, the rise in post-burn catecholamine levels leads to activation of adipose tissue lipolysis, mainly via β2 and β3 adrenergic stimulation [47, 48]. Lipolysis is defined as the enzymatic breakdown (hydrolysis) of triglycerides into free fatty acids (FFAs) and glycerol molecules. These substrates are then released into the circulation to be used as fuel by other tissues in the body through beta-oxidation, gluconeogenesis, and glycolysis [49]. Similar to glucose however, the amount of exogenous fat that can be utilized as an energy substitute after burn is limited [15, 50]. In fact, only 30% of FFAs at most is oxidized for fuel, while the remaining 70% is simply recycled. This is a marked difference from starvation during which 90% of lipolysis-derived FFAs are used for fuel [50]. Unfortunately, burn-induced lipolysis and FFA mobilization have been linked to a number of detrimental complications, including insulin resistance and multi-organ dysfunction. Specifically, increased FFA levels may overwhelm glucose transport activity after injury, which further impairs insulin-mediated glucose uptake contributing to post-burn insulin resistance [5, 50, 51]. This has been supported by research in type 2 diabetes, demonstrating that elevated FFA levels are predictive for the incidence and severity of the disease [52, 53].

Another major consequence of the post-burn lipolytic response is increased fatty infiltration into vital organs, especially the liver. Liver fatty infiltration and dysfunction, or hepatic steatosis, remain a leading cause of morbidity and mortality in burn patients [21]. A clinical analysis conducted by Kraft et al. demonstrated that a strong correlation exists between FFA and hepatic fat content after burn injury [54]. This data is in agreement with post-burn pathology examinations and spectroscopy reports showing that hepatic triglycerides are increased by three- to fivefold in severely burned children [55, 56]. In fact, these authors also found that in severely burned children, elevated triglycerides are associated with worsened organ function and glucose metabolism and increased incidence of infection, sepsis, and poor outcomes [54]. Thus, while adipose tissue was previously ignored for a long time, it is becoming increasingly evident that this organ plays a very central role in mediating post-burn hypermetabolic responses. Though this relationship is now clear, the mechanisms by which lipolysis-derived lipids induce these post-burn metabolic disturbances are still not entirely defined.

Protein Metabolism

The main source of fuel in the burned patient is protein/amino acids from skeletal muscle. Chronic catabolism of skeletal muscle is pathognomonic of severe burn trauma, which leads to marked wasting of muscle protein and consequently of lean body mass (LBM) within days after injury [7, 26, 44]. The prolonged erosion of LBM and resultant wasting leaves burn survivors cachectic and debilitated. This metabolic abnormality in turn significantly delays wound healing and contributes to long-term morbidity after injury [44]. While the specific mechanism is unclear, likely mediators are stress hormones, cytokines, and oxidants. The underlying pathophysiology was shown to be a substantial increase in muscle protein breakdown along with no or only a minor compensatory increase in muscle protein synthesis leading to muscle loss [56]. From a mechanistic view, burn injury induces a concurrent increase in both skeletal muscle protein synthesis (MPS) and breakdown (MPB) rates. However, MPB rates significantly surpass MPS rates, resulting in significant net loss of total body protein [56]. Moreover, increasing protein intake does not further increase muscle protein synthesis, indicating that the catabolic drive cannot be overcome with more substrate synthesis [57]. The exception would be addition of an anabolic agent, such as growth hormone or testosterone, which in fact would be more likely to overcome the net amino acid effect [57]. Medical management of hypermetabolic changes will be discussed in Management of Hypermetabolism: Pharmacological Intervention section.

Interestingly, recent evidence suggests that defects in skeletal muscle protein kinetics can persist for over a year after burn injury. Indeed, studies have shown that lean body mass is reduced for up to 2–3 years post-burn. In severely burn patients (>30% TBSA), this cachectic state can be observed for several years after injury [26]. The clinical consequences of persistent protein catabolism can be quite severe, depending on the degree of muscle protein loss [58]. A 10–15% loss in LBM has been shown to decrease wound healing, while a further increase in LBM loss ~30% is associated with significant increases in infection rates, profound weakness, pressure sores, and diminished wound healing [59, 60]. An LBM loss of 40% or greater usually becomes fatal [60]. Mortality in these burn patients is further augmented by severe muscle weakness, which can prolong mechanical ventilation requirements, inhibit sufficient cough reflexes, and delay mobilization in protein-malnourished patients [61]. Decreases in muscle mass may also be responsible for the delay in growth commonly observed in pediatric burn patients, even at 2 years post-burn [62]. Furthermore, given that skeletal muscle is responsible for 70–80% of whole-body insulin-stimulated glucose uptake, profound muscle wasting may further augment persistent insulin resistance after injury [20]. Modulation of this hypercatabolic response after burn injury is thus paramount for the restoration of normal metabolic structure and function in severely burned patients.

Targeting Organ Systems: Cardiac, Renal, Gastrointestinal, and Immune Systems

Cardiac

Burns are associated with poor myocardial function after injury as a result of impaired contractility and right heart overload [63, 64]. Increased systemic and pulmonary vascular resistance increases afterload for the left and right heart, respectively. While the left ventricle can compensate and sustain cardiac output due to post-burn adrenergic stimulation, the right ventricle lacks the capacity to compensate for the increased afterload. Burns greater than 45% TBSA can cause contractile issues and in severe conditions, desynchronization of the ventricles [65]. Aggressive early fluid resuscitation does not completely correct for left ventricular defects, suggesting that hypovolemia may not be the only mechanism of impaired post-burn cardiac function [63, 65, 66]. However, early, sufficient fluid therapy is important in ameliorating myocardial depression in burns, and animals given no resuscitation exhibit persistent myocardial depression [67]. Horton et al. demonstrated decreased left ventricular contractility in guinea pig hearts within 24 h post-burn, which was significantly reversed with adequate resuscitation [68–70].

The underlying mechanism by which post-burn shock impairs myocardial function is still unclear [71]. However, oxygen-derived free radicals may have a key role in myocardial cell membrane dysfunction. When given in conjunction with adequate fluid resuscitation (2–4 mL/kg/%TBSA), a combination infusion of superoxide dismutase and catalase (free radical scavengers) improves post-burn poor ventricular contractility. However, antioxidant infusion did not alter or obviate the volume needed for fluid resuscitation after burn [72].

Renal

Rebal function decreases due to reducedcardiac output and decresed renal blood flow leading to a reduced glommerular filtration rate. Additionally, stress-induced hormones that mediate fluid balance such as angiotensin, aldosterone, and antidiuretic hormone further limit renal blood flow and compound effects seen due to poor cardiac output. These changes result in oliguria that can worsen and culminate in acute tubular necrosis and ultimately, renal failure [71]. Furthermore, inflammatory mediators such as cytokines (e.g., TNF, IL-1), eicosanoids (e.g., prostaglandins), and platelet-activating factor are released early post-burn [73]. They increase vascular permeability and are involved in disseminated intravascular coagulation that results in formation of microthrombi in renal structures, further interfering with normal renal function. However, early, adequate resuscitation may decrease risk of renal failure, which parallels cardiac outcomes (e.g., improved cardiac function and output) [74].

Acute renal failure in burn patients is accompanied by increased morbidity and higher mortality rates and is detectable by reduced urine output despite adequate resuscitation in oliguric renal failure. Early renal support via incorporation of dialysis during the recovery period is key [75]. Dialysis regulates serum electrolytes and allows for large volumes of nutritional supplementation and removal of excess water or toxic substances when combined with hemofiltration in burn patients [75–77].

Gastrointestinal

Gastrointestinal (GI) changes in burns detrimentally impact nutritional status through several mechanisms. Burns induce mucosal atrophy within 12 h of injury directly proportional to burn size, increase intestinal permeability, and alter digestive absorption [78, 79]. The mucosal brush border undergoes atrophy and apoptosis of the epithelial lining, and cytoskeletal changes associated with apoptotic cell death are most pronounced at 18 h after injury [80]. Interruption in the intact mucosal barrier in turn enhances intestinal permeability to macromolecules, correlated with the extent of the burn [81, 82]. This includes enhanced permeability to molecules such as PEG3350, lactulose, and mannitol, and these effects are compounded by infection [83]. Importantly, altered permeability of the gut mucosa is closely related to blood flow. Systolic hypotension in severe burns (40% TBSA) and decreased intestinal blood flow after burn are associated with increased intestinal permeability early (5 h) after injury [84, 85]. In addition to increased permeability to dextrans, impaired intestinal blood flow and mucosal viability allow for augmented permeability to opportunistic agents such as *Candida* [85].

While burn injuries increase transport of the aforementioned, they are also accompanied by reduced glucose, amino acid, and fatty acid uptake and decreased brush border lipase activity within a few hours after injury [86]. These changes return to normal by 48–72 h after injury, which parallels mucosal atrophy. Thus, treating mucosal atrophy to ensure adequate nutrition for burn patients is vital. In order to ameliorate atrophy, early enteral nutrition and administration of glutamine and various antioxidants within 8–12 h can improve intestinal inflammation and function.

Immune System

Burns paradoxically cause systemic hyperinflammation and immune compromise, increasing risk for infectious complications such as bacterial, fungal, and viral infections. Impaired immune function is proportional to burn size in burns greater than 20% TBSA, and susceptibility to infection is a by-product of impaired activity of various immune cells including neutrophils, macrophages, and T and B lymphocytes [71]. Interestingly, neutrophil count is initially increased afterburn due to decreased apoptosis [87]. However, although neutrophil count is increased, these cells exhibit impaired diapedesis, chemotaxis, and phagocytosis. A deficiency in p47-phox and p67-phox oxidase components and associated impaired respiratory burst as well as compromised actin polymerization and depolymerization may account for the aforementioned outcomes [88, 89]. By 48–72 h, neutrophil counts decrease similar to macrophages, which are diminished after burn [90].

T lymphocyte function is similarly decreased after severe burns. This is due to polarization from the T-helper 1 (T_H1) to T_H2 response and is correlated with increased mortality rate [91, 92]. The T_H1 response is involved in cell-mediated immune defense while the T_H2 response is important for antibody responses and is characterized by increased interleukin-4 (IL-4) and IL-10 production. Interestingly, administration of anti-IL-10 antibodies and growth hormone partially reverses the T_H2 response and improves mortality rates in burn animal models [93, 94]. In addition to increased T_H2 responses, burn injury impairs cytotoxic T cell activity, which enhances infection risk. This can be ameliorated by early wound excision, which will be discussed in the subsequent section on management of post-burn hypermetabolism [95].

Adipose Tissue

Originally, adipose tissue was simply regarded as a passive energy reservoir, however research over the past two decades has led to a major shift in our understanding of its role in health and disease. Adipose tissue (AT) is now considered to be a remarkably complex endocrine organ capable of regulating a variety of diverse biological functions [96]. In addition to secreting a plethora of adipocyte-derived factors known as adipokines, AT plays a major part in inflammation, mechanical organ protection, and thermoregulation [96, 97]. Given its central role as a metabolic-endocrine-immune organ, adipose dysfunction is associated with a number of detrimental burn-related metabolic phenomena, and thus, understanding its biology appears crucial [98].

Traditionally, AT has been categorized into two distinct types, namely white adipose tissue (WAT) and brown adipose tissue (BAT) [98]. The main function of WAT is to store excess energy in the form of TGs (triacylglycerols), while BAT is specialized for thermogenesis and dissipates energy as heat through UCP1 (uncoupling protein 1)-mediated uncoupling of oxidative phosphorylation from ATP synthesis [99]. These distinct functions of the classic BAT and WAT are due, at least in part, to their different developmental origins. Based on lineage tracing experiments performed in mice, BAT seems to arise from Myf5 (myogenic factor 5)-expressing precursors—a property normally attributed to skeletal muscle [98]. Thus, brown preadipocytes express a skeletal muscle gene signature while white preadipocytes do not [98, 99]. In terms of morphology, classic brown adipocytes are characterized by a small multilocular lipid droplet structure, an abundance of mitochondria, and the expression of the mitochondrial brown fat marker, UCP1, which is produced in the inner mitochondrial membrane. Rodents and humans both possess BAT; however, whereas BAT depots remain throughout life in mice, human BAT diminishes with age. In contrast, WAT is found dispersed throughout the body in both humans and rodents, with the subcutaneous (inguinal in rodents) and visceral (epididymal) being the largest fat depots in the body [99]. These white adipocytes are characterized by unilocular morphology, reduced mitochondrial content, and the lack of UCP1 expression [99].

WAT has long been considered to only exist in the aforementioned classifications, and emerging evidence has revealed that a complex cellular heterogeneity exists even within a single fat pad [99]. Indeed, it was recently discovered that certain depots of WAT could adopt BAT characteristics when subjected to certain physiological stimuli in a process termed "browning" [100, 101]. This results in the recruitment of "brown-in-white," or beige adipocytes that are characterized by a multilocular appearance, increased mitochondrial biogenesis, and the expression of UCP1—the master regulator of non-shivering thermogenesis [98–100].

The dynamic nature of the adipose organ allows the body to adequately respond to both changes in nutrient supply and ambient temperature by mobilizing free fatty acids in periods of energy demand and storing excess as triglycerides when energy is no longer needed [98]. Owing to its high degree of plasticity, WAT browning has garnered significant attention over the past decade for its potential to be exploited for the treatment of obesity and type II diabetes [102, 103]. Numerous studies have demonstrated that enhanced thermogenesis in conditions of energy surplus (i.e., obesity) has beneficial effects on whole-body metabolic homeostasis including improved insulin sensitivity, increased resting energy expenditure, and enhanced weight loss [102]. While beneficial in obesity and diabetes, these attributes can be detrimental in cancer and burns [103]. In fact, in these hypermetabolic conditions, WAT browning has been shown to drive the progression of cancer-associated cachexia, a state characterized by severe weight loss and muscle catabolism [104]. Furthermore, evidence suggests that WAT browning may promote lipolysis and organ fatty infiltration in burn patients [105]. Indeed, hypermetabolic burn patients demonstrate elevated levels of circulating FFAs due to the constitutive activation of adipose tissue lipases, such as hormone sensitive lipase (HSL) following injury [106]. These findings were corroborated in a recent study from our group demonstrating browning-induced lipolysis facilitates hepatic steatosis and dysfunction in post-burn mice, thereby increasing morbidity and mortality [107].

Interestingly, in both conditions of cancer and burns where WAT browning has been implicated in persistent hypermetabolism and poor outcomes, the inflammatory cytokine IL-6 was identified as a major initiator of this pathological cascade of events [108–110]. In the context of burns, increased levels of bone marrow derived IL-6 have been shown to correlate with the magnitude of injury and organ failure, and genetic deletion of IL-6 in mice attenuates post-burn hypermetabolism via reductions in WAT browning and whole-body energy metabolism [111–114]. Despite all these findings that have implicated both WAT browning and IL-6 as major drivers of post-burn hypermetabolism, therapeutic agents that target these responses have lagged behind.

Central Nervous System

The central nervous system (CNS) has an integral role in activation of stress responses via relaying of afferent impulses from the site of injury to the hypothalamus [115]. As a result, hypothalamic inhibition of the pituitary is alleviated or alternatively, the hypothalamus produces hormones (e.g., corticotrophin-releasing hormone (CRH), growth hormone-releasing hormone (GHRH)) that stimulate production and release of pituitary hormones [115]. These include anterior pituitary corticotrophin (ACTH) and growth hormone (GH), which ultimately have important metabolic consequences. ACTH stimulates production of the stress hormone cortisol in the adrenal cortex, which promotes liver gluconeogenesis, hyperglycemia, and net muscle protein catabolism [116, 117]. Similar to cortisol, GH also increases blood glucose levels via stimulation of glycogenolysis, promoting post-burn hyperglycemia and long-term growth abnormalities in pediatric burn patients [115].

Importantly, the CNS has an integral role in driving the post-burn sympathetic response. Acetylcholine release at the splanchnic nerve-chromaffin cell junction provides a stimulus for catecholamine secretion for the adrenal medulla and binding to the respective receptors [118]. Epinephrine binds to $\alpha 1$, $\alpha 2$, $\beta 1$, and $\beta 2$ adrenergic receptors, norepinephrine binds to $\alpha 1$, $\alpha 2$, and $\beta 1$, and dopamine binds to D1 and D2 receptors [115]. Activation of post-burn sympathetic responses also may activate stress and inflammatory pathways including p38 mitogen-activated protein kinase (MAPK), JNK, and nuclear factor-kappa B (NF-kB), promoting inflammation and immunosuppression after burn [119]. Catecholamines also target various post-burn metabolic processes, driving the initial stages of the hypermetabolic response [120]. However, while elevated catecholamine levels after burn are associated with stress, inflammation, and hypermetabolism, the exact function of the CNS on burn-induced hypermetabolism is still unknown at this time.

Management of Hypermetabolism: Conservative Measures

Metabolic changes that occur after burn function in supplying energy support to preserve immune function, body tissues, and healing [121]. However, thermally injured patients exhibit prolonged, consistent whole-body and muscle catabolism, necessitating nutritional and medical support. Clinicians and scientists have targeted the post-burn hypermetabolic response utilizing several different therapeutic approaches, including conservative management and pharmacological intervention. Key nonpharmacological strategies include nutritional therapy and early mobilization and will be discussed in this section.

Nutrition—Calculating Energy Consumption and Nutrient Supplementation

Nutritional therapy aims to provide patients with sufficient energy, fluids, and nutrients (e.g., protein) to maintain vital organ and immune function and minimize further tissue loss. In the late twentieth century, high caloric feeding was a therapeutic strategy. Wilmore et al. suggested 8000 kcal/day, while Curreri proposed a 25 kcal/kg body weight plus 40 kcal/%TBSA burn [122, 123]. While the latter was the most frequently used formula between 1970 and 1980, Pennisi created a more comprehensive formula in 1976 which included an estimation of protein needs. Currently, there are several formulas developed for critically ill patients, including the Toronto, Schofield, American Society for Parenteral and Enteral Nutrition (ASPEN), and Ireton-Jones formulae (Table 2.1). However, comparison of supplementation values for a standardized patient (30 years old, 72 kg, 170 cm, 40%

TABLE 2.1 REE formulae and patient specifications

Reference	Specifications	Formula	
Harris & Benedict BMR	Male	BMR × Activity factor × Injury factor	
	Female	66 + (13.7 × weight (kg)) + (5 × height (cm)) − (6.8 × age)	
		665 + (9.6 × weight (kg)) + (1.8 × height (cm)) − (4.7 × age)	
		Activity factor –	Injury factor –
		Confined to bed: 1.2	<20% TBSA: 1.5
		Minimal ambulation: 1.3	20–40% TBSA: 1.6
			>40% TBSA: 1.7
Curreri	All patients	(25 kcal × weight (kg)) + (40 × %TBSA)	
Pennisi	*Adults*		
	Calories	(20 kcal × weight (kg)) + (70 kcal × %TBSA)	
	Protein	(1g × weight (kg)) + (3g × %TBSA)	
	Children		
	Calories	(60 kcal × weight (kg)) + (35 kcal × %TBSA)	
	Protein	(3g × weight (kg)) + (1g × %TBSA)	
Toronto Formula	All patients	[−4343 + (10.5 × %TBSA) + (0.23 × kcals) + (0.84 × Harris Benedict) + (114 × T(°C)) − (4.5 × days post-burn)] × Activity factors	
		Activity factor (non-ventilated) –	Activity factor (ventilated) − 1.2
		Confined to bed: 1.2	
		Minimal ambulation: 1.3	
Davies and Liljedahl		20 kcal (weight (kg)) + (70 × %TBSA)	

(continued)

TABLE 2.1 (continued)

Reference	Specifications	Formula
Modified Schofield	Male	BMR × Injury factor
		10–18 years = (0.074 × weight (kg)) + 2.754
		18–30 years = (0.063 × weight (kg)) + 2.896
		30–60 years = (0.048 × weight (kg)) + 3.653
		>60 years = (0.049 × weight (kg)) + 2.459
	Female	10–18 years = (0.056 × weight (kg)) + 2.898
		18–30 years = (0.062 × weight (kg)) + 2.036
		30–60 years = (0.034 × weight (kg)) + 3.538
		>60 years = (0.038 × weight (kg)) + 2.755
		Injury factors –
		<10% TBSA = 1.2
		11–20% TBSA = 1.3
		21–30% TBSA = 1.5
		31–50% TBSA = 1.8
		>50% TBSA = 2.0
ASPEN	All patients	25–35 kcal/kg/day
Ireton-Jones	Non-ventilated Ventilated	629 − (11 × yrs) + (25 × weight (kg)) − (609 × O)
		1784 − (11 × yrs) + (25 × weight (kg)) + (244 × S) + (239 × TR) + 804 × B)

Modified from Machado et al. (2011)
kcal: calorie intake in the past 24 h
Harris Benedict: calorie requirement using the Harris benedict formula with no stress or activity factors
T: body temperature
yrs: years
O: obesity = 1/absent = 0
S: male = 1/female = 0
TR: trauma present = 1/no trauma = 0
B: burn present = 1/no burn = 0

TBSA) using the different formulae demonstrated a wide range, from 2099 kcal/day (Ireton-Jones) to 5229 kcal/day (Modified Schofield) [124].

Currently, the appropriate caloric amount is still under debate as is the composition of nutritional support, and recent feeding regimens rely on resting energy expenditure (REE) in order to provide sufficient energy supply and nutrients [125–127]. Early enteral nutrition (within 12 hours) ameliorates post-burn catabolism and improves outcomes, but it is important to note that this is a delicate balance [128, 129]. Undernutrition reduces immunocompetence, delays healing, and increases dependency on mechanical ventilation and risk of infection while overfeeding (excess calories or protein) is associated with hyperglycemia, organ fatty infiltration, and azotemia. This underscores the need to estimate REE and accurately calculate caloric requirements [130]. REE can be estimated based on body mass, age, and gender although caloric requirements based on these factors can still be an overestimate [131, 132]. Energy requirements after burn fluctuate, and static formulas often result in underfeeding during high energy consumption and overfeeding later in the clinical course [133]. The gold standard for determining energy expenditure is indirect calorimetry, which can be used to confirm adequate nutritional support by calculating oxygen (O_2) consumption and carbon dioxide (CO_2) production [132, 134, 135]. The ratio of CO_2/O_2 (respiratory quotient (RQ)) is used to determine adequate feeding, and overfeeding results in an RQ >1.0 while normal metabolism is between 0.75 and 0.90 [136].

After determining a specific caloric goal, ratios of the key macronutrients (carbohydrates, proteins, lipids) need to be determined. Carbohydrates are an important nutrient source in burn patients due to their protein-sparing effects relative to high-fat diets, as highlighted in clinical studies [137]. However, high-carbohydrate diets are limited by the ability to oxidize and utilize glucose. Glucose administration >9 mg/kg/min cannot be oxidized sufficiently, and higher glucose administration rates can lead to hyperglycemia, glycosuria, and dehydration [116, 138]. Hence, higher carbohydrate supplementation may not be feasible although this may be lower than the estimated caloric expenditure.

Protein is also important in patients due to enhanced muscle catabolism in response to burns, necessitating supplementation to maintain adequate wound healing and immune function and allay lean body mass loss [139]. Administering supraphysiological doses improves protein synthesis and nitrogen balance although it does not eliminate catabolism [140]. It is important to note that protein (1.5–2.0 g/kg/day in adults, 2.5–4.0 g/kg/day in children) should be given with sufficient carbohydrates and fat to minimize use of protein as an energy source rather than as nutrients to maintain muscle mass and promote wound healing. In particular, glutamine and arginine were found to play an important role after burn. Glutamine provides energy for lymphocytes and enterocytes and serves as a precursor for the antioxidant glutathione. Clinically, glutamine supplementation improves burn patient outcomes and minimizes length of hospital stay (LOS) [141, 142]. Conversely, while arginine supplementation improves burn wound healing and immune responsiveness, it is potentially harmful overall and is not recommended in burn patients [143].

Lipolysis is enhanced after burn although utilization of lipids as an energy source is decreased [129, 144]. Rather, liberated FFAs accumulate in organs such as the liver. Lipid supplementations are recommended to minimize fatty acid deficiency but in limited doses (no more than 15% total calories) since increased fat consumption can worsen immune function. In addition to quantity, the fatty acid subtype needs to be taken into consideration. Omega-6-containing formulas can generate a pro-inflammatory response while formulas with a greater proportion of omega-3 are associated with an improved immune response, glycemic regulation, and patient outcomes [145, 146]. Some enteral formulas have an omega-6: omega-3 ratio from 2.5:1 to 6:1, while "immune enhancing" formulas have a more balanced composition of 1:1 [133]. It is important to note that although studies suggest that lower omega-6 levels and sufficient lipid supplementation are beneficial, there is still debate with regard to enteral formula composition and lipid quantity in burn patients [133].

In addition to macronutrients, micronutrient (vitamin and trace element) supplementation is also crucial after burns [147]. In particular, vitamins A and C improve epithelial growth and collagen cross-linking, respectively [148]. Vitamin D, which is involved in maintaining bone density, is decreased after burn resulting in bone demineralization [149]. Other nutrients that are lost in burns and have an integral role in wound healing and immunity are iron (Fe), copper (Cu), selenium (Se), and zinc (Zn) [150–152]. Fe and Cu serve as a cofactor for oxygen scavengers such as superoxide dismutase and other forms of endogenous antioxidant defense [153]. Cu is necessary for collagen production and wound healing, and Cu deficiency and corresponding decreased levels of its transporter ceruloplasmin are implicated in immune dysfunction, arrythmias, and poor wound healing in burn patients [154, 155]. Zn also has a function in wound healing and at the molecular level, protein synthesis, DNA replication, and immune cell function. Se similarly is involved in cell-mediated immunity, and dietary Se influences leukocyte functions such as adherence, migration, and cytokine secretion [156]. Additionally, several selenoproteins can regulate cellular redox processes and immune cell activation [156]. Taken together, micro- in addition to macronutrient supplementation is important in burn patient management.

Environment, Early Excision, and Exercise

Hypermetabolism may be an adaptive response to generate energy to offset heat loss. Thus, raising ambient temperature from 25 °C to 33 °C may obviate the need to increase core body temperate, which increases by 2 °C after major burn. In patients with burns >40% TBSA, increasing ambient temperature can diminish REE from a 2.0 to 1.4-fold increase [157]. In addition to environmental modulation, patient factors are also important in managing post-burn hypermetabolism. In particular, early excision (within 72 h) and wound coverage decrease burn-induced inflammation and activation of stress responses. This in turn substantially reduces REE and hypermetabolism, improving mortality rates [7, 158, 159].

A key component of severe burns and accompanying hypermetabolism is persistent skeletal muscle catabolism, which is further exacerbated by prolonged bed rest and physical inactivity. Rehabilitation programs are implemented although muscle catabolism and poor muscle strength can persist. However, resistance exercise programs can increase muscle strength and hypertrophy and be safely incorporated into routine burn care, mitigating frailty [132, 160]. In a study in burned children, resistance exercise over a 12-week period decreased REE and may attenuate sympathetic responses [161]. This was accompanied by increased lean body mass by over 20-fold in addition to enhanced muscle strength, total work, and power [161]. Ultimately, enhanced muscle strength and ability to do work allow for more rapid rehabilitation and return to normal activities of daily leaving, improving outcomes.

Management of Hypermetabolism: Pharmacological Intervention

Although non-pharmacologic interventions are employed to combat hypermetabolism, implementation of several key medical interventions is critical for clinical efficacy. Currently, there are various pharmaceutical agents used in burn care, including propranolol, growth hormone (GH), insulin-like growth factor 1 (IGF-1), insulin-like growth factor binding protein-3 (IGFBP-3), insulin, metformin, and oxandrolone. These therapeutics strategies are utilized to minimize catabolism and promote anabolism, ultimately improving burn patient morbidity and mortality.

Propranolol

Prolonged, substantial catecholamine production is a hall-mark of thermal injuries that ultimately contributes to the hypermetabolic response. Increased catecholamine levels contribute to generalized post-burn catabolism in addition to increased REE, lipolysis, and muscle catabolism via stimulation of α and β receptors [40]. The non-specific β-blocker propranolol is ideally administered post-resuscitation (3–10 days after burn) to minimize pronounced catecholamine-dependent changes [162]. Directly targeting sympathetic pathways can reduce cardiac work by decreasing heart rate by 15–20% and mitigates blood loss during grafting [13, 48, 163]. Moreover, treatment has supplementary benefits in addition to directly targeting sympathetic pathways. For example, propranolol is associated with improved wound healing, decreased healing time, and shorter hospital LOS [163].

Studies have shown that propranolol is a potent anti-catabolic agent and yields positive outcomes when combined with recombinant human growth hormone (rhGH), which will be discussed subsequently [137]. Combination therapy can ameliorate hypermetabolism and inflammation while eliminating the deleterious effects of rhGH monotherapy [164]. In addition to anti-catabolic effects, propranolol has an anabolic function as well. Treatment in severely burned children increases muscle protein balance by 82% above baseline in concert with upregulation of genes involved in muscle metabolism [48]. Long-term (1 year) treatment in pediatric patients significantly reduces bone loss, heart rate, and REE without compromising immune function and increasing infection incidence [137].

Although there is a risk that enhanced endogenous catecholamine production combined with β-blockade could result in unopposed α-adrenergic activity, vasoconstriction, and ischemia, this has not been unequivocally demonstrated in burn patients [165]. Other potential side effects, including hypotension and bradycardia, can easily be diagnosed and managed in a burn intensive care unit. Despite potential negative effects, there is sufficient evidence in pediatric burn populations regarding efficacy of propranolol treatment. While there are fewer studies establishing propranolol in adult and elderly burn hypermetabolism management, clinical trials are currently ongoing [166, 167]. However, it is important to note that propranolol administration is not simple and effectively dosing is a challenge. Pediatric patients are typically given 1–4 mg/kg/day, while adults usually start at 10 mg QID. The adult dose is increased in order to maintain heart rate below 100 bpm while maintaining blood pressure.

Recombinant Human Growth Hormone

Human GH is an endogenous anabolic hormone produced by the pituitary gland that has receptors and binding proteins in various tissues. Burn patients may exhibit disruptions in the GH/IGF-1/IGFBP-3 axis likely as a consequence of excessive pro-inflammatory cytokine production, favoring catabolism. Thus, rhGH injection could be a possible therapeutic strategy.

In adults, a 3-month rhGH regimen enhanced lean body mass and muscle power while positively regulating IGF-1 and adiponectin levels [168]. Other studies in children yielded similar beneficial effects with regard to recovery of lean body mass. As mentioned earlier, Hart et al. investigated long-term (1 year) therapy with propranolol and rhGH after burn in children, indicating that rhGH increases lean body mass, height and weight gain, and bone mineral density compared to placebo [169]. Importantly, long-term treatment increases thyroid hormone-binding sites, ameliorating post-burn growth arrest in children [170]. Similar results were seen in another study by Branski et al. with the added finding of a diminished hypermetabolic response [171]. Jeschke et al. also demonstrated that rhGH administration in children significantly decreases hypermetabolic and hyperinflammatory responses especially when combined with propranolol [164].

Beyond beneficial effects in muscle protein kinetics, rhGH treatment induces more rapid healing in children and adults alike and minimizes scarring while improving outcomes such as decreased hospital LOS [171, 172].

However, a key adverse event associated with rhGH treatment is hyperglycemia, which is of concern in burn patients. Interestingly, beneficial outcomes seen with rhGH are not reproducible in non-burn, critically ill patients. In fact, these patients have hyperglycemia and insulin resistance associated with a 40% increase in morbidity and mortality [173]. Therefore, while rhGH has an anabolic effect, care should be taken prior to implementation in patients. Currently, rhGH is not a standard of care in burn or critically ill patients.

Insulin-Like Growth Factor 1/Insulin-Like Growth Factor Binding Protein-3

Kim et al. demonstrated that rhGH treatment enhanced IGF-1 levels, which is produced in the liver in response to endogenous or exogenous GH. Therefore, the beneficial effects of rhGH could be attributed to IGF-1 upregulation. Similar to proinsulin, IGF-1 is a polypeptide whose principal binding protein is IGFBP-3 [174]. IGF-1 in animal models exhibits anti-inflammatory and anabolic effects and alleviates stress responses. However, because of the side effects, IGF-1 is given as a complex with IGFBP-3 in a 1:1 molar ratio. This complex improves protein metabolism and diminishes catabolism without significantly impacting glucose levels (unlike rhGH-associated hyperglycemia) [175]. The beneficial effects on muscle maintenance can, in part, be attributed to improved immune function and attenuated acute phase and inflammatory responses [57, 175–177].

However, similar to rhGH, IGF-1 alone is not effective in critically ill, non-burn patients. This indicates that IGF-1 (and by extension, rhGH) is primarily effective when administered in conditions of significant IGF-1 deficiency; for example, hypermetabolism-induced increased IGF-1 turnover. This could be accounted for by lower levels of IGFBPs, especially IGFBP-3, which is seen for up to 3 years post-burn in pediatric patients and is associated with severe growth arrest [21]. Exogenous IGF-1/IGFBP-3 treatment functions by partly reversing depressed T_H1 and exaggerated T_H2 cytokine responses after burns, balancing pro- and anti-inflammatory cytokines and improving organ function [178]. Treatment also attenuates the hepatic acute phase response, indirectly affecting serum levels of proteins that influence the hypercatabolic response [176, 177, 179, 180].

Although IGF-1 could be used to mitigate post-burn hypermetabolism and catabolism, currently its use is limited due to side effects such as hypoglycemia and poor efficacy with IGF-1 monotherapy in critically ill, non-burn patients [181, 182]. Dual therapy with IGF-1 and IGFBP-3 shows some promise with regard to reduction in catabolism and fewer hypoglycemic episodes [183]. However, IGF-1/IGFBP-3 administration is associated with adverse events such as neuropathies. At this point, further work is needed to optimize IGF-1 or IGF-1/IGFBP-3 complex prior to implementation for management of post-burn hypermetabolism [4].

Insulin

The hyperinsulinemic, hyperglycemic state after burn is associated with adverse clinical outcomes, and tight glycemic control decreases infection and sepsis rates and improves organ function [184, 185]. Insulin is an effective anti-hyperglycemic agent that is utilized in severely burned patients due to its additional anabolic and anti-catabolic effects. Insulin can attenuate hypermetabolism, evidenced by decreased lean body mass loss, which serves as a marker to monitor the hypermetabolic response [186]. Although the mechanisms underlying its anti-catabolic effects have not been elucidated as of yet, administration in burn patients unequivocally increases muscle protein synthesis and attenuates lean body mass loss [20, 127].

Gore et al. demonstrated that hyperinsulinemia in burn patients improves leg blood flow and muscle protein synthesis [184, 187]. Potentially, insulin mitigates hypermetabolism by increasing IGF-1 and IGFBP-3, which facilitates suppression of proteolysis and activation of protein synthesis [188, 189]. Additionally, insulin may exert anabolic effects by suppressing IGFBP-1, thus increasing availability of IGF-1. While high doses of insulin restore anabolism in critically ill surgical patients, this introduces the risk of hypoglycemia [190]. However, submaximal doses are sufficient to elicit anabolic effects while minimizing hypoglycemic episodes [191]. In addition to these beneficial effects, insulin is more cost effective than rhGH or IGF-1 and has a clearly established safety profile. If glucose levels are carefully monitored, insulin can be administered to manage post-burn hypermetabolism.

Metformin

Metformin is a primary alternative to insulin for hyperglycemic regulation in severely injured patients. Similar to insulin, metformin functions as both an anti-hyperglycemic and an anabolic agent. Although the mechanisms underlying muscle protein balance are still unclear, Gore et al. demonstrated a relationship between elevated glucose levels and protein catabolism [192]. Metformin likely regulates glucose levels by diminishing synthesis of cyclic AMP, which is elevated after burns and is a key potential mechanism in development of post-burn hyperglycemia and insulin resistance [193]. By improving insulin receptor sensitivity and attenuating post-burn hyperglycemia, metformin may diminish net muscle protein catabolism. Indeed, metformin treated patients exhibit increased fractional synthetic rate of muscle protein and improved net muscle protein balance [192, 194].

Metformin is compatible with insulin with regard to glycemic regulation and anabolic effects [195]. Additional advantages include cost-effectiveness and oral formulations, with the added benefit that glucose levels need to be monitored less frequently once glucose and medication levels are stabilized. However, metformin can possibly induce lactic acidosis and worsening of renal failure in high-risk patients [196]. Therefore, it should not be given to patients with poor lactate elimination, such as those with renal or hepatic failure [197]. However, safety and efficacy trials in severely burned patients indicate no significant worsening of renal or hepatic function or lactic acidosis with metformin treatment [198].

Oxandrolone

The anabolic agent oxandrolone is a testosterone analog that improves muscle protein catabolism via increased protein synthesis and muscle mass gain and decreased weight loss. Interestingly, oxandrolone has primarily anti-catabolic effects in adults and anabolic effects in children [199]. Pediatric burn patients treated with oxandrolone demonstrate upregulation in several genes (e.g., transcription factors, muscle-associated proteins, stress response proteins) and increased muscle protein balance [200, 201]. In adults, oxandrolone also restored lean body mass in the acute and rehabilitation phase, augmented hepatic protein synthesis, and shortened hospital LOS and donor site healing time [188, 202, 203]. Long-term administration decreases REE and hypermetabolism, increases lean body mass by 6, 9, and 12 months post-burn, and increases bone mineral content at 12 months compared to controls [204]. Moreover, evidence suggests that oxandrolone may have effects that persist for up to 5 years after burn [205].

Although it is as effective in mitigating weight loss and has similar benefits to agents such as rhGH, oxandrolone has an improved side effect profile. Compared to rhGH, oxandrolone has less hyperglycemia and an attenuated hypermetabolic response [206]. Currently, the most common side effect reported is hepatotoxicity although studies in burn patients indicate no significant differences in liver dysfunction and only a mild increase in transaminase levels in pediatric patients [207–209].

Testosterone

The hypothalamic–pituitary–gonadal (HPA) axis reduces the signal for production of testosterone under conditions of severe stress such as burns [210]. In theory, testosterone replacement should enable skeletal muscle anabolism. In a study by Ferrando et al., exogenous testosterone administration in severely burned male patients resulted in a two-fold reduction in muscle catabolism primarily due to reduction in breakdown rather than alterations in protein synthetic rate [211]. However, pediatric patients demonstrate an alternative mechanism of action of testosterone therapy. In these patients, short-term testosterone treatment enhances protein synthesis rather than impacting catabolism [212, 213].

   In spite of these beneficial effects, there are limitations to testosterone use in burn patients primarily due to the side effect profile. This includes increased risk of cardiovascular events, hepatotoxicity, erythrocytosis, and prostatic and dermatologic disorders [214]. Also, testosterone use is limited in women due to potential androgenic effects. Due to its side effect profile and the fact that there are no oral formulations, alternative agents are used such as oxandrolone.

Conclusion

Hypermetabolism is an important response that has an integral role in burn patient outcomes. While it may initially be an adaptive mechanism for post-burn survival, there are several negative outcomes associated with it. Although these consequences have been identified, hypermetabolism is still not completely understood. Delineating the mechanisms underpinning this complex response is imperative in order to successfully manage burn patients in the clinical setting. Clinical features of the hypermetabolic response include hyperglycemia and insulin resistance, hyperinflammation, catecholamine fluctuations, and whole-body catabolism, and contribute to adverse outcomes. These detrimental effects target multiple organ systems including cardiopulmonary, renal, gastrointestinal, and immune systems and contribute to organ failure. While several conservative and pharmacological advances in clinical management focus on regulating hypermetabolism, accurately determining and preserving nutritional status and developing a consensus therapeutic approach is still challenging.

Early excision and wound closure is an important initial strategy that significantly improves burn patient mortality rate. Important additional measures include environmental temperature modulation and incorporation of resistance exercises to aid in recovery and maintain lean body mass. However, despite utility of conservative strategies, pharmacological intervention is a vital tool. Pharmacological agents such as the β-blocker propranolol attenuate post-burn hypermetabolism and inflammation and have a significant anti-catabolic effect, especially when combined with agents such as rHGH. Other important drugs include blood glucose regulators. Insulin administration to maintain blood glucose levels below 130 mg/dL significantly reduces morbidity, while metformin reduces muscle catabolism with the added benefit of lower risk of hypoglycemic episodes.

Taken together, we show the broad long-term effects of the hypermetabolic response after burns. Although the exact initiating cause is not entirely defined, altered production of stress-related mediators (catecholamines, glucocorticoids, glucagon) can stimulate and maintain hypermetabolism, which results in a profound catabolic state if not treated with appropriate agents. While the conservative and pharmacological strategies discussed in this chapter are promising, further investigation is required at this point to elaborate and improve burn care (Table 2.2).

TABLE 2.2 Summary of interventions

Intervention	Summary	Reference
Propranolol	Anti-catabolic and anabolic agent, beneficial when combined with rhGH. Combination therapy ameliorates hypermetabolism and inflammation. Treatment in children increases muscle protein balance by 82%, long-term treatment reduces bone loss, cardiac work (heart rate), and REE without compromising immune function and increasing infection incidence. Administration is not simple, and effective dosing is a challenge. Side effects such as hypotension and bradycardia can easily be diagnosed but needs to be managed in a burn intensive care unit. Despite negative effects, sufficient evidence showing efficacy in pediatric burns. Clinical trials are currently ongoing in adults.	Arbabi et al. (2004) Breitenstein et al. (1990) Mohammadi et al. (2009) Herndon et al. (2001) Flores et al. (2016)
Recombinant Human Growth Hormone	RhGH diminishes the hypermetabolic response, enhances lean body mass and muscle power in adults, increases bone mineral density, height, and weight in children. A key adverse event is hyperglycemia. RhGH is currently not a standard of care in burn or critically ill patients and should not be given if the patient has an ongoing infection or is septic.	Takala et al. (1999) Hart et al. (2002) Connolly et al. (2003) Jeschke et al. (2008) Branski et al. (2009) Kim et al. (2016)

TABLE 2.2 (continued)

Intervention	Summary	Reference
Insulin	Effective anti-hyperglycemic. Attenuates hypermetabolism, (decreased lean body mass loss, increased muscle protein synthesis). More cost effective than rhGH or IGF-1 and has a clearly established safety profile. However, high doses increase hypoglycemia risk. If glucose levels are carefully monitored, insulin can be administered to manage post-burn hypermetabolism.	Gore et al. (2002) Gore et al. (2004) Van den Berghe (2004) Jeschke et al. (2007) Pidcoke et al. (2014)
Metformin	Anti-hyperglycemic and anabolic agent. Compatible with insulin with regards to glycemic regulation and anabolic effects. Cost-effective, oral formulations available, glucose needs to be monitored less frequently once medication levels are stabilized. Can induce lactic acidosis and worsening of renal failure. Should not be given to patients with poor lactate elimination (renal or hepatic failure). No significant worsening of renal/ hepatic function or lactic acidosis in burn patients. Attractive strategy to manage burn-induced hypermetabolism.	Salpeter et al. (2003) Gore et al. (2005) Riesenman et al. (2007) Sears and Perry (2015)

(continued)

TABLE 2.2 (continued)

Intervention	Summary	Reference
Oxandrolone	Acute and long-term administration decreases REE and hypermetabolism, increases lean body mass and bone mineral content. Improved side effect profile compared to rhGH (less hyperglycemia, hypermetabolic response). Most common side effect is hepatotoxicity, although no significant differences in liver dysfunction and only mild increase in transaminase levels in children. Hepatic function monitoring is recommended.	Barrow et al. (2003) Wolf et al. (2003) Demling (2005) Jeschke et al. (2007) Pham et al. (2008) Miller and Btaiche (2009) Porro et al. (2012) Cochran et al. (2013)
Testosterone	Administration in severely burned adult male patients decreases muscle catabolism and enhances protein synthesis in pediatric patients. Limitations due to the side effect profile (cardiovascular events, hepatotoxicity, erythrocytosis, and prostatic and dermatologic disorders) and androgenic effects. Alternative testosterone derivatives preferred.	Ferrando (1999) Spratt (2001) Ferrando et al. (2007) Basaria et al. (2010)

References

1. Jeschke MG, Gauglitz GG, Kulp GA, Finnerty CC, Williams FN, Kraft R, Suman OE, Mlcak RP, Herndon DN. Long-term persistance of the pathophysiologic response to severe burn injury. PloS One. 2011;6(7):e21245. https://doi.org/10.1371/journal.pone.0021245. Epub 2011 Jul 18.

2. Brigham PA, McLoughlin E. Burn incidence and medical care use in the United States: estimates, trends, and data sources. J Burn Care Rehabil. 1996;17(2):95–107. https://doi.org/10.1097/00004630-199603000-00003.

3. Banfield J, Rehou S, Gomez M, Redelmeier DA, Jeschke MG. Healthcare costs of burn patients from homes without fire sprinklers. J Burn Care Res. 2015;36(1):213–7. https://doi.org/10.1097/BCR.0000000000000194.

4. Jeschke MG. Postburn hypermetabolism: past, present, and future. J Burn Care Res. 2016;37(2):86–96. https://doi.org/10.1097/BCR.0000000000000265.

5. Long CL, Schaffel N, Geiger JW, Schiller WR, Blakemore WS. Metabolic response to injury and illness: estimation of energy and protein needs from indirect calorimetry and nitrogen balance. JPEN J Parenter Enteral Nutr. 1979;3(6):452–6. https://doi.org/10.1177/014860717900300609.

6. Dev R, Hui D, Chisholm G, Delgado-Guay M, Dalal S, Del Fabbro E, Brurera E. Hypermetabolism and symptom burden in advanced cancer patients evaluated in a cachexic clinic. J Cachexia Sarcopenia Muscle. 2015;6(1):95–8. https://doi.org/10.1002/jcsm.12014.

7. Herndon DN, Tompkins RG. Support of the metabolic response to burn injury. Lancet. 2004;363(9424):1895–902. https://doi.org/10.1016/S0140-6736(04)16360-5.

8. Jeschke MG, Chinkes DL, Finnerty CC, Kulp G, Suman OE, Norbury WB, Branski LK, Gauglitz GG, Mlcak RP, Herndon DN. Pathophysiologic response to severe burn injury. Ann Surg. 2008;248(3):387–401. https://doi.org/10.1097/SLA.0b013e3181856241.

9. Wilmore DW, Aulick LH. Metabolic changes in burned patients. Surg Clin North Am. 1978;58(6):1173–87. https://doi.org/10.1016/s0039-6109(16)41685-3.

10. Gore DC, Chinkes D, Heggers J, Herndon DN, Wolf SE, Desai M. Association of hyperglycemia with increased mortality after severe burn injury. J Trauma. 2001;51(3):540–4. https://doi.org/10.1097/00005373-200109000-00021.

11. Gore DC, Chinkes DL, Hart DW, Wolf SE, Herndon DN, Sanford AP. Hyperglycemia exacerbates muscle protein catabolism in burn-injured patients. Crit Care Med. 2002;30(11):2438–42. https://doi.org/10.1097/00003246-200211000-00006.

12. Hemmila MR, Taddonio MA, Arbabi S, Maggio PM, Wahl WL. Intensive insulin therapy is associated with reduced

infectious complications in burn patients. Surgery. 2008;144(4):629–35. https://doi.org/10.1016/j.surg.2008.07.001; discussion 635-7. Epub 2008 Aug 29.

13. Jeschke MG, Kulp GA, Kraft R, Finnerty CC, Mlcak R, Lee JO, Herndon DN. Intensive insulin therapy in severely burned pediatric patients: a prospective randomized trial. Am J Respir Crit Care Med. 2010;182(3):351–9. https://doi.org/10.1164/rccm.201002-0190OC. Epub 2010 Apr 15

14. Wolfe RR, Herndon DN, Jahoor F, Miyoshi H, Wolfe M. Effect of severe burn injury on substrate cycling by glucose and fatty acids. N Engl J Med. 1987;317(7):403–8. https://doi.org/10.1056/NEJM198708133170702.

15. Demling RH, Seigne P. Metabolic management of patients with severe burns. World J Surg. 2000;24(6):673–80. https://doi.org/10.1007/s002689910109.

16. Hill GL, Jonathan E, Lecture R. Body composition research: implications for the practice of clinical nutrition. JPEN J Parenter Enteral Nutr. 1992;16(3):197–218. https://doi.org/10.1177/0148607192016003197.

17. Smith A, Barclay C, Quaba A, Sedowofia K, Stephen R, Thompson M, Watson A, McIntosh N. The bigger the burn, the greater the stress. Burns. 1997;23(4):291–4. https://doi.org/10.1016/s0305-4179(96)00137-4.

18. Calvano SE, Xiao W, Richards DR, Felciano RM, Baker HV, Cho RJ, Chen RO, Brownstein BH, Cobb JP, Tschoeke SK, Miller-Graziano C, Moldawer LL, Mindrinos MN, Davis RW, Tompkins RG, Lowry SF, Inflamm and Host Response to Injury Large Scale Collab. Res. Program. A network-based analysis of systemic inflammation in humans. Nature. 2005;437(7061):1032–7. https://doi.org/10.1038/nature03985. Epub 2005 Aug 31. Erratum in: Nature. 2005 Dec 1;438(7068):696.

19. Xiao W, Mindrinos MN, Seok J, Cuschieri J, Cuenca AG, Gao H, Hayden DL, Hennessy L, Moore EE, Minei JP, Bankey PE, Johnson JL, Sperry J, Nathens AB, Billiar TR, West MA, Brownstein BH, Mason PH, Baker HV, Finnerty CC, Jeschke MG, López MC, Klein MB, Gamelli RL, Gibran NS, Arnoldo B, Xu W, Zhang Y, Calvano SE, McDonald-Smith GP, Schoenfeld DA, Storey JD, Cobb JP, Warren HS, Moldawer LL, Herndon DN, Lowry SF, Maier RV, Davis RW, Tompkins RG. Inflammation and Host Response to Injury Large-Scale Collaborative Research Program. A genomic storm in critically

injured humans. J Exp Med. 2011;208(13):2581–90. https://doi.org/10.1084/jem.20111354. Epub 2011 Nov 21.

20. Diaz EC, Herndon DN, Lee J, Porter C, Cotter M, Suman OE, Sidossis LS, Børsheim E. Predictors of muscle protein synthesis after severe pediatric burns. J Trauma Acute Care Surg. 2015;78(4):816–22. https://doi.org/10.1097/TA.0000000000000594.

21. Gauglitz GG, Herndon DN, Kulp GA, Meyer WJ 3rd, Jeschke MG. Abnormal insulin sensitivity persists up to three years in pediatric patients post-burn. J Clin Endocrinol Metab. 2009;94(5):1656–64. https://doi.org/10.1210/jc.2008-1947. Epub 2009 Feb 24

22. Hart DW, Wolf SE, Mlcak R, Chinkes DL, Ramzy PI, Obeng MK, Ferrando AA, Wolfe RR, Herndon DN. Persistence of muscle catabolism after severe burn. Surgery. 2000;128(2):312–9. https://doi.org/10.1067/msy.2000.108059.

23. Monk DN, Plank LD, Franch-Arcas G, Finn PJ, Streat SJ, Hill GL. Sequential changes in the metabolic response in critically injured patients during the first 25 days after blunt trauma. Ann Surg. 1996 Apr;223(4):395–405. https://doi.org/10.1097/00000658-199604000-00008.

24. Coss-Bu JA, Jefferson LS, Walding D, David Y, Smith EO, Klish WJ. Resting energy expenditure and nitrogen balance in critically ill pediatric patients on mechanical ventilation. Nutrition. 1998;14(9):649–52. https://doi.org/10.1016/s0899-9007(98)00050-1.

25. Williams FN, Jeschke MG, Chinkes DL, Suman OE, Branski LK, Herndon DN. Modulation of the hypermetabolic response to trauma: temperature, nutrition, and drugs. J Am Coll Surg. 2009;208(4):489–502. https://doi.org/10.1016/j.jamcollsurg.2009.01.022.

26. Porter C, Herndon DN, Børsheim E, Bhattarai N, Chao T, Reidy PT, Rasmussen BB, Andersen CR, Suman OE, Sidossis LS. Long-Term Skeletal Muscle Mitochondrial Dysfunction is Associated with Hypermetabolism in Severely Burned Children. J Burn Care Res. 2016;37(1):53–63. https://doi.org/10.1097/BCR.0000000000000308.

27. Yo K, Yu YM, Zhao G, Bonab AA, Aikawa N, Tompkins RG, Fischman AJ. Brown adipose tissue and its modulation by a mitochondria-targeted peptide in rat burn injury-induced hypermetabolism. Am J Physiol Endocrinol

Metab.   2013;304(4):E331–41.   https://doi.org/10.1152/ajpendo.00098.2012. Epub 2012 Nov 20

28. Sheridan RL. A great constitutional disturbance. N Engl J Med. 2001;345(17):1271–2. https://doi.org/10.1056/NEJM200110253451710.

29. Mlcak RP, Jeschke MG, Barrow RE, Herndon DN. The influence of age and gender on resting energy expenditure in severely burned children. Ann Surg. 2006;244(1):121–30. https://doi.org/10.1097/01.sla.0000217678.78472.d3.

30. Przkora R, Barrow RE, Jeschke MG, Suman OE, Celis M, Sanford AP, Chinkes DL, Mlcak RP, Herndon DN. Body composition changes with time in pediatric burn patients. J Trauma. 2006;60(5):968–71s. https://doi.org/10.1097/01.ta.0000214580.27501.19.

31. Przkora R, Herndon DN, Suman OE, Jeschke MG, Meyer WJ, Chinkes DL, Mlcak RP, Huang T, Barrow RE. Beneficial effects of extended growth hormone treatment after hospital discharge in pediatric burn patients. Ann Surg. 2006;243(6):796–801.; discussion 801-3. https://doi.org/10.1097/01.sla.0000219676.69331.fd.

32. Dolecek R. Endocrine changes after burn trauma--a review. Keio J Med 1989;38(3):262-276. doi: https://doi.org/10.2302/kjm.38.262.

33. Jeffries MK, Vance ML. Growth hormone and cortisol secretion in patients with burn injury. J Burn Care Rehabil. 1992;13(4):391–5. https://doi.org/10.1097/00004630-199207000-00001.

34. Jeschke MG, Klein D, Herndon DN. Insulin treatment improves the systemic inflammatory reaction to severe trauma. Ann Surg. 2004;239(4):553–60. https://doi.org/10.1097/01.sla.0000118569.10289.ad.

35. Goodall M, Stone C, Haynes BW Jr. Urinary output of adrenaline and noradrenaline in severe thermal burns. Ann Surg. 1957;145(4):479–87. https://doi.org/10.1097/00000658-195704000-00004.

36. Coombes EJ, Batstone GF. Urine cortisol levels after burn injury. Burns Incl Therm Inj. 1982;8(5):333–7. https://doi.org/10.1016/0305-4179(82)90033-x.

37. Norbury WB, Herndon DN. Modulation of the hypermetabolic response after burn injury. In: Herndon DN, editor. Total Burn Care. 3rd ed. New York: Saunders Elsevier; 2007. p. 420–33.

38. Jeevanandam M, Ramias L, Shamos RF, Schiller WR. Decreased growth hormone levels in the catabolic phase of severe injury. Surgery. 1992;111(5):495–502.

39. Plymate SR, Vaughan GM, Mason AD, Pruitt BA. Central hypogonadism in burned men. Horm Res. 1987;27(3):152–8. https://doi.org/10.1159/000180803.
40. Pereira C, Murphy K, Jeschke M, Herndon DN. Post burn muscle wasting and the effects of treatments. Int J Biochem Cell Biol. 2005;37(10):1948–61. https://doi.org/10.1016/j.biocel.2005.05.009.
41. Gearhart MM, Parbhoo SK. Hyperglycemia in the critically ill patient. AACN Clin Issues. 2006;17(1):50–5. https://doi.org/10.1097/00044067-200601000-00007.
42. Robinson LE, van Soeren MH. Insulin resistance and hyperglycemia in critical illness: role of insulin in glycemic control. AACN Clin Issues. 2004;15(1):45–62. https://doi.org/10.1097/00044067-200401000-00004.
43. Wolfe RR, Jahoor F, Herndon DN, Miyoshi H. Isotopic evaluation of the metabolism of pyruvate and related substrates in normal adult volunteers and severely burned children: effect of dichloroacetate and glucose infusion. Surgery. 1991;110(1):54–67.
44. Porter C, Tompkins RG, Finnerty CC, Sidossis LS, Suman OE, Herndon DN. The metabolic stress response to burn trauma: current understanding and therapies. Lancet. 2016;388(10052):1417–26. https://doi.org/10.1016/S0140-6736(16)31469-6.
45. Jeschke MG, Klein D, Thasler WE, Bolder U, Schlitt HJ, Jauch KW, Weiss TS. Insulin decreases inflammatory signal transcription factor expression in primary human liver cells after LPS challenge. Mol Med. 2008;14(1–2):11–9. https://doi.org/10.2119/2007-00062.Jeschke.
46. Pham TN, Warren AJ, Phan HH, Molitor F, Greenhalgh DG, Palmieri TL. Impact of tight glycemic control in severely burned children. J Trauma. 2005;59(5):1148–54. https://doi.org/10.1097/01.ta.0000188933.16637.68.
47. Herndon DN, Nguyen TT, Wolfe RR, Maggi SP, Biolo G, Muller M, Barrow RE. Lipolysis in burned patients is stimulated by the beta 2-receptor for catecholamines. Arch Surg. 1994;129(12):1301–4; discussion 1304-5. https://doi.org/10.1001/archsurg.1994.01420360091012.
48. Herndon DN, Hart DW, Wolf SE, Chinkes DL, Wolfe RR. Reversal of catabolism by beta-blockade after severe burns. N Engl J Med. 2001;345(17):1223–9. https://doi.org/10.1056/NEJMoa010342.
49. Galster AD, Bier DM, Cryer PE, Monafo WW. Plasma palmitate turnover in subjects with ther-

mal injury. J Trauma. 1984;24(11):938–45. https://doi. org/10.1097/00005373-198411000-00003.

50. Cree MG, Wolfe RR. Postburn trauma insulin resistance and fat metabolism. Am J Physiol Endocrinol Metab. 2008;294(1):E1– 9. https://doi.org/10.1152/ajpendo.00562.2007. Epub 2007 Oct 23

51. Cree MG, Aarsland A, Herndon DN, Wolfe RR. Role of fat metabolism in burn trauma-induced skeletal muscle insulin resistance. Crit Care Med. 2007;35(9 Suppl):S476–83. https:// doi.org/10.1097/01.CCM.0000278066.05354.53.

52. Shah P, Vella A, Basu A, Basu R, Adkins A, Schwenk WF, Johnson CM, Nair KS, Jensen MD, Rizza RA. Effects of free fatty acids and glycerol on splanchnic glucose metabolism and insulin extraction in nondiabetic humans. Diabetes. 2002;51(2):301–10. https://doi.org/10.2337/diabetes.51.2.301.

53. Boden G, Chen X, Ruiz J, Heifets M, Morris M, Badosa F. Insulin receptor down-regulation and impaired antilipolytic action of insulin in diabetic patients after pancreas/kidney transplantation. J Clin Endocrinol Metab. 1994;78(3):657–63. https://doi.org/10.1210/jcem.78.3.8126138.

54. Kraft R, Herndon DN, Finnerty CC, Hiyama Y, Jeschke MG. Association of postburn fatty acids and triglycerides with clinical outcome in severely burned children. J Clin Endocrinol Metab. 2013;98(1):314–21. https://doi.org/10.1210/jc.2012-2599. Epub 2012 Nov 12.

55. Cree MG, Newcomer BR, Herndon DN, Qian T, Sun D, Morio B, Zwetsloot JJ, Dohm GL, Fram RY, Mlcak RP, Aarsland A, Wolfe RR. PPAR-alpha agonism improves whole body and muscle mitochondrial fat oxidation, but does not alter intracellular fat concentrations in burn trauma children in a randomized controlled trial. Nutr Metab (Lond). 2007;4:9. https://doi. org/10.1186/1743-7075-4-9.

56. Jahoor F, Desai M, Herndon DN, Wolfe RR. Dynamics of the protein metabolic response to burn injury. Metabolism. 1988;37(4):330–7. https://doi.org/10.1016/0026-0495(88)90132-1.

57. Herndon DN, Ramzy PI, DebRoy MA, Zheng M, Ferrando AA, Chinkes DL, Barret JP, Wolfe RR, Wolf SE. Muscle protein catabolism after severe burn: effects of IGF-1/IGFBP-3 treatment. Ann Surg. 1999;229(5):713–20; discussion 720–2. https://doi.org/10.1097/00000658-199905000-00014.

58. Kinney JM, Long CL, Gump FE, Duke JH Jr. Tissue composition of weight loss in surgical patients. I. Elective operation. Ann Surg. 1968;168(3):459–74. https://doi. org/10.1097/00000658-196809000-00013.

59. Pollack SV. Wound healing: a review. III. Nutritional factors affecting wound healing. J Dermatol Surg Oncol. 1979;5(8):615–9. https://doi.org/10.1111/j.1524-4725.1979.tb00733.x.

60. Windsor JA, Hill GL. Weight loss with physiologic impairment. A basic indicator of surgical risk. Ann Surg. 1988;207(3):290–6. https://doi.org/10.1097/00000658-198803000-00011.

61. Arora NS, Rochester DF. Respiratory muscle strength and maximal voluntary ventilation in undernourished patients. Am Rev Respir Dis. 1982;126(1):5–8. https://doi.org/10.1164/arrd.1982.126.1.5.

62. DeFronzo RA, Jacot E, Jequier E, Maeder E, Wahren J, Felber JP. The effect of insulin on the disposal of intravenous glucose. Results from indirect calorimetry and hepatic and femoral venous catheterization. Diabetes. 1981;30(12):1000–7. https://doi.org/10.2337/diab.30.12.1000.

63. Adams HR, Baxter CR, Izenberg SD. Decreased contractility and compliance of the left ventricles as complications of thermal trauma. Am Heart J. 1984;108:1477–87. https://doi.org/10.1016/002-8703(84)90695-1.

64. Martyn J, Wilson RS, Burke IF. Right ventricular function and pulmonary hemodynamics during dopamine infusion in burned patients. Chest. 1986;89:357–60. https://doi.org/10.1378/chest.89.3.357.

65. Merriman TW Jr, Jackson R. Myocardial function following thermal injury. Circ Res. 1962;11:669–73. https://doi.org/10.1161/01.RES.11.4.669.

66. Horton JW, White J, Baxter CR. Aging alters myocardial response during resuscitation in burn shock. Surg Forum. 1987;38:249–51.

67. Cioffi WG, DeMeules JE, Gamelli RL. The effects of burn injury and fluid resuscitation on cardiac function in vitro. J Trauma. 1986;26(7):638–42. https://doi.org/10.1097/00005373-198607000-00008.

68. Horton JW, Baxter CR, White J. Differences in cardiac response to resuscitation from burn shock. Surg Gynecol Obstet. 1989;168(3):201–13.

69. Horton JW, White DJ, Baxter CR. Hypertonic saline dextran resuscitation of thermal injury. Ann Surg. 1990;211(3):301–11.

70. Horton JW, Garcia NM, White DJ, et al. Postburn cardiac contractile and biochemical markers of postburn cardiac injury. J Am Coll Surg. 1995;181:289–98.

71. Jeschke MG, Gauglitz GG. Pathophysiology of burn injuries. In: Jeschke M, Kamolz LP, Sjöberg F, Wolf S, editors.

Handbook of burns Volume 1. Cham: Springer; 2020. https://doi. org/10.1007/978-3-030-18940-2_18.

72. Horton JW, Baxter CR, White DJ. The effects of aging on the cardiac contractile response to unresuscitated thermal injury. J Burn Care Rehabil. 1988;9(1):41–51. https://doi. org/10.1097/00004630-198801000-00011.

73. Kowal-Vern A, Walenga JM, Sharp-Pucci M, Hoppensteadt D, Gamelli RL. Postburn edema and related changes in interleukin-2, leukocytes, platelet activation, endothelin-1, and C1 esterase inhibitor. J Burn Care Rehabil. 1997;18(2):99–103. https://doi.org/10.1097/00004630-199703000-00002.

74. Wolf SE, Rose JK, Desai MH, Mileski JP, Barrow RE, Herndon DN. Mortality determinants in massive pediatric burns. An analysis of 103 children with > or = 80% TBSA burns (> or =70% full-thickness). Ann Surg. 1997;225(5):554–65. https://doi. org/10.1097/00000658-199705000-00012.

75. Emara SS, Alzaylai AA. Renal failure in burn patients: a review. Ann Burns Fire Disasters. 2013;26(1):12–5.

76. Ansermino M, Hemsley C. Intensive care management and control of infection in burned patients. BMJ. 2004;329(7459):220–3. https://doi.org/10.1136/bmj.329.7459.220.

77. Leblanc M, Thibeault Y, Quérin S. Continuous haemofiltration and haemodiafiltration for acute renal failure in severely burned patients. Burns. 1997;23(2):160–5. https://doi. org/10.1016/s0305-4179(96)0085-x.

78. LeVoyer T, Cioffi WGJ, Pratt L, Shippee R, McManus WF, Mason AD Jr, Pruitt BA Jr. Alterations in intestinal permeability after thermal injury. Arch Surg. 1992;127(1):26–9. https://doi. org/10.1001/archsurg.1992.01420010032005.

79. Wolf SE, Ikeda H, Matin S, Debroy MA. Cutaneous burns increases apoptosis in the gut epithelium of mice. J Am Coll Surg. 1999;188(1):10–6. https://doi.org/10.1016/ s1072-7515(98)00260-9.

80. Ezzell R, Carter EA, Yarmush ML, Tompkins RG. Thermal injury-induced changes in the rat intestine brush border cytoskeleton. Surgery. 1993;114:591–7.

81. Deitch EA. Intestinal permeability is increased in burn patients shortly after injury. Surgery. 1990;107(4):411–6. https://doi. org/10.1002/bjs.1800770541.

82. Deitch EA, Rutan R, Waymack JP. Trauma, shock, and gut translocation. New Horiz. 1996;4(2):289–99.

83. Berthiaume F, Ezzell RM, Toner M, Yarmush ML, Tompkins RG. Transport of fluorescent dextrans across the rate ileum after cutaneous thermal injury. Crit Care Med. 1994;22(3):455–64. https://doi.org/10.1097/00003246-199403000-00016.

84. Horton JW. Bacterial translocation after burn injury: the contribution of ischemia and permeability changes. Shock. 1994;1(4):286–90.

85. Gianotti L, Alexander JW, Pyles T, James L, Babcock GF. Relationship between extent of burn injury and magnitude of microbial translocation from the intestine. J Burn Care Rehabil. 1993;14(3):336–42. https://doi.org/10.1097/00004630-199305000-00004.

86. Carter EA, Udall JN, Kirkham SE, Walker WA. Thermal injury and gastrointestinal function. I. Small intestine nutrient absorption and DNA synthesis. J Burn Care Rehabil. 1986;7(6):469–74. https://doi.org/10.1097/00004630-198611000-00004.

87. Chitnis D, Dickerson C, Munster AM, Winchurch RA. Inhibition of apoptosis in polymorphonuclear neutrophils from burn patients. J Leukoc Biol. 1996;59(6):835–9. https://doi.org/10.1002/jlb.59.6.835.

88. Rosenthal J, Thurman GW, Cusack N, Peterson VM, Malech HL, Ambruso DR. Neutrophils from patients after burn injury express a deficiency of the oxidase components p47-phox and p67-phox. Blood. 1996;88(11):4321–9.

89. Vindenes HA, Bjerknes R. Impaired actin polymerization and depolymerization in neutrophils from patients with thermal injury. Burns. 1997;23(2):131–6. https://doi.org/10.1016/s0305-4179(96)00121-0.

90. Shoup M, Weisenberger JM, Wang JL, Pyle J, Gamelli RL, Shankar R. Mechanisms of neutropenia involving myeloid maturation arrest in burn sepsis. Ann Surg. 1998;228(1):112–22. https://doi.org/10.1097/00000658-199807000-00017.

91. Hunt JP, Hunter CT, Brownstein MR, Giannopoulos A, Hultman CS, deSerres S, Bracey L, Frelinger J, Meyer AA. The effector component of the cytotoxic T-lymphocyte response has a biphasic pattern after burn injury. J Surg Res. 1998;80(2):243–51. https://doi.org/10.1006/jsre.1998.5488.

92. Zedler S, Bone RC, Baue AE, von Donnersmarch GH, Faist E. T-cell reactivity and its predictive role in immunosuppression after burns. Crit Care Med. 1999;27(1):66–72. https://doi.org/10.1097/00003246-199901000-00028.

93. Kelly JL, Lyons A, Soberg CC, Mannick JA, Lederer JA. Anti-interluekin-10 antibody restores burn-induced defects in T-cell function. Surgery. 1997;122(2):146–52. https://doi.org/10.1016/s0039-6060(97)90003-9.

94. Takagi K, Suzuki F, Barrow RE, Wolf SE, Herndon DN. Recombinant human growth hormone modulates Th1 and Th2 cytokine response in burned mice. Ann Surg. 1998;228(1):106–11. https://doi.org/10.1097/00000658-199807000-00016.

95. Hultman CS, Yamamoto H, deSerres S, Frelinger JA, Meyer AA. Early but not late burn wound excision partially restores viral-specific T lymphocyte cytotoxicity. J Trauma. 1997;43(3):441–7. https://doi.org/10.1097/00005373-199709000-00009.

96. Rosen ED, Spiegelman BM. Adipocytes as regulators of energy balance and glucose homeostasis. Nature. 2006;444(7121):847–53. https://doi.org/10.1038/nature05483.

97. Zechner R, Zimmermann R, Eichmann TO, Kohlwein SD, Haemmerle G, Lass A, Madeo F. FAT SIGNALS—lipases and lipolysis in lipid metabolism and signaling. Cell Metab. 2012;15(3):279–91. https://doi.org/10.1016/j.cmet.2011.12.018.

98. Abdullahi A, Jeschke MG. White adipose tissue browning: a double-edged sword. Trends Endocrinol Metab. 2016;27(8):542–52. https://doi.org/10.1016/j.tem.2016.06.006. Epub 2016 Jul 5.

99. Schoettl T, Fischer IP, Ussar S. Heterogeneity of adipose tissue in development and metabolic function. J Exp Biol. 2018;221(Pt Suppl 1):jeb162958. https://doi.org/10.1242/jeb.162958.

100. Sidossis LS, Porter C, Saraf MK, Børsheim E, Radhakrishnan RS, Chao T, Ali A, Chondronikola M, Mlcak R, Finnerty CC, Hawkins HK, Toliver-Kinsky T, Herndon DN. Browning of subcutaneous white adipose tissue in humans after severe adrenergic stress. Cell Metab. 2015;22(2):219–27. https://doi.org/10.1016/j.cmet.2015.06.022.

101. Patsouris D, Qi P, Abdullahi A, Stanojcic M, Chen P, Parousis A, Amini-Nik S, Jeschke MG. Burn induces browning of the subcutaneous white adipose tissue in mice and humans. Cell Rep. 2015;13(8):1538–44. https://doi.org/10.1016/j.celrep.2015.10.028. Epub 2015 Nov 12.

102. Villarroya F, Cereijo R, Gavalda-Navarro A, Villarroya J, Giralt M. Inflammation of brown/beige adipose tissues in obesity and metabolic disease. J Intern Med. 2018;284:492–504.

103. Abdullahi A, Jeschke MG. Taming the flames: targeting white adipose tissue browning in hypermetabolic conditions. Endocr Rev. 2017;38(6):538–49. https://doi.org/10.1210/er.2017-00163.

104. Petruzzelli M, Schweiger M, Schreiber R, Campos-Olivas R, Tsoli M, Allen J, Swarbrick M, Rose-John S, Rincon M, Robertson G, Zechner R, Wagner EF. A switch from white to brown fat increases energy expenditure in cancer-associated cachexia. Cell Metab. 2014;20(3):433–47. https://doi.org/10.1016/j.cmet.2014.06.011. Epub 2014 Jul 17.

105. Barayan D, Vinaik R, Auger C, Knuth CM, Abdullahi A, Jeschke MG. Inhibition of lipolysis with acipimox attenuates postburn white adipose tissue browning and hepatic fat infiltration. Shock. 2020;53(2):137–45. https://doi.org/10.1097/SHK.0000000000001439.

106. Diao L, Patsouris D, Sadri AR, Dai X, Amini-Nik S, Jeschke MG. Alternative mechanism for white adipose tissue lipolysis after thermal injury. Mol Med. 2016;21(1):959–68. https://doi.org/10.2119/molmed.2015.00123. Epub 2015 Dec 29.

107. Abdullahi A, Samadi O, Auger C, Kanagalingam T, Boehning D, Bi S, Jeschke MG. Browning of white adipose tissue after a burn injury promotes hepatic steatosis and dysfunction. Cell Death Dis. 2019;10(12):870. https://doi.org/10.1038/s41419-019-2103-2.

108. Abdullahi A, Auger C, Stanojcic M, Patsouris D, Parousis A, Epelman S, Jeschke MG. Alternatively activated macrophages drive browning of white adipose tissue in burns. Ann Surg. 2019;269(3):554–63. https://doi.org/10.1097/SLA.0000000000002465.

109. Ando K, Takahashi F, Kato M, Kaneko N, Doi T, Ohe Y, Koizumi F, Nishio K, Takahashi K. Tocilizumab, a proposed therapy for the cachexia of Interleukin6-expressing lung cancer. PloS One. 2014;9(7):e102436. https://doi.org/10.1371/journal.pone.0102436.

110. Abdullahi A, Chen P, Stanojcic M, Sadri AR, Coburn N, Jeschke MG. IL-6 signal from the bone marrow is required for the browning of white adipose tissue post burn injury. Shock. 2017;47(1):33–9. https://doi.org/10.1097/SHK.0000000000000749.

111. Hager S, Foldenauer AC, Rennekampff HO, Deisz R, Kopp R, Tenenhaus M, Gernot M, Pallua N. Interleukin-6 serum levels correlate with severity of burn injury but not with gender. J Burn Care Res. 2018;39(3):379–86. https://doi.org/10.1097/BCR.0000000000000604.

112. Biffl WL, Moore EE, Moore FA, Peterson VM. Interleukin-6 in the injured patient. Marker of injury or mediator of inflammation? Ann Surg. 1996;224(5):647–64. https://doi.org/10.1097/00000658-199611000-00009.

113. Gebhard F, Pfetsch H, Steinbach G, Strecker W, Kinzl L, Brückner UB. Is interleukin 6 an early marker of injury severity following major trauma in humans? Arch Surg. 2000;135(3):291–5. https://doi.org/10.1001/archsurg.135.3.291.

114. Yeh FL, Lin WL, Shen HD, Fang RH. Changes in circulating levels of interleukin 6 in burned patients. Burns. 1999;25(2):131–6. https://doi.org/10.1016/s0305-4179(98)00150-8.

115. Finnerty CC, Mabvuure NT, Ali A, Kozar RA, Herndon DN. The Surgically Induced Stress Response. JPEN. 2013;37:21S–9S. https://doi.org/10.1177/0148607113496117.

116. Gore DC, Jahoor F, Wolfe RR, Herndon DN. Acute response of human muscle protein to catabolic hormones. Ann Surg. 1993;218(5):679–84.

117. Raju R. Immune and metabolic alterations following trauma and sepsis—an overview. Biochim Biophys Acta. 2017;1863(10): 2523–5. https://doi.org/10.1016/j.bbadis.2017.08.008.

118. Perlman RL, Chalfie M. Catecholamine release from the adrenal medulla. Clin Endocrinol Metab. 1977;6(3):551–76. https://doi.org/10.1016/s0300-595x(77)80071-6.

119. Ballard-Croft C, Maass DL, Sikes P, White J, Horton J. Activation of stress-responsive pathways by the sympathetic nervous system in burn trauma. Shock. 2002;18:38–45. https://doi.org/10.1097/00024382-200207000-00008.

120. Bakhtyar N, Sivayoganathan T, Jeschke MG. Therapeutic approaches to combatting hypermetabolism in severe burn injuries. J Crit Care. 2015;1(16):1–12. https://doi.org/10.21767/2471-8505.10006.

121. Cartwright MM. The metabolic response to stress: a case of complex nutrition support management. Crit Care Nurs Clin North Am. 2004;16(4):467–87. https://doi.org/10.1016/j.ccell.2004.07.001.

122. Wilmore DW, Curreri PW, Spitzer KW, Spitzer ME, Pruitt BA. Supranormal dietary intake in thermally injured hypermetabolic patients. Surg Gynecol Obstet. 1971;132(5):881–6.

123. Curreri PW. Assessing nutritional needs for the burned patient. J Trauma. 1990;30(12):S20–3. https://doi.org/10.1097/00005373-199012001-00007.

124. Machado NM, Gragnani A, Ferreira LM. Burns, metabolism and nutritional requirements. Nutr Hosp. 2011;26(4):692–700. https://doi.org/10.3305/nh.2011.26.4.5217.

125. Hall KL, Shahrokhi S, Jeschke MG. Enteral nutrition support in burn care: a review of current recommendations as instituted in

the Ross Tilley Burn Centre. Nutrients. 2012;4:1554–65. https://doi.org/10.3390/nu4111554.

126. Rodriquez NA, Jeschke MG, Williams FN, Kamolz LP, Herndon DN. Nutrition in burns: Galveston contributions. JPEN. 2011;35(6):704–14. https://doi.org/10.1177/0148607111417446.

127. Williams FN, Branski LK, Jeschke MG, Herndon DN. What, how, and how much should patients with burns be fed? Surg Clin North Am 2011;9(3)1:609-629. doi: https://doi.org/10.1016/j.suc.2011.03.002.

128. Gore DC, Chinkes D, Sanford A, Hart DW, Wolfe SE, Herndon DN. Influence of fever on the hypermetabolic response in burn-injured children. Arch Surg. 2003;138(2):169–74. https://doi.org/10.1001/archsurg.138.2.169.

129. Mochizuki H, Trocki O, Dominioni L, Brackett KA, Joffe SN, Alexander JW. Mechanism of prevention of post-burn hypermetabolism and catabolism by early enteral feeding. Ann Surg. 1984;200(3):297–310. https://doi.org/10.1097/00000658-198409000-00007.

130. Saffle JR, Graves C, Herndon DN. Nutritional support of the burned patient. Total burn care. 2007, 3rd ed. London Saunders Elsevier:389-419.

131. Gore DC, Rutan RL, Hildreth M, Desai MH, Herndon DN. Comparison of resting energy expenditures and caloric intake in children with severe burns. J Burn Care Rehabil. 1990;11(5):400–4. https://doi.org/10.1097/00004630-1999009000-00005.

132. Suman OE, Mlcak RP, Chinkes DL, Herndon DN. Resting energy expenditure in severely burned children: analysis of agreement between indirect calorimetry and prediction equations using the Bland-Altman method. Burns. 2006;32(3):335–42.

133. Clark A, Imran J, Madni T, Wolf SE. Nutrition and metabolism in burn patients. Burns Trauma. 2017;5:11. https://doi.org/10.1186/s41038-017-0076-x.

134. Gottschlich MM, Jenkins ME, Mayes T, Khoury J, Kagan RJ, Warden GD. The 2002 Clinical Research Award. An evaluation of the safety of early vs. delayed enteral support and effects on clinical, nutritional, and endocrine outcomes after severe burns. J Burn Care Rehabil. 2002;23(6):401–15. https://doi.org/10.1097/01.BCR.0000036588.09166.F1.

135. Peck MD, Kessler M, Cairns BA, Chang YH, Ivanova A, Schooler W. Early enteral nutrition does not decrease hyperme-

tabolism with burn injury. J Trauma. 2004;57(6):1143–8. https://doi.org/10.1097/01.ta.0000145826.84657.38.

136. Graf S, Pichard C, Genton L, Oshima T, Heidegger CP. Energy expenditure in mechanically ventilated patients: the weight of body weight! Clin Nutr. 2017;36(1):224–8. https://doi.org/10.1016/j.clnu.2015.11.007.

137. Hart DW, Wolf SE, Beauford RB, Lal SO, Chinkes DL, Herndon DN. Determinants of blood loss during primary burn excision. Surgery. 2001;130(2):396–402. https://doi.org/10.1067/msy.2001.116916.

138. Burke JF, Wolfe RR, Mullany CJ, Mathews DE, Bier DM. Glucose requirements following burn injury. Parameters of optimal glucose infusion and possible hepatic and respiratory abnormalities following excessive glucose intake. Ann Surg. 1979;190(3):274–85. https://doi.org/10.1097/00000658-197909000-00002.

139. Wolfe RR. Metabolic response to burn injury: nutritional implications. Semin Nephrol. 1993;13(4):382–90.

140. Patterson BW, Nguyen T, Pierre E, Herndon DN, Wolfe RR. Urea and protein metabolism in burned children: effect of dietary protein intake. Metabolism. 1997;46(5):573–8. https://doi.org/10.1016/S0026-0495(97)90196-7.

141. Gore DC, Jahoor F. Glutamine kinetics in burn patients. Comparison with hormonally induced stress in volunteers. Arch Surg. 1994;129(12):1318–23. https://doi.org/10.1001/archsurg.1994.01420360108015.

142. Windle EM. Glutamine supplementation in critical illness: evidence, recommendations, and implications for clinical practice in burn care. J Burn Care Res. 2006;27(6):764–72. https://doi.org/10.1097/01.BCR.0000245417.47510.9C.

143. Heyland DK, Samis A. Does immunonutrition in patients with sepsis do more harm than good? Intensive Care Med. 2003;29(5):669–71. https://doi.org/10.1007/s00134-003-1719-6.

144. Garrel DR, Razi M, Larivière F, Jobin N, Naman N, Empotoz-Bonneton A, Pugeat MM. Improved clinical status and length of care with low-fat nutrition support in burn patients. JPEN. 1995;19(6):482–91. https://doi.org/10.1177/0148607195019006482.

145. Alexander JW, Gottschlich MM. Nutritional immunomodulation in burn patients. Crit Care Med. 1990;18(2S):S149–53.

146. Alexander JW, Saito T, Trocki O, Ogle CK. The importance of lipid type in the diet after burn injury. Ann Surg. 1986;204(1):1–8. https://doi.org/10.1097/00000658-198607000-00001.

147. Gamliel Z, DeBiasse MA, Demling RH. Essential microminerals and their response to burn injury. J Burn Care Rehabil. 1996;17(3):264–72.

148. Rock CL, Dechert RE, Khilnani R, Parker PS, Rodriguez JL. Carotenoids and antioxidant vitamins in patients after burn injury. J Burn Care Rehabil. 1997;18(3):269–78. https://doi.org/10.1097/00004630-199705000-00018.

149. Klein GL. Burns: where has all the calcium (and vitamin D) gone? Adv Nutr. 2011;2(6):457–62. https://doi.org/10.3945/an.111.000745.

150. Berger MM, Shenkin A. Trace element requirements in critically ill burned patients. J Trace Elem Mol Biol. 2007;21(S1):44–8. https://doi.org/10.1016/j.jtemb.2007.09.013.

151. Berger MM, Binnert C, Chiolero RL, Taylor W, Raffoul W, Cayeux M-C, Benethan M, Shenkin A, Tappy L. Trace elements supplementation after major burns increases burned skin trace element concentrations and modulates local protein metabolism but not whole-body substrate metabolism. Am J Clin Nutr. 2007;85(5):1301–6.

152. Gottschlich MM, Mayes T, Khoury J, Warden GD. Hypovitaminosis D in acutely injured pediatric burn patients. J Am Diet Assoc. 2004;104(6):931–41. https://doi.org/10.1016/j.jada.2004.03.020.

153. Berger MM. Antioxidant micronutrients in major trauma and burns: evidence and practice. Nutr Clin Pract. 2006;21(5):438–49. https://doi.org/10.1177/0115426506021005438.

154. Sampson B, Constantinescu MA, Chandarana I, Cussons PD. Severe hypocupraemia in a patient with extensive burn injuries. Ann Clin Biochem. 1996;33(Pt 5):462–4. https://doi.org/10.1177/000456329603300513.

155. Cunningham JJ, Lydon MK, Emerson R, Harmatz PR. Low ceruloplasmin levels during recovery from major burn injury: Influence of open wound size and copper supplementation. Nutrition. 1996;12(2):83–8. https://doi.org/10.1016/0899-9007(96)90704-2.

156. Huang Z, Rose AH, Hoffman PR. The role of selenium in inflammation and immunity: from molecular mechanisms to therapeutic opportunities. Antioxid Redox Signal. 2012;16(7):705–43. https://doi.org/10.1089/ars.2011.4145.

157. Wilmore DW, Mason AD, Johnson DW, Pruitt BA. Effect of ambient temperature on heat production and heat loss in

burn patients. J Appl Physiol. 1975;38(4):593–7. https://doi.org/10.1152/jappl.1975.38.4.593.

158. Herndon DN, Hawkins HK, Nguyen TT, Pierre E, Cox R, Barrow RE. Characterization of growth hormone enhanced donor site healing in patients with large cutaneous burns. Ann Surg. 1995;221(6):649–56. https://doi.org/10.1097/00000658-199506000-00004.

159. Solomon JR. Early surgical excision and grafting of burns including tangential excision. Prog Pediatr Surg. 1981;14:133–49.

160. Kraemer WJ, Deschenes MR, Fleck SJ. Physiological adaptations to resistance exercise. Implications for athletic conditioning. Sports Med. 1988;6(4):246–56. https://doi.org/10.2165/00007256-198806040-00006.

161. Suman OE, Spies RJ, Celis MM, Mlcak RP, Herndon DN. Effects of a 12-wk resistance exercise program on skeletal muscle strength in children with burn injuries. J Appl Physiol. 2001;91(3):1168–75. https://doi.org/10.1152/jappl.2001.91.3.1168.

162. Breitenstein E, Chioléro RL, Jéquier E, Dayer P, Krupp S, Schutz Y. Effects of beta-blockade on energy metabolism following burns. Burns. 1990;16(4):259–64. https://doi.org/10.1016/0305-4179(90)900136-K.

163. Mohammadi AA, Bakhshaeekia A, Alibeigi P, Hasheminasab MJ, Tolide-ei HR, Tavakkolian AR, Mohammadi MK. Efficacy of propranolol in wound healing for hospitalized burn patients. J Burn Care Res. 2009;30(6):1013–7. https://doi.org/10.1097/BCR.0b013e3181b48600.

164. Jeschke MG, Finnerty CC, Kulp GA, Przkora R, Mlcak RP, Herndon DN. Combination of recombinant human growth hormone and propranolol decreases hypermetabolism and inflammation in severely burned children. Pediatr Crit Care Med. 2008;9(2):209–16. https://doi.org/10.1097/PCC.0b013e318166d414.

165. Martinez R, Rogers A, Numanoglu A, Rode H. Fatal non-occlusive mesenteric ischemia and the use of propranolol in pediatric burns. Burns. 2016;42(4):e70–3. https://doi.org/10.1016/j.burns.2015.08.015.

166. Arbabi S, Ahrns KS, Wahl WL. Beta-blocker use is associated with improved outcomes in adult burn patients. J Trauma. 2004;56(2):265–9. https://doi.org/10.1097/01.TA.0000109859.91202.C8.

167. Flores O, Stockton K, Robers JA. The efficacy and safety of adrenergic blockade after burn injury: a systematic review and

meta-analysis. J Trauma Acute Care Surg. 2016;80(1):146–55. https://doi.org/10.1097/TA.0000000000000887.

168. Kim JB, Cho YS, Jang KU, Joo SY, Choi JS, Soo CH. Effects of sustained release growth hormone treatment during the rehabilitation of adult severe burn survivors. Growth Horm IGF Res. 2016;27:1–6. https://doi.org/10.1016/j.ghir.2015/12.009.

169. Hart DW, Wolf SE, Chinkes DL, Lal SO, Ramzy PI, Herndon DN. β-Blockade and growth hormone after burn. Ann Surg. 2002;236(4):450–7. https://doi.org/10.1097/00000658-200210000-00007.

170. Connolly CM, Barrow RE, Chinkes DL, Martinez JA, Herndon DN. Recombinant human growth hormone increases thyroid hormone-binding sites in recovering severely burned children. Shock. 2003;19(5):399–403. https://doi.org/10.1097/01.shk.0000051758.08171.bc.

171. Branski LK, Herndon DN, Barrow RE, Kulp GA, Klein GL, Suman OE, Przkora R, Meyer W 3rd, Huang T, Lee JO, Chinkes DL, Mlcak RP, Jeschke MG. Randomized controlled trial to determine the efficacy of long-term growth hormone treatment in severely burned children. Ann Surg. 2009;250(4):514–23. https://doi.org/10.1097/SLA.0b013e3181b8f9ca.

172. Breederveld RS, Tuinebreijer WE. Recombinant human growth hormone for treating burns and donor sites (Cochrane Systematic Review). Cochrane Database Syst Rev. 2014;(9):CD008990.

173. Takala J, Ruokonen E, Webster NR, Nielsen MS, Zandstra DF, Vundelinckx G, Hinds CJ. Increased mortality associated with growth hormone treatment in critically ill adults. NEJM. 1999;341:785–92. https://doi.org/10.1056/NEJM199909093411102.

174. Lang CH, Frost RA. Role of growth hormone, insulin-like growth factor-I, and insulin-like growth factor binding proteins in the catabolic response to injury and infection. Curr Opin Clin Nutr Metab Care. 2002;5(3):271–9. https://doi.org/10.1097/00075197-2000205000-00006.

175. Cioffi WG, Gore DC, Rue LW 3rd, Carrougher G, Guler HP, McManus WF, Pruitt BA Jr. Insulin-like growth factor-1 lower protein oxidation in patients with thermal injury. Ann Surg. 1994;220(3):310–6. https://doi.org/10.1097/00000658-199409000-00007.

176. Jeschke MG, Barrow RE, Herndon DN. Recombinant human growth hormone treatment in pediatric burn patients and its role during the hepatic acute phase

response. Crit Care Med. 2000;28(5):1578–84. https://doi.org/10.1097/00003246-200005000-00053.

177. Spies M, Wolf SE, Barrow RE. Modulation of types I and II acute phase reactants with insulin-like growth factor-1/binding protein-3 complex in severely burned children. Crit Care Med. 2002;30(1):83–8.

178. Wolf SE, Woodside KJ, Ramirez RJ, Kobayashi M, Suzuki F, Herndon DN. Insulin-like growth factor-1/insulin-like growth factor binding protein-3 alters lymphocyte responsiveness following severe burn. J Surg Res. 2004;117(2):255–61. https://doi.org/10.1016/S0022-4804(03)00305-6.

179. Jeschke MG, Barrow RE, Herndon DN. Insulin-like growth factor I plus insulin-like growth factor binding protein 3 attenuates the proinflammatory acute phase response in severely burned children. Ann Surg. 2000;231(2):246–52. https://doi.org/10.1097/00000658-200002000-00014.

180. Jeschke MG, Barrow RE, Suzuki F, Rai J, Benjamin D, Herndon DN. IGF-1/IGFBP-3 equilibrates ratios of pro- to anti-inflammatory cytokines, which are predictors for organ function in severely burned pediatric patients. Mol Med. 2002;8(5):238–46.

181. Hasselbren PO. Burns and metabolism. J Am Coll Surg. 1999;188(2):98–103.

182. Van den Berghe G. On the neuroendocrinopathy of critical illness. Am J Respir Crit Care Med. 2016;194(11):1337–48.

183. Debroy MA, Wolf SE, Zhang XJ, Chinkes DL, Ferrando AA, Wolfe RR, Herndon DN. Anabolic effects of insulin-like growth factor in combination with insulin-like growth factor binding protein-3 in severely burned adults. J Trauma. 1999;47(5):904–10.

184. Gore DC, Wolfe SE, Herndon DN, Wolfe RR. Relative influence of glucose and insulin on peripheral amino acid metabolism in severely burned patients. JPEN. 2002;26(5):272–7. https://doi.org/10.1177/0148607102026005271.

185. Pham TN, Warren AJ, Phan HH. Impact of tight glycemic control in severely burned children. J Trauma. 2005;59:1148–54. https://doi.org/10.1097/01.ta.0000188933.16637.68.

186. Pidcoke HF, Baer LA, Wu X, Wolf SE, Aden JK, Wade CE. Insulin effects on glucose tolerance, hypermetabolic response, and circadian-metabolic protein expression in a rat burn and disuse model. Am J Physiol Regul Integr

Comp Physiol. 2014;307(1):R1–R10. https://doi.org/10.1152/ajpregu.00312.2013.

187. Gore DC, Wolf SE, Sanford AP. Extremity hyperinsulinemia stimulates muscle protein synthesis in severely injured patients. Am J Physiol Endocrinol Metab. 2004;286(4):E529–34. https://doi.org/10.1152/ajpendo.00258.2003.

188. Jeschke MG, Boehning DF, Finnerty CC, Herndon DN. Effect of insulin on the inflammatory and acute phase response after burn injury. Crit Care Med. 2007;35(9S):S519–23.

189. Van den Berghe G. How does blood glucose control with insulin save lives in intensive care? J Clin Invest. 2004;114(9):1187–225. https://doi.org/10.1172/JCI23506.

190. Codère-Maruyama T, Schricker T, Shum-Tim D, Wykes L, Nitschmann E, Guichon C, Kristof AS, Hatzakorzian R. Hyperinsulinemic-normoglycemic clamp administered together with amino acids induces anabolism after cardiac surgery. Am J Physiol Regul Integr Comp Physiol. 2016;311(6):1085–92. https://doi.org/10.1152/ajpregu.000334.2016.

191. Ferrando AA, Chinkes DL, Wolfe SE, Matin S, Herndon DN, Wolfe RR. A submaximal dose of insulin promotes net skeletal muscle protein synthesis in patients with severe burns. Ann Surg. 1999;229(1):11–8. https://doi.org/10.1097/00000658-199901000-00002.

192. Gore DC, Wolf SE, Sanford A, Herndon DN, Wolfe RR. Influence of metformin on glucose intolerance and muscle catabolism following severe burn injury. Ann Surg. 2005;241(2):334–42. https://doi.org/10.1097/01.sla.0000152013.23032.d1.

193. Miller RA, Chu Q, Xie J, Foretz M, Viollet B, Birnbaum MJ. Biguanides suppress hepatic glucagon signaling by decreasing production of cyclic AMP. Nature. 2013;494(7436):256–60. https://doi.org/10.1038/nature11808.

194. Gore DC, Herndon DN, Wolfe RR. Comparison of peripheral metabolic effects of insulin and metformin following severe burn injury. J Trauma. 2005;59(2):316–23. https://doi.org/10.1097/01.ta.0000180387.34057.5a.

195. Auger C, Samadi O, Jeschke MG. The biochemical alterations underlying post-burn hypermetabolism. Biochim Biophys Acta. 2017;1863(10):2633–44. https://doi.org/10.1016/j.bbadis.2017.02.019.

196. Salpeter SR, Greyber E, Pasternak GA, Salpeter EE. Risk of fatal and nonfatal lactic acidosis with metformin use in type 2

diabetes mellitus: a systematic review and meta-analysis. Arch Intern Med. 2003;163(21):2594–602.

197. Riesenman PJ, Braithwaite SS, Cairns BA. Metformin-associated lactic acidosis in a burn patient. J Burn Care Res. 2007;28(2):342–7. https://doi.org/10.1097/BCR.0B013E318031A1FE.

198. Sears B, Perry M. The role of fatty acids in insulin resistance. Lipids Health Dis. 2015;14:121. https://doi.org/10.1186/s12944-015-0123-1.

199. Di Girolamo FG, Situlin R, Biolo G. What factors influence protein synthesis and degradation in critical illness? Curr Opin Clin Nutr Metab Care. 2017;20(2):124–30.

200. Barrow RE, Dasu MR, Ferando AA, Spies M, Thomas SJ, Perez-Polo JR, Herndon DN. Gene expression patterns in skeletal muscle of thermally injured children treated with oxandrolone. Ann Surg. 2003;237(3):422–8. https://doi.org/10.1097/01.SLA.0000055276.10357.FB.

201. Wolf SE, Thomas SJ, Dasu MR, Ferrando AA, Chinkes DL, Wolfe RR, Herndon DN. Improved net protein balance, lean mass, and gene expression changes with oxandrolone treatment in the severely burned. Ann Surg. 2003;237(6):801–11. https://doi.org/10.1097/01.SLA.0000071562.12637.3E.

202. Cochran A, Thuet W, Holt B, Faraklas I, Smout RJ, Horn SD. The impact of oxandrolone on length of stay following major burn injury: a clinical practice evaluation. Burns. 2013;39(7):1374–9. https://doi.org/10.1016/j.burns.2013.04.002.

203. Jeschke MG, Norbury WB, Finnerty CC, Branski LK, Herndon DN. Propranolol does not increase inflammation, sepsis, or infections episodes in severely burned children. J Trauma. 2007;62(3):676–81. https://doi.org/10.1097/TA/0b013e318031afd3.

204. Pham TN, Klein MB, Gibran NS, Arnolod BD, Camelli RL, Silver GM, Jeschke MG, Finnerty CC, Tompkins RG, Herndon DN. Impact of oxandrolone treatment on acute outcomes after severe burn injury. J Burn Care Res. 2008;29(6):902–6. https://doi.org/10.1097/BCR.0b013e31818ba14d.

205. Porro LJ, Herndon DN, Rodriguez NA. Five-year outcomes after oxandrolone administration in severely burned children: a randomized clinical trial of safety and efficacy. J Am Coll Surg. 2012;214(4):489–502. https://doi.org/10.1016/j.jamcollsurg.2011.12.038.

206. Demling RH. The role of anabolic hormones for wound healing in catabolic states. J Burns Wounds. 2005;4:46–62.

207. Jeschke M, Finnerty CC, Suman OE. The effect of oxandrolone on the endocrinologic, inflammatory, and hypermetabolic responses during the acute phase postburn. Ann Surg. 2007;246(3):351–62. https://doi.org/10.1097/SLA.0b013e318146980e.

208. Miller JT, Btaiche IF. Oxandrolone treatment in adults with severe thermal injury. Pharmacotherapy. 2009;29(2):213–26. https://doi.org/10.1592/phco.29.2.213.

209. McCullough MC, Namias N, Schulman C, Gomez E, Manning R, Goldberg S, Pizano L, Ward GC. Incidence of hepatic dysfunction is equivalent in burn patients receiving oxandrolone and controls. J Burn Care Res. 2007;28(3):412–20. https://doi.org/10.1087/BCR.0B013E318053D257.

210. Ferrando AA, Sheffield-Moore M, Wolfe SE, Herndon DN, Wolfe RR. Testosterone administration in severe burn patients ameliorates muscle catabolism. Crit Care Med. 2001;29(10):1936–42. https://doi.org/10.1097/00003246-200110000-00015.

211. Ferrando AA. Anabolic hormones in critically ill patients. Curr Opin Clin Nutr Metab Care. 1999;2(2):171–5. https://doi.org/10.1097/00075197-199903000-00014.

212. Ferrando AA, Wolfe RR. Restoration of hormonal action and muscle protein. Crit Care Med. 2007;35(9S):S630–4. https://doi.org/10.1097/01.CCM.0000278529.44899.57.

213. Spratt DI. Altered gonadal steroidogenesis in critical illness: is treatment with anabolic steroids indicated? Best Pract Res Clin Endocrinol Metab. 2001;15(4):479–94. https://doi.org/10.1053/beem.2001.0165.

214. Basaria S, Coviello AD, Travison TG, et al. Adverse events associated with testosterone administration. N Engl J Med. 2010;363(2):109–22. https://doi.org/10.1056/NEJMoa1000485.

Chapter 3
Initial Assessment of Burn Patient

Matthew A. DePamphilis and Robert L. Sheridan

Introduction

One of the first documented initial assessments of a burn patient was by the Harvard anesthesiologist Henry K. Breecher in description of his first impression when caring for victims of the Coconut Grove Fire [1] in Boston, Massachusetts on November 28, 1942 [2]. This historic tragedy led to a new era of burn research focused on optimizing patient survival and long-term outcome. Since then, a four

M. A. DePamphilis
Boston Shriners Hospital for Children, Boston, MA, USA

Boston University Chobanian and Avedisian School of Medicine, Boston, MA, USA

Division of Burns, Massachusetts General Hospital, Boston, MA, USA
e-mail: mdepamph@bu.edu

R. L. Sheridan (✉)
Boston Shriners Hospital for Children, Boston, MA, USA

Division of Burns, Massachusetts General Hospital, Boston, MA, USA

Department of Surgery, Harvard Medical School, Boston, MA, USA
e-mail: rsheridan@mgh.harvard.edu

© The Author(s), under exclusive license to Springer Nature Switzerland AG 2023
J. O. Lee (ed.), *Essential Burn Care for Non-Burn Specialists*,
https://doi.org/10.1007/978-3-031-28898-2_3

clinical phase approach to burn care has been formulated and specialized burn centers have been established [3]. The first phase of burn care encompasses initial assessment, triage, and fluid resuscitation, which is typically completed over the first 72 hours post-injury. A methodical initial assessment accompanied with an effectively implemented triage and referral system can help shorten hospital stay, reduce costs, and most importantly, have a long-lasting impact on a patient's recovery. In this chapter, the authors will describe how to perform the initial assessment of burn care in terms of careful evaluation of the patient, thorough assessment of the burn wounds, and appropriate determination of when specialty referral is needed. Basic principles of prehospital care and initial assessment considerations for special situations are also reviewed.

First Aid and Prehospital Considerations

The main priorities of prehospital care include removing the patient from the burn source, addressing any immediate life-threatening conditions, maintaining normothermia, and appropriately transporting the patient to a medical facility (Fig. 3.1). On arrival to the injury site and prior to initiating care, emergency responders should take a moment to assess the scene, ensuring that it is safe to approach and that they will not be putting their own lives at risk. If the patient is still at the burn source, then a provider should cautiously extricate the patient and stop the burning process. The patient's clothing should be removed to prevent further burn injury. Any belts or jewelry should also be removed as they may produce a tourniquet-like effect resulting in vascular compromise with onset of edema.

During prehospital care, first responders have the option of applying cool water (15–25 °C) to the burn wounds in attempt to limit the extent of burn injury and reduce pain. This practice is a topic of controversy because of the risk of inducing systemic hypothermia due to impaired thermoregulation in burn patients. Generally, immediate cooling is only advised in instances when the providers arrive within a few minutes of injury for minor burns less than 10% of the body surface. Ice or icepacks should not be used as a topical cool-

First Aid and Prehospital Measures	Comments and Considerations
Extricate the patient and stop the burning process	• Always first assess scene safety • Carefully approach with the necessary protective equipment
Remove the patient's clothing and jewelry	• This step can help prevent further injury • Do not attempt to remove any material that has adhered to the patient's skin, cut around it
Immediately cool the burn wounds by application of water	• The patient's condition and risk of hypothermia must be considered, typically cooling is only beneficial within minutes of minor burns • Water should be 15°C to 25°C and applied briefly (3-5 minutes) • Ice or icepacks should not be used
Assess the patient and address any life-threatening conditions	• Primary survey (ABCs of trauma management) • Secondary survey (when applicable)
Obtain and document a detailed history	• Especially related to the events and circumstances of injury from personnel who will not be available to the receiving facility • Emergency providers should clearly document all interventions administered
Appropriately triage and transport	• Consult regional protocols: most patients are first transported to the nearest emergency department for stabilization, some patients may be eligible for direct burn center admission • Notify family members of the transport decision (when applicable) • Fluid administration may be necessary for transport times greater than 1 hour
Maintain the patient's body temperature	• Patients with burn injuries are at high risk for hypothermia • The transporting vehicle should be heated • The patient should be wrapped in dry, clean, sheets or blankets • Wet dressings or any topical home remedies should not be used

FIGURE 3.1 A checklist of important measures that first responders should address during prehospital care of a burn patient

ing measure. During transport, the patient should be kept in a warm and dry environment to prevent hypothermia. Transporting vehicles should be heated and the patient should be wrapped in dry, clean, sheets, and blankets. Wet dressings should be avoided and may even be hazardous due to the significant risk of hypothermia and infection.

Standard prehospital triage of a burn patient typically follows a system of first transporting the patient to the best available care facility for assessment, stabilization, and subsequent referral determination. Appropriate options are often the nearest emergency department or local general hospital. There are some instances where an amalgamation of factors such as age, past medical history, burn severity, and mechanism may warrant direct admission to a specialized burn center.

Initial Assessment

At some point in their career, non-burn specialists may be called upon to perform an initial assessment on a patient that sustained a burn injury. Most commonly, patients will present to a non-burn specialist with superficial wounds that are uncomplicated, necessitating a non-intensive initial assessment. However, in some instances, a patient may present with severe burns accompanied with serious multisystem injury requiring high-level evaluation. Following an organized approach to the initial assessment with attention to certain burn-specific issues, as described in this section, can have a profound impact on the patient's survival and long-term recovery [4, 5].

Primary Survey

The initial assessment of a burn patient begins with the primary survey, which is similar to that of a trauma patient. It should follow the format that has been developed by the American College of Surgeons Committee on Trauma and taught in the Advanced Trauma Life Support program [6]. The American Burn Association has also established guidelines that are covered in the Advanced Burn Life Support courses [7]. The main principle of the primary survey is to identify and immediately address life-threatening injuries related to airway, breathing, circulation, disability, and exposure (the ABCs). There are some salient burn-specific circumstances that should be highlighted.

Airway security is of utmost importance and can be especially challenging to maintain in burn patients (see Chap. 5) [8, 9]. Inhalation injury or burns to the face and neck can threaten airway patency and breathing, sometimes requiring prophylactic endotracheal intubation if obstructive mucosal edema evolves. This is especially true for young children as they have proportionally smaller airways that can be rapidly occluded by progressive edema [10]. Indications that should raise concern for impending airway loss include: (1) a history of smoke exposure or enclosed space entrapment, (2) progressive stridor, wheezing, or hoarseness, (3) singed nasal vibrissae, (4) soot in the airway, (5) carbonaceous debris in the mouth, pharynx, or sputum, or (6) hypoxia. Following

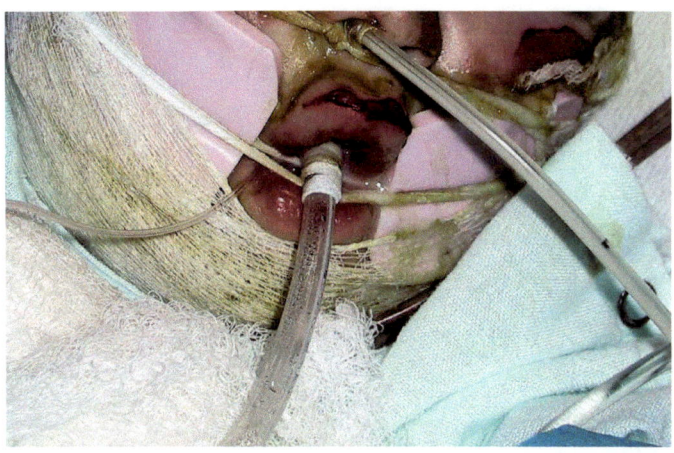

FIGURE 3.2 Examining the airway is an essential component of the initial assessment for a burn patient. Patients with facial burns or suspected inhalation injury may require intubation. Following intubation, it is crucial to properly secure and frequently monitor the endotracheal tube as extensive airway edema formation can make reintubation increasingly difficult. A twill-tie harness system overprotective pads, as assembled for this patient, can reliably secure the endotracheal tube and reduce injury to the oral commissures

intubation, it is critical to properly secure and monitor the endotracheal tube, which can be reliably accomplished with a harness system using umbilical ties or other commercial devices (Fig. 3.2). Improper management of a threatened airway or an unplanned extubation can be severely problematic as evolving edema may complicate intubation or reintubation efforts [11].

Following airway control, effective breathing and symmetrical air entry should be assessed. Any thick or circumferential eschar considerably hindering chest wall compliance may require escharotomy to improve ventilation. Bronchospasm can typically be treated with nebulized β-adrenergic agonists. Achieving reliable vascular access and beginning initial fluid infusion are important priorities for patients with visibly large

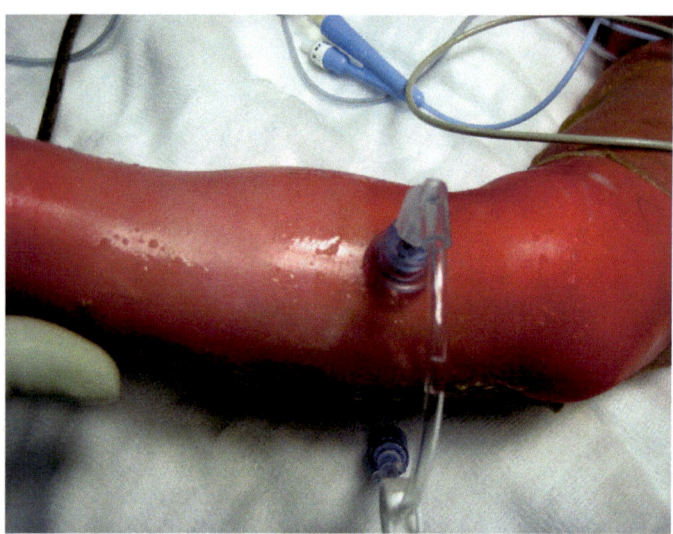

FIGURE 3.3 Obtaining stable vascular access is of critical importance for patients with severe burns. When central or peripheral access is difficult to secure, intraosseous access is a sufficient alternative that can support initial resuscitation. In emergencies, placing the device through burned skin is acceptable. These devices should be removed or replaced at an unburned site when appropriate

burns. The optimal access option is central venous line placement through intact skin. In emergencies, placing peripheral or intraosseous lines through burns is acceptable (Fig. 3.3). As the final component of the primary survey, it is imperative to perform a quick neurological assessment for all burn patients to assess level of consciousness (AVPU scale ["Awake, Verbal, Pain, Unresponsive"] and Glasgow Coma Scale).

Burn-Specific Secondary Survey

Obtaining a Burn-Specific History

One of the priorities of the secondary survey should be eliciting and documenting a detailed history from the patient (when possible) concerning the patient's past medical history

All Burn Patients		Special Situations	
Past Medical History	Circumstances of Burn Injury	Chemical Injury	Electrical Injury
• Allergies • Medications • Previous illnesses or injuries • Last oral intake • Immunization status (especially tetanus) • Pre-injury weight • Any vital signs, fluids, or procedures performed by prior providers	• Mechanism • Date and time of injury • Closed space exposure • Extrication time • Loss of consciousness • Presence of smoke or toxic gases • Potential for nonaccidental injury	•Substance(s) involved •Quantity and concentration of the agents •Duration of exposure •Suspected occular involvement •Any prior decontamination efforts	•Voltage and amperage of source •Type of circuit (AC/DC) •Points of contact •Duration of contact •Any falls or potential trauma •Ignition of clothing or presence of flame
		Cold Injury	Nonaccidental Injury: Child Maltreatment
		•If mechanism was influenced by societal factors (home insecurity, substance misuse, mental illness) •Duration of exposure •Any prior rewarming efforts	•Tap water temperature (scald) •Caretakers involved •Conflicting reports from involved caretakers •Timeline (delay in seeking treatment)

FIGURE 3.4 A checklist of the pertinent history points that should be gathered at the beginning of the secondary survey. Significant information related to the patient's past medical history and the circumstances of injury should be collected from all patients that present with burn wounds. For special burn situations, there are additional etiology-specific details that should be gathered. Thorough documentation of all relevant history information is essential

and circumstances surrounding the burn injury (Fig. 3.4). A directed effort should also be made to interview any family members or witnesses that were present at the time of injury as well as any emergency response personnel or medical providers involved in prior care. This is a crucial component of the initial assessment as an accurate history can provide insight into factors that might influence burn care and management decisions.

Burn Patient Assessment

A more detailed head-to-toe assessment is an essential component of the secondary survey and should precede examination of the burn wounds. This patient assessment component of the secondary survey is similar to that of any trauma patient. At this stage, the patient should have a reliable airway and should be hemodynamically stabilized. Careful assessment should identify any associated medical illness or traumatic injury as approximately 5–7% of burn patients may also present with non-thermal trauma [12]. Physical examination should be supplemented with appropriate use of laboratory testing and diagnostic imaging driven by mechanism of injury. There are some common concomitant clinical issues that may present with burn injuries that should be discussed.

Neurologic

A comprehensive neurological evaluation is paramount and can become exceedingly difficult as patients with serious burn injuries can typically enter an obtunded state over the succeeding hours. Central nervous system trauma such as intracranial injury or any spinal and ligamentous disruption should be excluded. A computed tomographic scan of the head and spine should be ordered for any mechanism that is consistent with head injury. Toxic gas poisoning may occur in patients with inhalation injury or a history consistent with enclosed space exposure. Mental status abnormalities should prompt suspicion of carbon monoxide poisoning, which can be detected by measurement of carboxyhemoglobin levels. Additionally, there should be an early multidisciplinary effort to devise a strategy for safely managing the patient's inevitable pain and anxiety (see Chap. 16). For most burn patients, pain and anxiety are often best initially controlled by titrating small doses of narcotic analgesics and benzodiazepines.

Ophthalmologic

An ocular examination is another necessary component of the secondary survey. The globes should be assessed early for injury because progressive edema and adnexal swelling will make this challenging. Deep ocular burns resulting in corneal epithelial loss may cause the cornea to have a cloudy appear-

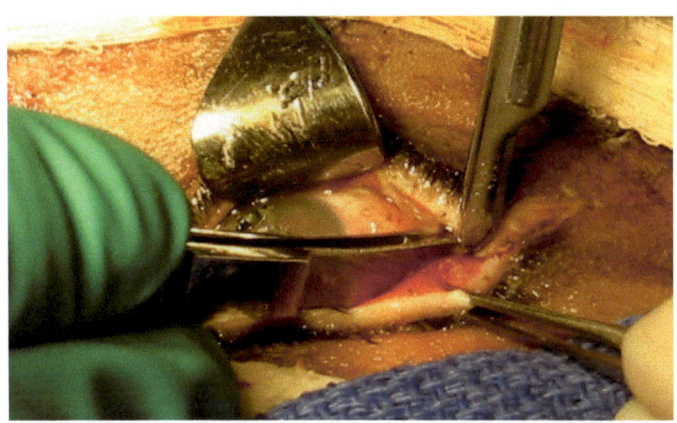

FIGURE 3.5 An early ocular examination is an important part of the secondary survey for a burn patient. Although rare, deep burns to the face and orbit may result in diffuse edema formation that can elevate intraocular pressure and threaten vision. Critically high intraocular pressures can be diagnosed by tonometry and decompressed by lateral canthotomy, as demonstrated in this patient. Note the cornea's clouded appearance, indicating serious globe burns

ance. More subtle ocular injuries can be detected using fluorescein staining. At this time, tarsorrhaphy is rarely necessary as eyelid edema typically provides sufficient globe coverage. Deep facial burns in patients with large surface area burns and diffuse edema can be associated with vision-threatening intraocular hypertension. In such scenarios, early ophthalmologic consultation with tonometry is indicated. If demonstrated, lateral canthotomy can immediately normalize intraocular pressure and preserve retinal blood flow (Fig. 3.5).

Otolaryngologic

The otolaryngology assessment begins with palpation of the head, face, and neck for signs of trauma or fractures. The possibility of inhalation injury should be reevaluated through physical examination of the throat and nose. Fiberoptic bronchoscopy, CT scanning, and radionuclide imaging have been proposed as adjuncts for inhalation injury severity stratification, but in most cases diagnostic accuracy is adequate with history and physical examination [12, 13]. When applicable, the position and security of the endotracheal tube should be reassessed. Although rare, the neck and face should be examined for any deep, circumferential eschar that may impair venous return and addressed accordingly with escharotomy.

Chest and Abdomen

There are several objectives of the chest and abdominal secondary survey. The torso and abdomen should be examined for any associated trauma. Inappropriate resuscitative volume requirements may be a sign of an occult intra-abdominal injury. Ulcer prophylaxis and nasogastric tube placement are indicated for all patients with serious burn injuries. Radiographs can help rule out any concomitant trauma and confirm catheter or tube placement. The chest should be reassessed to ensure adequate and symmetric ventilation. The evolving need for chest or abdominal decompression should be evaluated. Intra-abdominal hypertension can develop in patients with large burns, diffuse anasarca, and delayed resuscitation causing hypotension, impaired ventilation, and oliguria. In such patients, abdominal decompression may be required to restore hemodynamics, ventilation, and renal perfusion (Fig. 3.6).

Genitourinary

In addition to documenting injury, the primary genitourinary concern of the secondary survey is ensuring that a Foley catheter is placed for patients requiring fluid resuscitation. For uncircumcised male patients, the foreskin should be reduced over the bladder catheter to prevent paraphimosis as a result of progressive edema.

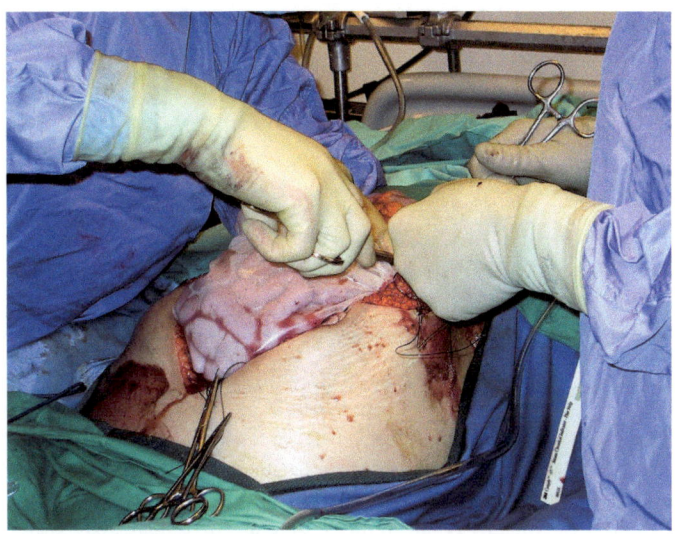

FIGURE 3.6 When assessing the abdomen, significant distention in the presence of oliguria should raise concern for abdominal compartment syndrome. This syndrome can be confirmed with bladder pressure measurements and treated with decompressive laparotomy, as illustrated in this patient

Extremity

Evaluation of the extremities centers on excluding non-burn injuries and monitoring peripheral perfusion. Radiographs can be helpful to identify any extremity fractures. Fractured and burned extremities should initially be stabilized with splints. Elevating the affected extremities may help reduce swelling. The evolving need for escharotomy should be carefully examined by frequently assessing extremity temperature, pliability, voluntary motion, pain with passive motion, named vessel pulsations, and low-pressure blood flow with the use of capillary refill and Doppler signals in the digital vessels (Fig. 3.7). In instances when escharotomy does not

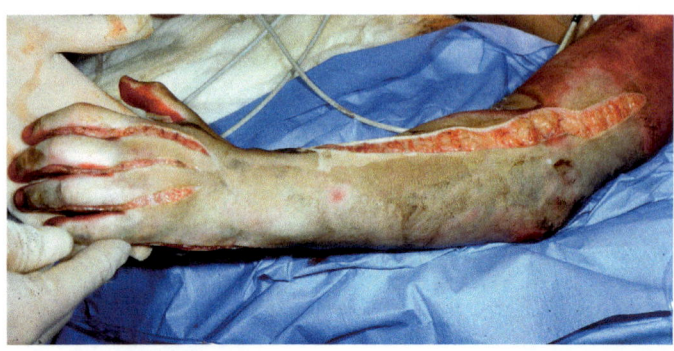

FIGURE 3.7 In patients with deep circumferential burns, edema may form beneath eschar, which can result in vascular comprise and impaired function. During the initial assessment, clinicians should identify any burn wounds that require close monitoring or decompression by escharotomy. Promptly and properly performed escharotomy will typically result in immediate improvement in perfusion, as demonstrated in this example of an upper extremity (including hand and digits) escharotomy. Use of electrocautery and topical clotting agents can help control bleeding

restore peripheral perfusion, fasciotomy should be considered; most common with very deep burns or high-voltage electrical injuries (Fig. 3.8).

Evaluation of the Burn Wound

A fundamental aspect of initial burn care is knowing how to accurately evaluate a patient's burn injuries. Burn wounds are highly quantifiable, and these calculations are critical as they will help guide resuscitation requirements, referral determination, and prognosis. Focus should be shifted to examining the burn wounds only after the patient's overall condition has been thoroughly assessed and stabilized. Important burn wound assessment measures include (1) depth, (2) extent, (3) circumferential components, and (4) infectious colonization.

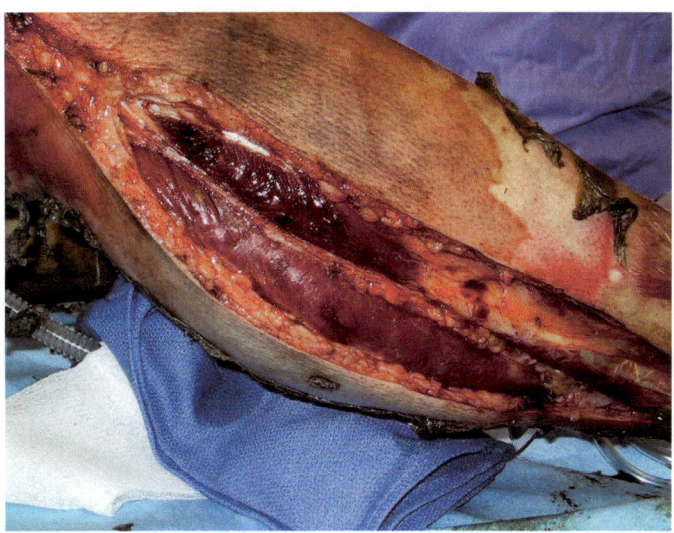

FIGURE 3.8 In instances of very deep burns or high-voltage electrical injury, edema may collect within extremity muscle compartments that can result in limb ischemia. In these cases, escharotomy alone may not be sufficient, requiring fasciotomy to release tension and restore perfusion. Fasciotomies can be performed through the initial escharotomy incisions, as portrayed in this lateral view of a decompressed lower extremity that sustained deep flame burns

Burn wound depth (or the propensity of a burned area to heal) drives surgical and non-surgical care planning (Fig. 3.9). Burn depth follows a classification system that categorizes the degree of tissue penetration from superficial to full-thickness (more commonly known as first-degree to fourth-degree) (Figs. 3.10 and 3.11). Burn wound extent influences resuscitation and transport decisions and is calculated by determining the percentage of total body surface area (%TBSA) that is involved in a burn. Superficial burns (first-degree burns) are the most benign and should not be included in %TBSA calculations.

Level of Burn Injury			Clinical Characteristics				
Burn Thickness	Common Classification	Depth of Involved Tissues	Color and Texture	Blisters	Intact Hair Follicles	Capillary Refill	Sensation
Superficial	First-degree	Epidermis only	Pink to red; dry	No	Yes	Blanches quickly with pressure	Hypersensitive; painful
Superficial partial-thickness	Superficial second-degree	Papillary dermis (entire epidermis and superficial dermis)	Homogeneous pink to red; wet	Yes	Yes	Blanches with pressure	Hypersensitive; very painful
Deep partial-thickness	Deep second-degree	Reticular dermis (entire epidermis and deeper portions of the dermis)	Mottled red and white; dry	Yes or No	No, hair removes easily	Reduced blanching with pressure	Intact but decreased sensation; variable in pain
Full-thickness	Third-degree, fourth-degree	Entire cutaneous layer (third-degree), and may extend through subcutaneous tissue involving fascia, muscle, and/or bone (fourth-degree)	Waxy white, brown, and/or black; leathery, charred, and/or inelastic; dry	No	No	Does not blanch	Insensate; any pain is typically caused by surrounding burned tissue of lesser depth

Figure 3.9 A summary of the clinical characteristics at each burn depth level

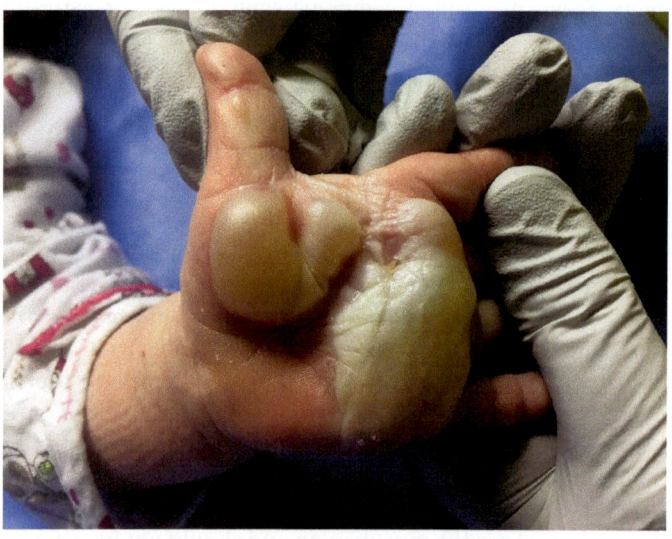

Figure 3.10 An example of a superficial partial-thickness contact burn to the hand. Note the characteristic blister and fluid formation. When blisters are removed, the underlying wound is pink, wet, and hypersensitive

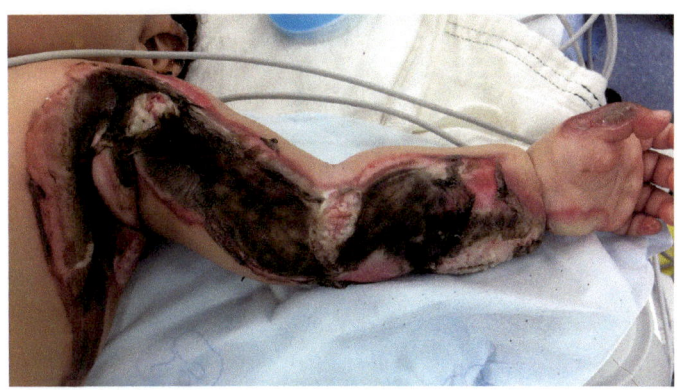

FIGURE 3.11 An example of a deep full-thickness burn to the upper extremity. Note the charred and dry surface appearance with areas of thick, black eschar

Several clinical evaluation methods exist to help guide %TBSA measurements including the "Rule of Nines" [14], the "Rule of Palms" [15], and the Lund-Browder Chart [16]. The "Rule of Nines" is the quickest guide as it divides anatomic regions into distinct sections that are equivalent to multiples of 9% TBSA. However, this method is usually the most inaccurate and should not be used for children because it fails to account for different body size ratios. The "Rule of Palms" considers the palmar surface of the patient's hand (including digits) as 1% TBSA and is especially advantageous for irregularly shaped burns that are not confluent. Overall, the Lund-Browder chart is the most preferred method because it accounts for changes in body proportions across different age groups, making it the most reliable. For the Lund-Browder method, a 2D diagram that mimics the patient is utilized to shade in the burn and then an associated table helps to calculate the %TBSA. A Lund-Browder diagram should be carefully completed and documented for all patients with major burns.

Unfortunately, in many cases, burn wound depth and extent are difficult to ascertain on initial examination, especially for

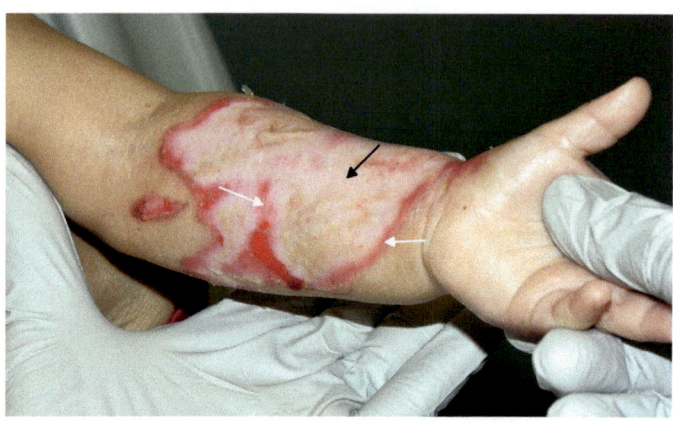

FIGURE 3.12 Burn depth can be difficult to ascertain on initial encounter. In some cases, variable burn depth may not be apparent until after initial wound cleansing and debridement. Note the scattered and surrounding areas of partial-thickness injury (*white arrows*) within this majority full-thickness burn wound (*black arrow*)

those who are non-burn specialists (Fig. 3.12) [17]. For any questionable burn wounds, a non-burn provider should consider consulting by telemedicine with a burn specialist to help make an accurate wound assessment and craft an appropriate plan [18]. Even by specialists, burn wounds are often underestimated in depth and overestimated in extent at initial encounter [19, 20]. Therefore, there have been ongoing efforts to develop non-invasive technology to precisely determine extent and depth of a burn wound. Various wound mapping applications are currently available to assist with extent determination [21, 22]. A number of adjuncts have been devised to help estimate burn wound depth including fluorescence [23], thermography [24], ultrasound imaging [25], and laser Doppler imaging [26]. Each of these technologies has weaknesses and none have become standard of care. If used, these adjuncts should supplement, not replace, clinical evaluation.

In addition to depth and extent examination, burn wounds that have circumferential nature should be identified, closely monitored, and decompressed with escharotomy when necessary (see Burn Patient Assessment section). Pertinent locations include the extremities, torso, abdomen, and neck. Wounds should also be inspected for signs of infection including unusual color, drainage, or odor. Suspicions of infection should be confirmed with wound and blood cultures.

Triage, Referral, and Transfer Determination

At the conclusion of the secondary survey, a determination needs to be reached as to who should be treated as an outpatient, who should be treated in a local general hospital, and who should be referred to a specialized burn center. It is as important to properly assess a burn patient as it is to recognize those wounds and patients that require specialty care [27]. Appropriate and early referral determination can have a large impact on optimizing a patient's outcome and reducing costs [28, 29].

Treatment of minor burns can be successfully achieved through close outpatient clinic follow-up (predominately uncomplicated and small superficial to superficial partial-thickness burns) (see Chap. 17). Although, there are some circumstances when hospital admission for minor burns is acceptable. Moderate burns may be treated by an experienced physician as an inpatient at a general hospital or can be referred to a burn center (generally partial-thickness to small full-thickness burns). If the burns are major (large or deep burns, any special type of burn, and any burn complicated by inhalation injury, circumferential nature, critical area involvement [face, hands, feet, genitalia, perineum, or major joints], associated non-burn injuries, preexisting conditions, or the patient's age), then the patient should be transferred to a specialized regional burn care facility. The American Burn Association has promulgated guidelines that outline specific burn injuries that typically require specialty burn center referral [7].

Using a "common sense" approach when contemplating whether a patient should be transferred is always advisable, honestly considering local resources and care team expertise.

Regardless of disposition decision, detailed coordination is essential. Frequent and ongoing communication should be facilitated between the referring and receiving centers. When in doubt, the best practice is to consult a specialist at a local burn center to help guide the decision process [18].

Tertiary Survey

The last phase of the initial assessment for a burn patient is the tertiary survey, which occurs over a period of 24–72 h post-admission. The tertiary survey is applicable to patients that cannot be transferred within 24 h or if a determination has been made to continue treatment at a general hospital. At this point in care, fluid resuscitation and initial wound management should already have commenced (see Chap. 4). The main focus of this stage is reevaluation, accomplished through both serial physical examination and one final thorough patient assessment. For serious burns, there should be an ongoing effort to reasonably exclude all potential injuries. The importance of this phase cannot be underestimated [30]. Several issues that may have been overlooked or appear subtle during previous stages of the initial assessment can quickly become catastrophic and life threatening over time.

In addition to regularly monitoring the patient's condition, the burn wounds should be serially examined. Progressive edema formation beneath eschar or fascial compartments is common in burn patients and is especially prominent throughout the initial resuscitative period for those with large, deep, or circumferential wounds. Failure to identify at-risk compartments can result in impaired ventilation or irreversible tissue necrosis. Therefore, the evolving need for or the effectiveness of previous decompression should be frequently assessed throughout initial care. Also, a continuous effort to reevaluate the burn wounds for depth and extent should be instituted. Burns are dynamic and may continue to progress for days after injury; especially common with chemical and electrical injuries, which are notorious for underestimation. This step is essential because it may trigger adjustments to initial resuscitation requirements or initial management strategies.

Another necessary component of the tertiary survey is a planned meticulous head-to-toe patient examination supplemented with focused diagnostic testing. The main objective of this repeat thorough assessment is to identify concomitant injuries that were either minor or missed during the chaos of previous stages of the initial assessment. Common examples that clinicians should be on the lookout for are any extremity fractures, small lacerations of the scalp, subtle eye injuries, or abdominal visceral injuries. Taking the time for this additional assessment is critically important as early discovery of these injuries can have a significant impact on minimizing the patient's suffering and long-term morbidity [31].

Prehospital and Initial Assessment Considerations for Special Situations

Chemical Injury

Chemical burn injuries (see Chap. 14) are typically caused from exposure to strong acid or alkalis [32]. The first priority of prehospital care should be ensuring that all providers have the appropriate equipment to protect against harmful contact with the involved agents. All contaminated clothing should be carefully removed from the patient. If there is any residual dry chemical or powder agent, it can be brushed away. Following mechanical removal, or for liquid agents, the affected areas should be irrigated with copious amounts of water for 30 min to dilute the contaminating agent. In the majority of cases, attempts to neutralize chemicals are contra-indicated as the neutralization reaction may produce heat as a by-product which can inflict further tissue damage. Throughout the prehospital management process, special attention should be given to limit spread of the agent to unaffected regions.

There are specific components of the initial assessment that are essential for patients who are present with chemical injuries. The clinician must obtain a focused history to identify the substance(s) involved, quantity and concentration of the agent(s), and the duration of exposure as these may provide insight to the severity of injury. Poison control centers should be consulted if there is a suspected risk of systemic toxicity. In particular, hydrofluoric acid injuries may result in dangerous hypocalcemia [33]. For all chemical exposures, the potential for fume inhalation or ocular injury should be assessed during the primary and secondary survey. For these injuries, it is also especially important to perform serial wound examination as chemical burns are insidious for progressing over prolonged periods. Consequently, all chemical burns should be considered deep partial-thickness or full-thickness during initial evaluation until proven otherwise. Depending on the initial assessment findings, chemical burns meet the criteria and should typically be referred to a specialized burn center.

Cold Injury

Cold induced injuries (frostbite) (see Chap. 24) typically occur to the distal extremities or exposed areas of the face to those with decreased ability to respond to cold or those involved in expeditions (Fig. 3.13) [34]. During the initial assessment, patients with cold injuries should always be evaluated for hypothermia and managed accordingly. The involved frozen tissues should be rewarmed with water that is at 37–40 °C. However, the affected regions should not be rewarmed if there is a risk of refreeze (in instances when rewarming is performed during prehospital care) as freeze-thaw-refreeze may result in worse injury. A cold injury-specific wound evaluation of the secondary survey should assess for the following clinical features as they may provide insight to the stage of injury: burning, numbness, or pallor followed by erythema and discomfort in response to

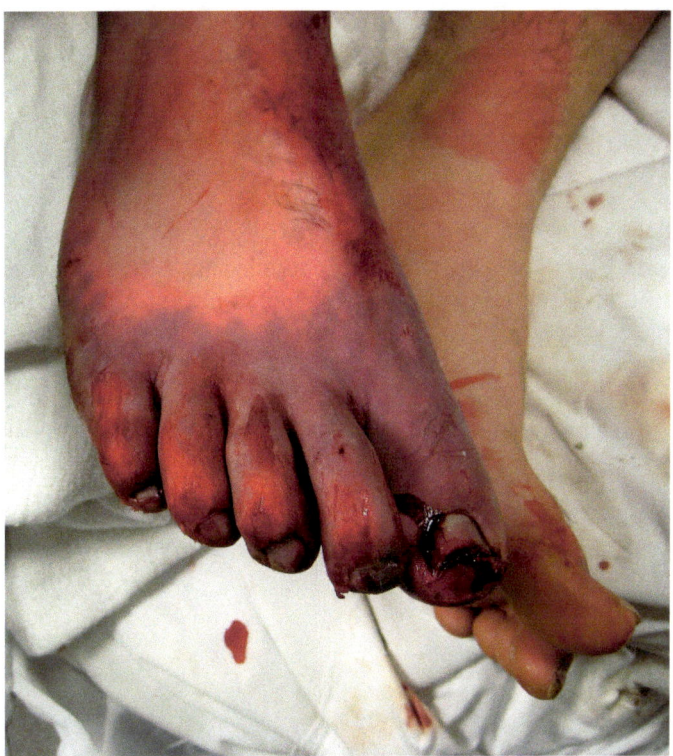

FIGURE 3.13 An example of a cold injury to the foot that has been rewarmed. Cold injuries commonly occur to exposed areas of the face or distal extremities, such as fingers or toes (as in this case). Careful assessment of clinical features following rewarming efforts is essential. In a select group of patients with ischemic wounds that do not reperfuse after rewarming, diagnostic angiography and fibrinolytic therapies may be warranted

warming (stage 1); insensate or pallid followed by blistering and pain with restored perfusion in response to warming (stage 2); insensate, pallid, or hard followed by hemorrhagic blisters and variable pain or perfusion in response to warming (stage 3) [35]. Depending on the status of reperfusion after thaw, fibrinolytic therapies may be indicated [36].

Early burn center consultation can facilitate prompt decision-making in equivocal cases.

Electrical Injury

Electrical injuries (see Chap. 13) are classified as either high voltage (>1000 V) or low voltage (<1000 V) [37]. Contact with a low-voltage source may cause locally destructive burn wounds at the contact site but uncommonly result in systemic sequelae (Fig. 3.14). High-voltage exposure is rare but requires meticulous attention due to the potential for massive underlying tissue damage and multisystem trauma [38]. Emergency personnel should extricate the patient from the scene of an electrical exposure with a non-conducting mate-

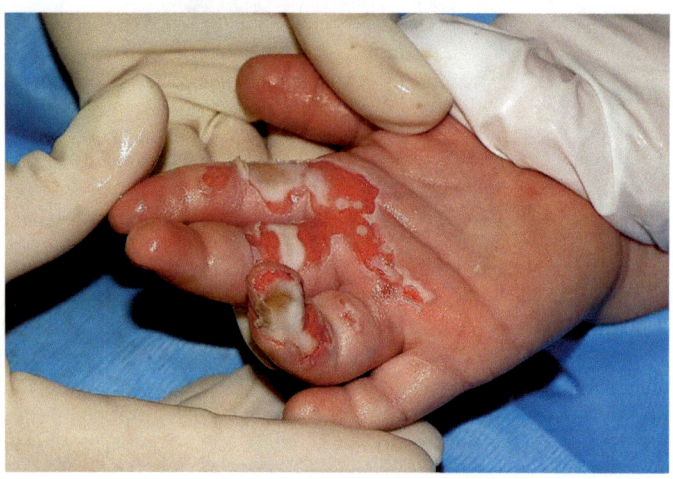

FIGURE 3.14 A mid-range electrical injury sustained from contact with a 220-volt power source. Following direct contact with an energy source, current will travel the path of least resistance, generating heat that inflicts deep thermal injury. In this case, contact resulted in locally destructive burn wounds to the hand and digits of deep-partial thickness (tissues with mottled cherry red and white appearance) and full-thickness injury (waxy, white surface)

rial, only once they have been assured that the electrical current has been turned off.

Patients that present with electrical injuries require a vigilant initial assessment, which typically results in referral to a specialized burn center. When collecting an electrical injury-specific history, it is important to gather information related to the voltage and amperage of the source, type of circuit (AC/DC), points of contact, duration of contact, potential for trauma, and any presence of flame or ignition of clothing. Depending on the extent of electrical exposure, a patient may have burn wounds that are accompanied with a set of concomitant injuries or complications. During the secondary survey, special attention is warranted for the following common examples including compartment syndromes, myocardial injury, musculoskeletal injuries, neurologic sequelae, ocular sequelae, myoglobinuria, and renal failure.

Clinicians should be on high alert for concomitant trauma or complications in all patients that present with high-voltage exposure. For these patients cardiac rhythm should be monitored for 24–72 hours post-injury, thorough neurological and ocular examinations should be completed, creatine kinase and renal markers should be followed closely, and Foley catheters should be placed to track pigmenturia. Injured extremities should be assessed frequently for intracompartmental edema [39]. Muscle compartments are especially at risk and may require prompt fasciotomy. In some instances, amputation may also be necessary but this decision should be deferred to the specialists at the receiving burn center. A baseline ophthalmologic examination for late development of cataracts is advisable in patients with high-voltage injuries.

Non-accidental Injury

Non-accidental injuries include suspected cases of abuse, negligence, assault, self-inflicted harm, or substance abuse. Non-accidental injury is not only limited to children. Any patient should be admitted to the hospital if there is suspicion of non-accidental injury, even if the injury itself is of little physiologic significance. During the initial assessment, clinicians should ensure that they have detailed documentation of the stated history and of the wound presentation. Burn diagrams should be carefully completed, and photographic documentation is ideal. These injuries will often require special social/emotional support. Psychosocial services and social work should be consulted immediately. Suspicious non-accidental injuries must be filed with the appropriate local and state agencies.

Approximately 20% of burns in young children are associated with maltreatment although this can occur in any age group [40]. The potential for abuse or neglect should be considered for every child. When applicable, important history information that should be gathered as part of the initial assessment include water temperature, duration of contact, caretakers involved, documentation of conflicting reports from involved caretakers, delay in seeking treatment, and prior injuries. Subsequently, during burn wound evaluation of the secondary survey, the following points should be evaluated and documented including the uniformity of burn depth, absence of splash marks, sharply defined wound margins, porcelain-contact sparing, flexor sparing, stocking or glove patterns, dorsal location of contact burns of the hand, and localized very deep contact burns (Fig. 3.15).

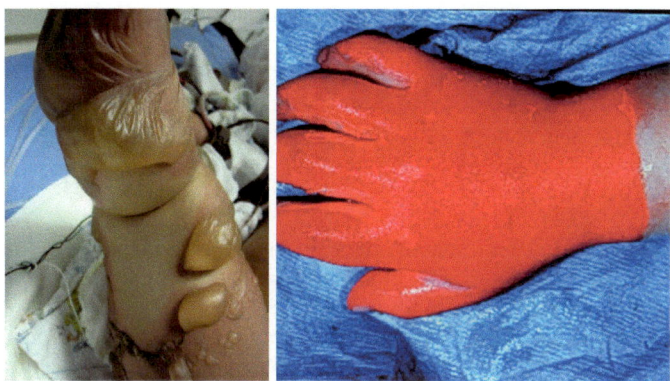

FIGURE 3.15 When assessing a child with burn injuries, it is imperative to be familiar with burn patterns that are indicative of child
maltreatment. Immersion scald burns secondary to child abuse will
typically present with uniform burn depth, defined wound margins,
porcelain-contact sparing, flexor sparing, and/or absence of splash
marks. Flexor sparing can be detected by the presence of a striped
"zebra" pattern of burned-unburned-burned zones at a flexor surface, signifying a tightly flexed position at the time of burn. Note the
popliteal flexor sparing pattern in this case example, suggesting child
abuse tub immersion of the lower extremity (*left*). Maltreatment
should also be considered in cases of contact burns, such as in this
case example of an immersion contact burn sustained from a heated
iron (*right*). Note the uniform burn depth with glove pattern distribution and well-demarcated margins that are located on the dorsal
surface of the child's hand, a burn pattern consistent with child
abuse. Detailed documentation and photography of any evidence
consistent with maltreatment are essential. All suspicious cases must
be filed with the appropriate local and state agencies

References

1. Faxon NW, Churchill ED. The cocoanut grove disaster in boston:
   a preliminary account. JAMA. 1942;120(17):1385–8.
2. Beecher HK. Resuscitation and sedation of patients with burns
   which include the airway: some problems of immediate therapy.
   Ann Surg. 1943;117(6):825–33.

3. Sheridan RL. Burn care: results of technical and organizational progress. JAMA. 2003;290(6):719–22.

4. Sheridan R, Weber J, Prelack K, Petras L, Lydon M, Tompkins R. Early burn center transfer shortens the length of hospitalization and reduces complications in children with serious burn injuries. J Burn Care Rehabil. 1999;20(5):347–50.

5. Greenhalgh DG. Management of burns. N Engl J Med. 2019;380(24):2349–59.

6. Committee on Trauma, American College of Surgeons. Advanced Trauma Life Support Student Course Manual. 10th ed. Chicago: American College of Surgeons; 2018.

7. ABLS Advisory Committee. Advanced Burn Life Support Course Provider Manual. Chicago: American Burn Association; 2018.

8. Cancio LC. Initial assessment and fluid resuscitation of burn patients. Surg Clin North Am. 2014;94(4):741–54.

9. Bittner EA, Shank E, Woodson L, Martyn JA. Acute and perioperative care of the burn-injured patient. Anesthesiology. 2015;122(2):448–64.

10. Sheridan RL. Recognition and management of hot liquid aspiration in children. Ann Emerg Med. 1996;27(1):89–91.

11. Fidkowski CW, Fuzaylov G, Sheridan RL, Cote CJ. Inhalation burn injury in children. Paediatr Anaesth. 2009;19(Suppl 1):147–54.

12. Sheridan RL. Fire-Related Inhalation Injury. N Engl J Med. 2016;375(5):464–9.

13. Ryan CM, Fagan SP, Goverman J, Sheridan RL. Grading inhalation injury by admission bronchoscopy. Crit Care Med. 2012;40(4):1345–6.

14. Wallace AB. The exposure treatment of burns. Lancet. 1951;1(6653):501–4.

15. Rossiter ND, Chapman P, Haywood IA. How big is a hand? Burns. 1996;22(3):230–1.

16. Lund CC, Browder NC. The estimation of areas of burns. Surg Gynecol Obstet. 1944;79:352–8.

17. Goverman J, Bittner EA, Friedstat JS, Moore M, Nozari A, Ibrahim AE, et al. Discrepancy in initial pediatric burn estimates and its impact on fluid resuscitation. J Burn Care Res. 2015;36(5):574–9.

18. Saffle JR, Edelman L, Theurer L, Morris SE, Cochran A. Telemedicine evaluation of acute burns is accurate and cost-effective. J Trauma. 2009;67(2):358–65.

19. Monstrey S, Hoeksema H, Verbelen J, Pirayesh A, Blondeel P. Assessment of burn depth and burn wound healing potential. Burns. 2008;34(6):761–9.
20. Jaspers MEH, van Haasterecht L, van Zuijlen PPM, Mokkink LB. A systematic review on the quality of measurement techniques for the assessment of burn wound depth or healing potential. Burns. 2019;45(2):261–81.
21. Benjamin NC, Lee JO, Norbury WB, Branski LK, Wurzer P, Jimenez CJ, et al. Accuracy of currently used paper burn diagram vs a three-dimensional computerized model. J Burn Care Res. 2017;38(1):e254–e60.
22. Parvizi D, Giretzlehner M, Wurzer P, Klein LD, Shoham Y, Bohanon FJ, et al. BurnCase 3D software validation study: Burn size measurement accuracy and inter-rater reliability. Burns. 2016;42(2):329–35.
23. McUmber H, Dabek RJ, Bojovic B, Driscoll DN. Burn depth analysis using indocyanine green fluorescence: a review. J Burn Care Res. 2019;40(4):513–6.
24. Burmeister DM, Cerna C, Becerra SC, Sloan M, Wilmink G, Christy RJ. Noninvasive techniques for the determination of burn severity in real time. J Burn Care Res. 2017;38(1):e180–e91.
25. Sen CK, Ghatak S, Gnyawali SC, Roy S, Gordillo GM. Cutaneous imaging technologies in acute burn and chronic wound care. Plast Reconstr Surg. 2016;138(3 Suppl):119S–28S.
26. Burke-Smith A, Collier J, Jones I. A comparison of non-invasive imaging modalities: Infrared thermography, spectrophotometric intracutaneous analysis and laser Doppler imaging for the assessment of adult burns. Burns. 2015;41(8):1695–707.
27. Vercruysse GA, Alam HB, Martin MJ, Brasel K, Moore EE, Brown CV, et al. Western Trauma Association critical decisions in trauma: preferred triage and initial management of the burned patient. J Trauma Acute Care Surg. 2019;87(5):1239–43.
28. Palmieri TL, Taylor S, Lawless M, Curri T, Sen S, Greenhalgh DG. Burn center volume makes a difference for burned children. Pediatr Crit Care Med. 2015;16(4):319–24.
29. Al-Mousawi AM, Jeschke MG, Herndon DN. Invited commentary on "The demographics of modern burn care: should most burns be cared for by non-burn surgeons?". Am J Surg. 2011;201(1):97–9.
30. Hajibandeh S, Hajibandeh S, Idehen N. Meta-analysis of the effect of tertiary survey on missed injury rate in trauma patients. Injury. 2015;46(12):2474–82.

31. Grigorian A, Nahmias J, Schubl S, Gabriel V, Bernal N, Joe V. Rising mortality in patients with combined burn and trauma. Burns. 2018;44(8):1989–96.

32. Palao R, Monge I, Ruiz M, Barret JP. Chemical burns: pathophysiology and treatment. Burns. 2010;36(3):295–304.

33. Stuke LE, Arnoldo BD, Hunt JL, Purdue GF. Hydrofluoric acid burns: a 15-year experience. J Burn Care Res. 2008;29(6):893–6.

34. McIntosh SE, Hamonko M, Freer L, Grissom CK, Auerbach PS, Rodway GW, et al. Wilderness Medical Society practice guidelines for the prevention and treatment of frostbite. Wilderness Environ Med. 2011;22(2):156–66.

35. Sheridan RL, Greenhalgh D. Special problems in burns. Surg Clin North Am. 2014;94(4):781–91.

36. Sheridan RL, Goldstein MA, Stoddard FJ Jr, Walker TG. Case records of the Massachusetts General Hospital. Case 41-2009. A 16-year-old boy with hypothermia and frostbite. N Engl J Med. 2009;361(27):2654–62.

37. Arnoldo BD, Purdue GF. The diagnosis and management of electrical injuries. Hand Clin. 2009;25:46979.

38. Depamphilis MA, Cauley RP, Sadeq F, Lydon M, Sheridan RL, Driscoll DN, et al. Surgical management and epidemiological trends of pediatric electrical burns. Burns. 2020;46:1693–9.

39. Friedstat J, Brown DA, Levi B. Chemical, electrical, and radiation injuries. Clin Plast Surg. 2017;44(3):657–69.

40. Wibbenmeyer L, Liao J, Heard J, Kealey L, Kealey G, Oral R. Factors related to child maltreatment in children presenting with burn injuries. J Burn Care Res. 2014;35(5):374–81.

Chapter 4
Initial Management and Resuscitation

Leopoldo C. Cancio and Jill M. Cancio

Introduction

Successful initial care of a patient with extensive burns sets the stage for a long recovery process. Although there are many steps on the way to recovery, the first step is one of the most important. Mistakes made during the resuscitation phase of care may cause irreversible damage, leading to loss of life, limb, or eyesight. In this chapter, we will review how to successfully traverse this most important phase of care, focusing on the care of the critically ill burn patient. A key message is that early care of a burn patient should be undertaken, whenever possible, in consultation with a burn center.

Big Problem or Little Problem?

An accurate determination of burn size is a key initial step in caring for any burn patient, but burn size is often overestimated by referring hospitals by a factor of 100% or more

L. C. Cancio (✉) · J. M. Cancio
US Army Institute of Surgical Research, Fort Sam Houston, San Antonio, TX, USA
e-mail: leopoldo.c.cancio.civ@health.mil; jill.m.cancio.civ@health.mil

© The Author(s), under exclusive license to Springer Nature Switzerland AG 2023
J. O. Lee (ed.), *Essential Burn Care for Non-Burn Specialists*, https://doi.org/10.1007/978-3-031-28898-2_4

[1]. There are several reasons why this is problematic. Burn size is a major determinant of fluid resuscitation requirements. Burn size also influences the decision to intubate, or not to intubate, a burn patient (see below). Burn size, along with age and the presence of inhalation injury, is an independent predictor of postburn mortality risk [2] and thus is used in triage decisions.

The Rule of Nines can provide a quick estimate of burn size (Fig. 4.1). Also, the Rule of Hands is very helpful for small and irregularly shaped burns. It states that at any age, a patient's hand (palm and fingers) equals about 1% of their total body surface area (TBSA). This initial estimate should then be refined using the Lund-Browder diagram, which divides the body into smaller areas than does the Rule of Nines, and which also takes age-related changes into account. With an accurate burn size estimate in hand, one may then determine whether a patient should be considered for burn center referral. The American Burn Association (ABA) guidelines, in brief, recommend referral of patients who meet the following criteria [3]:

- Burn size of 10% TBSA or greater
- Special mechanisms: inhalation, chemical, electric
- Full-thickness burns
- Functionally significant burns, e.g., hand or face
- Patients with special medical or psychosocial needs

Furthermore, burn size helps determine who should be admitted to an intensive care unit (ICU). All patients with burn size of 20% or greater, and those with possible inhalation injury, are admitted to the ICU. Previously healthy young persons with burns in the 10–19% TBSA range might be orally resuscitated on a burn ward. On the other hand, those in the 10–19% range who are children, who are elderly, or who have complex medical problems belong in the ICU.

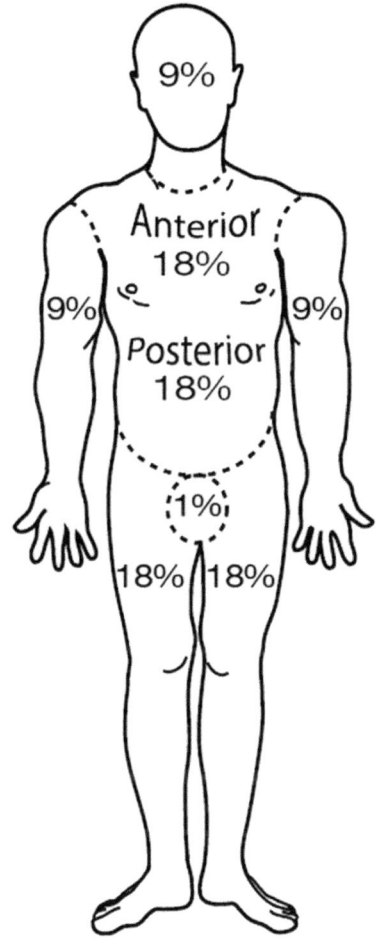

FIGURE 4.1 The Rule of Nines can be used to provide a quick initial estimate of burn size. Reproduced from Emergency War Surgery: Fifth United States Edition. Fort Sam Houston, TX: Borden Institute, 2018

Airway: Who Needs to be Intubated, and How?

It is well recognized that a patient with symptomatic inhalation injury, to include respiratory distress, cough, hoarseness, or stridor, should be expeditiously intubated. While it is true that the patient with minimal signs and symptoms of inhalation injury can be safely monitored in a critical care setting, prophylactic intubation before ambulance or aeromedical transport is often prudent. Even patients without inhalation injury, but whose burn size is 40% or greater, should be intubated simply because progressive edema during the first 24–48 h places the airway at risk (and makes intubation more difficult as time goes on). These patients may develop rapid airway obstruction soon after injury, or more insidiously during the course of the first 24–48 h postburn [4, 5].

Induction of general anesthesia in patients who are hypovolemic because of burn shock may precipitate hypotension. Ketamine is considered a good choice for induction, because it generally maintains the blood pressure by increasing sympathetic outflow from the central nervous system. But even ketamine, which also has a myocardial depressant effect, may cause hypotension in the maximally "catecholamine-depleted" burn shock patient [6]. Thus, the provider must be prepared to support the blood pressure pharmacologically during intubation.

The endotracheal tube must be secured in a manner which precludes dislodgement. Adhesive tape does not stick to the burned or edematous face in burn patients and should not be used. Rather, a umbilical tie (or similar technique) should be used to secure the tube circumferentially around the head and neck. Once placed, the endotracheal tube should be religiously suctioned as often as necessary, removing sloughed cellular debris, fibrinous exudate, and mucus, thus maintaining and ensuring patency. If not, patients with inhalation injury may experience complete tube obstruction and may require emergency exchange [4].

It is reasonable to follow low-tidal-volume (ARDSNet) recommendations in the mechanical ventilation of intubated burn patients, with three caveats. First, patients with suspected inhalation injury should receive 100% oxygen until carbon monoxide poisoning can be ruled out by means of co-oximetry (direct measurement of the carboxyhemoglobin level, or, alternatively, until 6 h have passed) [7].

FIGURE 4.2 Location of escharotomy incisions. The bold lines indicate the importance of including the eschar overlying any involved joints in the incisions. Reproduced from Emergency War Surgery: Fifth United States Edition. Fort Sam Houston, TX: Borden Institute, 2018

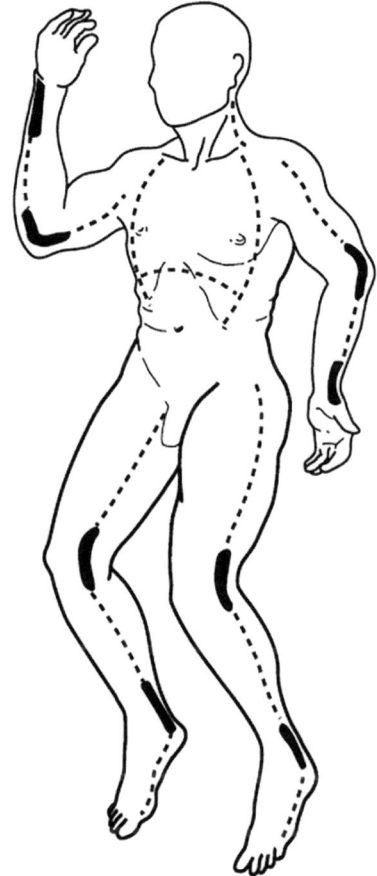

   Second, patients with circumferential, deep burns of the torso may develop a thoracic eschar syndrome. In these patients, the tight inelastic eschar and the formation of edema fluid beneath the eschar progressively impede chest excursion. These patients require emergency escharotomy of the chest in order to permit respiration (Fig. 4.2). Escharotomy is performed expeditiously at the bedside. A Bovie electrocautery device is used to incise through the full thickness of the skin and into the subcutaneous tissue. Successful chest escharotomy results in rapid restoration of chest excursion and a decrease in peak airway pressures.

Third, we have shown the superiority of high-frequency percussive ventilation (Volumetric Diffusive Respiration [VDR], Percussionaire, Sandpoint, ID) to low-tidal volume ventilation, particularly in inhalation injury patients—reflecting the underlying pathophysiology of this patient population [8].

Fluid Resuscitation: Why and How?

After managing the airway, fluid resuscitation is the main goal of therapy during the first 48 h postburn. Patients with burn size greater than 20% TBSA—and many patients with burn size greater than 10% TBSA, such as children and the elderly—require formal burn resuscitation. Burn shock features three elements:

- *Hypovolemia* caused by loss of fluid from the intravascular space into the interstitial space in response to changes in the Starling forces across the microvasculature (often summarized as "leaky capillaries") [9, 10]. In patients with larger burns, this occurs in both burned and unburned tissues [11].
- Increased *systemic vascular resistance*, reflecting massive catecholamine release [12].
- Decreased myocardial *contractility*, which is more commonly evident in older patients and in those with medical comorbidities [13, 14].

Of these factors, the first one, hypovolemia, is the primary target of most of our resuscitative efforts. Replacement of ongoing plasma volume losses, in order to restore cardiac output and maintain vital-organ perfusion, is the main goal of resuscitation. But the time course of burn shock is more gradual than that of hemorrhagic shock, and there is no intervention (analogous to surgery to repair a blood vessel) which can rapidly repair the diffuse microvascular permeability of burn injury. Rather, the purpose of burn resuscitation is gradually to replace ongoing plasma volume losses while waiting for the body to recover its microvascular integrity. Meanwhile, as fluids leak out of the vascular space into the interstitium, they cause edema, both locally (in the burn wound) and systemically. Careful titration of fluid input is required in order to prevent excessive edema on the one hand, and inadequate vital-organ perfusion on the other.

The most commonly used fluid for IV burn resuscitation is lactated Ringer's solution (LR). Other balanced crystalloid solutions, such as Plasma-Lyte A, are also used. The use of crystalloids instead of colloids is predicated on the concept that increased microvascular permeability makes the use of colloids ineffective during the early postburn hours [15]. The exact time at which such permeability begins to be repaired (making colloids more effective) is a matter of debate, may range between 8 and 24 h postburn, occurs sooner in unburned tissues than in burned tissues, and is probably patient-specific [11, 15]. 5% albumin is often used during the 2nd 24 h postburn (hours 25–48), or earlier as a "rescue" strategy (see below) [16–18]. Recently, there has been a renewed interest in the use of plasma for resuscitation, not merely because of its colloidal properties, but also with the intent of restoring the endothelial glycocalyx [19].

Peripheral IV access (through unburned skin, through burned skin if necessary) is adequate for initiation of burn shock resuscitation. It is common practice to place a central venous catheter (and an arterial catheter) under sterile conditions to permit multiple infusions and monitoring in patients with larger burns. These lines must be securely sutured in place to prevent dislodgement.

After IV access is obtained, a controlled infusion of LR should be started at an age-based rate: 500 mL/h for adults, 250 mL/h for children, 125 mL/h for small children. This buys time while the burn size is measured and one of the formulas is calculated (see below). The temptation to give an initial bolus (except for profound hypotension) should be avoided [20]. During the hyperpermeable phase of early burn shock, the likely fate of a bolus is rapid loss into the interstitium and increased edema formation, with no lasting benefit.

Given the need for careful fluid dosing in burn resuscitation, a variety of formulas have been used to help estimate the starting rate for IV infusion. The traditional burn shock resuscitation formulas take into account the patient's burn size and weight. Thus, the modified Brooke formula estimates that patients should receive 2 mL/kg/TBSA burn of LR during the first 24 h postburn [15], whereas the Parkland formula estimates 4 mL/kg/TBSA burn [21]. Under the Brooke formula, for example, an 80-kg adult with a 40% burn would be programmed to receive 2 mL*80 kg*40% = 6400 mL over the first 24 h postburn, with half of this, or 3200 mL, scheduled for infusion over the first 8 h postburn, and half over the next 16 h postburn. Thus the starting rate under the Brooke formula would be 3200 mL/8 h or 400 mL/h.

The Parkland formula would estimate twice as much: 4*80 kg*40% = 12,800 mL over the first 24 h, with half of this given over the first 8 h postburn, or 800 mL/h. Particularly in patients with large burn sizes, the amount of fluid predicted by the Parkland formula can be massive and potentially hazardous (see Complications, below). Furthermore, many patients, whether started on the Brooke or the Parkland formulas, experience an increase in the volume delivered in excess of the formula predictions [22–24]. Accordingly, the Advanced Burn Life Support (ABLS) course now recommends the Brooke formula, that is, 2 mL/kg/TBSA burn [20].

Since there is a certain amount of math involved in the above calculations, a simpler burn formula was introduced called the "ISR Rule of Tens" for adults. The Rule of Tens states that the initial fluid resuscitation rate is the burn size*10. For example, an adult with burn size of 40% would be started on resuscitation fluid at 40*10 = 400 mL/h. An adult with a burn size of 60% would be started at 60*10 = 600 mL/h. This formula usually gives predictions which are between those of the Brooke and Parkland formulas. (In addition, patients with weight over 80 kg receive an additional 100 mL/h for each additional 10 kg. Thus, a 100 kg person with a 40% burn would receive 400 mL/h + 200 mL/h = 600 mL/h). The Rule of Tens is the formula we now use at the US Army Burn Center [25].

The Rule of Tens formula only applies to patients with weight greater than 40 kg; for smaller patients, a weight-based formula must be used. Furthermore, children have a greater surface-area-to-weight ratio. Thus, they are estimated to require more than the Brooke formula, that is, 3 mL/kg/TBSA burn. Again, half of this is programmed for the first 8 h [26].

In addition to receiving resuscitation fluid, smaller children (< 30 kg) also need a maintenance fluid rate. This serves two purposes. First, the amount of fluid predicted by the formulas may be less than maintenance for small children with small burns. Second, small children may deplete their glycogen stores and become hypoglycemic during burn shock. To prevent this, an exogenous glucose source is helpful. The maintenance fluid of choice for children is D5LR or D5½NS. The rate should be that calculated by the 4-2-1 rule (4 mL/kg for the first 10 kg, 2 mL/kg for the next 10 kg, 1 mL/kg for the subsequent kilograms). Normally, this rate is not adjusted during resuscitation—it runs in the background while the resuscitation fluid is titrated according to physiologic response [20].

Monitoring

It is important to realize that all of these formulas only provide a starting rate; there is no sudden change in the fluid infusion rate at the eighth postburn hour in actual practice; and the hourly infusion rate has to be titrated based on physiologic response. The patient must be continually reassessed during the 24–48 h postburn. The hourly urine output (UO) is the primary index of the adequacy of fluid resuscitation. Thus, a Foley catheter should be placed and the UO recorded hourly for patients undergoing IV resuscitation. The target UO for adults is 30–50 mL/h; for children it is 1.0 mL/kg/h [20]. (An exception is the patient with gross myoglobinuria due to high-voltage electric injury. As described in the chapter on that topic, the target UO in these patients is 70–100 mL/h for adults.) Reducing the fluid infusion rate when the UO is too high is just as important as increasing it when the UO is too low [24]. As needed, an increase or decrease of about 25% every hour or two is a reasonable rule of thumb.

Nevertheless, the UO alone is often insufficient for monitoring. The accuracy of the UO should be questioned in patients with renal failure, diuretic use, or alcohol intoxication, and other indices of resuscitation should be considered. Furthermore, in all patients with burn shock, the following should be monitored as well:

- *Heart rate.* Because of increased sympathetic nervous system (SNS) activity and catecholamine release, a previously healthy person undergoing burn resuscitation normally has an elevated heart rate (100–120/min in adults). A further increase, even in the absence of hypotension, suggests hypovolemia.
- *Blood pressure.* Again because of SNS and catecholamine effects, hypotension is a late finding during burn shock resuscitation. A normal blood pressure, *per se*, is not very reassuring. The non-invasive blood pressure, particularly on burned extremities, may be inaccurate, and an arterial catheter is often placed when patients are undergoing IV fluid resuscitation.
- *Lactate.* Burn shock patients typically develop a lactic acidosis which resolves with successful resuscitation [27]. Lactate correlates with postburn mortality, but how best to use it is ill-defined [28, 29]. Certainly, an increasing lactate should prompt a reexamination of whether the patient's shock state is worsening.
- *Arterial base deficit.* Patients also typically develop a base deficit, which also correlates with postburn mortality [30]. This does not exactly mirror the lactate and may represent other consequences of shock such as renal tubular acidosis secondary to acute kidney injury [28].
- *Fluids* (hourly fluid infusion rate [mL/h] and cumulative fluid volume [mL/kg]). Awareness of these variables is

extremely important during resuscitation, since the volume infused during the first 24 h correlates with complications such as abdominal compartment syndrome that must be avoided if at all possible (see below) [31].

• *Vasoactive drug infusion rates* (if any).

Finally, data from invasive cardiac output monitoring devices may be useful. These methods include the pulmonary artery (PA) catheter; those which estimate cardiac output from analysis of the arterial blood pressure waveform; those which perform transpulmonary indicator dilution; and echocardiography. The data from these devices must be interpreted with reference to the values expected at that point in the resuscitation process. That is, burn shock is a dynamically changing phenomenon. The successfully resuscitated burn patient passes through 3 stages (Table 4.1) [15].

One impact of this concept of "stages" is the following. Early attempts to make intravascular volume and cardiac output normal (or worse, supranormal) not only are unnecessary (because successfully resuscitated patients tolerate a period of relative hypovolemia and low cardiac output), but also risk failure by driving up intravascular volume and edema formation precisely when the microvasculature is at its most permeable [32].

Echocardiography can be particularly helpful in assessing the etiology of low cardiac output. Previously healthy patients demonstrate increased contractility and hypovolemia during the early phases of burn shock [14]. Less commonly, echocardiography may reveal impaired contractility, indicating a potential role for an inotrope.

Because burn injury results in a rapid and sustained increase in SNS activity and catecholamine production [12, 33], for many years the use of vasoactive medications to treat hypotension during burn shock was discouraged in favor of volume loading. This is no longer the case. A recent European Society of Intensive Care Medicine (ESICM) Burn ICU working group survey stated that 80% of respondents use vasopressors to reduce volume administration during the first 48 hours postburn [34]. But how best to use vasopressors is

Table 4.1 Time course of key variables during a typical successful resuscitation

Stage	Postburn hour	Cardiac output	SVR	Plasma volume	Urine output	Fluid infusion rate
1	0–12	Rapidly reaches nadir	Rapidly reaches peak	Decreases at its most rapid rate	Oliguria is common	May increase to peak at hour 8–10
2	12–36	Slightly less than normal	Decreases toward normal	Nadir at hour 12–18, then slowly increases	Adequate	Slowly decreases
3	36–beyond	Supranormal	Subnormal	Normal	Often above target	Reaches a maintenance rate

SVR Systemic vascular resistance

undefined. The 2008 U.S. Joint Theater Trauma System guidelines for burn resuscitation described a stepwise approach to the hypotensive burn patient, as follows:

1. Vasopressin
2. Volume infusion to achieve central venous pressure (CVP) or pulmonary arterial wedge pressure (PAWP) targets
3. Norepinephrine up to 20 mcg/min
4. Epinephrine or phenylephrine. Meanwhile, these patients should be evaluated for missed injury, adrenal insufficiency, hypocalcemia, or other issues [35]

Our practice has evolved since that publication. Vasopressors are used more routinely. CVP is rarely monitored in the critically ill burn patient. Pulmonary artery catheters are placed less frequently, and use of predetermined CVP or PAWP targets is unusual. On the other hand, it is important to understand that the cavalier up-titration of alpha agonists during burn shock is potentially hazardous. An increasing requirement for such agents should prompt a comprehensive reevaluation of volume status, cardiac function, end-organ perfusion, and acid–base status. The risk/benefit ratio of volume vs. vasopressor infusions must be assessed.

Maintaining situational awareness of all the data that need to be monitored during a complicated burn resuscitation is challenging and starts with effective documentation. The Joint Trauma System flowsheet is one paper-based format, developed for the battlefield, that can be used to record the basic data [35]. Furthermore, decision support tools such as Burn Navigator (Arcos Medical, Houston, TX) can be used to document and display these data in a manner which was developed specifically for burn resuscitation. This system also makes recommendations on fluid infusion rates based on analysis of trends in the UO [36].

During hours 24–48 postburn, we routinely infuse 5% albumin in normal saline in accordance with the modified Brooke formula. The dose for this infusion is weight based, according to a sliding scale:

- 0.3 mL/kg/TBSA for burn size 30–49%
- 0.4 mL/kg/TBSA for burn size 50–69%
- 0.5 mL/kg/TBSA for burn size 70–100%

Thus, an 80 kg patient with a 70% burn would receive (80 *70*0.5 mL)/24 h = 2800 mL/24 h = 117 mL/h. This infusion is given over 24 h and is normally not titrated. Meanwhile, the LR infusion used during the first 24 h is weaned to off. As described below, initiation of an albumin infusion before the 24th postburn hour is sometimes used to rescue patients who are failing resuscitation.

Typically, burn patients spontaneously diurese their resuscitation volume over days 3–10 postburn. Increasingly, we have recognized the value of active "de-resuscitation" to offload this volume more quickly [37]. Beneficial effects of this strategy may include earlier extubation and, in patients who require excision of the burn wound, more successful healing of skin grafts [38]. De-resuscitation can be performed either pharmacologically using diuretics or by means of continuous renal replacement therapy.

Complicated Resuscitation

Not all patients respond to resuscitation successfully; historically, about 12% of burn patients who died, did so during the first 48 h despite full resuscitative efforts [39]. Indications of resuscitation failure, in patients who have already received a substantial volume of fluids, include the following:

- Progressive metabolic acidosis
- Acute kidney injury
- Refractory oliguria or anuria
- Escalating vasoactive pressor doses

In this setting, it is tempting to respond with a further escalation in crystalloid resuscitation volume. This may be reasonable at first, but as the cumulative infusion volume nears 250 mL/kg during the first 24 h (the "Ivy Index"), the risk of abdominal and other compartment syndromes mounts [31].

In our experience, abdominal compartment syndrome (ACS) in burn patients is associated with a mortality risk of nearly 100% if it requires decompressive laparotomy [40]. The group at UC Davis reported a 40% survival rate after decompressive laparotomy for ACS, but many of those patients were children who developed ACS in the setting of sepsis rather than burn shock [41]. Although a decompressive laparotomy may temporize ACS, it is often impossible to achieve timely abdominal closure, there is loss of domain, and the physiologic insult of an open abdomen compounds that of an extensive burn.

Thus, we aim to keep the resuscitation volume below 250 mL/kg/24 h. This requires ongoing awareness of the current infusion rate, the cumulative volume, and the projected 24-h volume. As a rule of thumb, an hourly infusion of 2000 mL or more is cause for concern, as is a sustained infusion rate of 1500 mL/h or more for several hours. By about 8–10 h postburn, it should be possible to extrapolate: the cumulative volume to the 24-h point, and to begin to make an assessment of the risk of exceeding 250 mL/kg/24 h (Fig. 4.3). Interventions to salvage patients who are headed toward resuscitation failure include:

- Reassess volume and cardiac status via enhanced monitoring (see above)
- Look for a missed injury, such as non-thermal trauma
- Measure bladder pressure; assess for ACS
- Initiate early albumin
- Initiate continuous renal replacement therapy (CRRT) or therapeutic plasma exchange (TPE)
- Initiate high-dose ascorbic acid therapy

Measurement of bladder pressure should be done routinely in patients whose predicted or actual infused volume exceeds 250 mL/kg. WSACS — the World Society of Abdominal Compartment Syndrome — defines ACS as a bladder pressure of 20 mmHg with new onset organ failure [42]. In burn patients, others have recommended decompressive laparotomy at a bladder pressure of 30 mmHg and signs of physio-

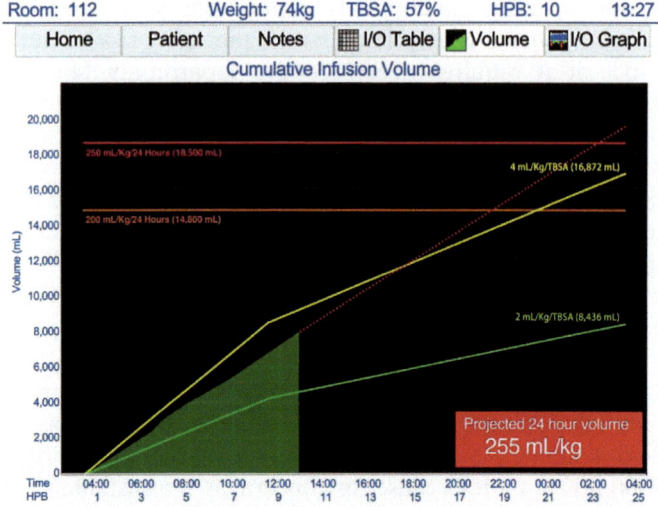

FIGURE 4.3 Screen shot from the Burn Navigator burn resuscitation decision support system. This graph shows the cumulative fluid volume. Extrapolation of the cumulative fluid volume curve to the 24th postburn hour allows an estimation of the risk of exceeding the Ivy index of 250 mL/kg by that hour. Reproduced with permission of Arcos Medical, Inc., Houston, TX

logic compromise [41]. Thus, a bladder pressure of 20–30 mmHg could be defined as a "warning zone." Short of decompressive laparotomy, burn patients with ACS may benefit from several interventions to include abdominal escharotomy, neuromuscular blockade, and paracentesis [43]. Placement of a diagnostic peritoneal lavage catheter into the abdomen may allow ongoing drainage to occur as resuscitation proceeds.

We routinely infuse 5% albumin in normal saline during hours 24–48 postburn, in accordance with the modified Brooke formula (see above). In light of evidence suggesting that microvascular permeability, at least in unburned tissues, begins to resolve around hours 8–12 postburn [11], we institute albumin before the 24th postburn hour in patients whose trajectory indicates that they are headed toward exceeding the Ivy Index. We have observed that it is possible to decrease the fluid infusion rate within about 3 h in many patients who receive early albumin [18].

At the US Army Burn Center, CRRT for the treatment of burn patients with sepsis-induced acute kidney injury (AKI) was associated with decreased 28-day and hospital mortality, in comparison with matched case controls [44]. Although that study did not examine the use of CRRT during burn shock, we now routinely provide CRRT to patients during burn shock resuscitation who develop AKI, to include hyperkalemia or metabolic acidosis refractory to medical management. CRRT also facilitates the off-loading of edema fluid during de-resuscitation. Another extracorporeal rescue strategy is TPE [45].

Finally, high-dose IV ascorbic acid (vitamin C) was studied by Tanaka and colleagues in Tokyo. In their randomized controlled single-center trial, patients were considered for enrollment if they were admitted within 2 h of injury. Vitamin C at a dose of 66 mg/kg/h was started as soon as possible after admission and was continued for the first 24 h postburn. It was associated with a decrease in resuscitation fluid requirements, weight gain, wound edema, serum malondialdehyde levels, and ventilator days [46]. Since the proposed mechanism of action of vitamin C in burn shock is its anti-oxidant properties, it makes sense to begin it as soon as possible after admission, rather than as a later rescue therapy.

Management of the Burned Extremity

One of the most challenging aspects of early burn care is the management of the burned extremity. Extremities with deep circumferential burns are at risk of ischemic injury via a process we term "extremity eschar syndrome." Whereas normal skin is elastic, full-thickness burns are inelastic. Furthermore, edema beneath the inelastic burn wound progressively squeezes the extremity, acting like a tourniquet, and impeding venous outflow, capillary blood flow, and ultimately arterial inflow. To decrease edema formation, burned extremities (especially upper extremities) should be elevated by any available means at a level above the heart throughout resuscitation; see below for more information on the role of the rehabilitation team in positioning.

Doppler flowmetry of circumferentially burned extremities is performed hourly during resuscitation. The arteries to be monitored are the radial and ulnar arteries at the wrist; the superficial palmar arch of the hand; and the dorsalis pedis and posterior tibial arteries at the ankle/foot. Loss or progressive diminution in the audible Doppler signal is an indication for escharotomy.

Escharotomy is an incision through the full thickness of the burn eschar and into the underlying subcutaneous tissue. Escharotomies of the extremities are performed along the mid-medial and/or mid-lateral joint lines (Fig. 4.2). Structures to avoid include the ulnar nerve at the elbow (place the incision anterior to the medial epicondyle) and the superficial radial nerve at the wrist (which becomes subcutaneous about 9 cm proximal to the radial styloid) [47]. Successful escharotomy results in restoration of the distal Doppler signal. Doppler flow must be rechecked after the procedure, and hourly thereafter till resuscitation is complete.

The deeply burned hand is a problem of great concern. The following procedures should be performed by qualified surgeons. In a patient with deep dorsal hand burns, loss of the palmar arch Doppler signal despite the presence of radial and ulnar flow is an indication for dorsal hand escharotomies via incisions over the second and fourth metacarpals, with care not to injure the extensor tendons. In addition, some authors recommend that interosseous (intrinsic) muscle fasciotomies should routinely accompany dorsal hand escharotomies [48, 49], although this has not been our usual practice.

Patients with deeply burned but still viable fingers who lose Doppler signal in the digital arteries may benefit from digital escharotomies. This is a matter of ongoing controversy in the burn literature with some advocating for digital escharotomies [49, 50], and some questioning the benefit [51]. There are limited studies, with one small prospective trial showing an improvement in the number of necrotic phalanges with digital escharotomies [52]. The incision for a digital escharotomy is performed along one side of the involved finger, between the neurovascular bundle (which lies at the level of the digital flexion crease) and the extensor tendon apparatus. This procedure can be bloody, and pinpoint electrocautery will likely be needed.

The advent of Nexobrid (MediWound Ltd, Industrial Zone Yavne, Israel), a rapidly acting, enzymatic debriding agent, may facilitate the prevention and treatment of extremity eschar syndromes, especially of the hands. At present, NexoBrid is recommended for use by trained specialists [53]. FDA approval for marketing in the US has been obtained.

The extremity eschar syndrome should not be confused with a true intramuscular compartment syndrome. In the former situation, the problem is edema beneath the burn eschar, and the remedy is an incision through the skin. In the latter situation, the problem is edema (or bleeding) beneath the investing fascia, and the treatment is a fasciotomy. To be sure, compartment syndrome does occur in burn patients, for example:

- With massive resuscitation, in either burned or unburned extremities
- Following delayed escharotomy, via an ischemia-reperfusion mechanism
- In the setting of concomitant mechanical trauma (e.g., crush, fracture, vascular ischemia-reperfusion)
- With burns that extend into the muscle
- Following high-voltage electrical injury

Thus, even patients who undergo apparently successful escharotomies must continue to receive monitoring of the Doppler signal and of the physical examination throughout the resuscitation period. In patients diagnosed with compartment syndrome, operative fasciotomy is required.

Wound Care and Pain Management

During first aid at the scene, immediate cooling of a burn wound with cool running water appears to be beneficial if it can be performed without causing hypothermia or delaying lifesaving interventions [54]. Any toxic chemicals must be rapidly decontaminated. Wound debridement is not an early priority in the management of a critically ill burn patient, but it should be completed during the first 24 h postburn. At the US Army Burn Center and many other centers, a special room is dedicated to showering burn patients while they are recumbent on a shower cart. In other settings, it may be advantageous to use the operating room for initial debridement. Burn wound debridement is often an aggressive process intended to remove all sloughed epidermis, debris, dirt, and other material. An antiseptic such as chlorhexidine gluconate is used. Once debridement has been completed, a topical antimicrobial or other burn dressing is applied as described in the Burn Wound Management chapter.

Adequate debridement requires adequate analgesia. Conscious sedation may be helpful, but general anesthesia is rarely needed. Analgesia may consist of intermittent IV boluses or a continuous rate infusion of narcotics and/or ketamine. Intravenous sedatives with a sympatholytic effect such as propofol may be poorly tolerated during burn shock. Intermittent low-dose lorazepam or an infusion of midazolam may be better tolerated during this phase of care.

Supportive Care

Because of increased blood flow to the injured surface of the body, impaired thermoregulation, and loss of the cutaneous barrier to evaporative water loss, burn patients are at high risk of hypothermia. During debridement and indeed throughout the resuscitation period, prevention of hypothermia is essential, and the primary method for accomplishing this is a warm environment.

Patients with burn size of 20% or greater, and those who are mechanically ventilated, require prophylaxis against stress gastroduodenal ulceration (Curling's ulcer). We use a proton-pump inhibitor for this purpose. We provide deep-venous-thrombosis prophylaxis with subcutaneous low-molecular weight or unfractionated heparin.

We aim to provide enteral nutrition within 24 h of injury, via a nasogastric or nasoduodenal tube [55]. Reasons for delay during the burn shock period may include a high vasopressor dose (e.g., norepinephrine >10 mcg/min) or lactic acidosis (e.g., lactate >3 mmol/L).

Care of the eyes during burn resuscitation includes evaluation upon admission for corneal injury and measurement of intraocular pressures. If undiagnosed and untreated, corneal injuries in burn patients may become infected, ulcerate, and perforate, leading to blindness. Like abdominal and extremity compartment syndromes, orbital compartment syndrome (OCS) is more likely in patients who receive >250 mL/kg during the first 24 h postburn. However, it can also occur in patients with facial burns who receive no fluid resuscitation at all [56]. OCS, another vision-threatening complication, is easily treated with lateral canthotomy and cantholysis. This speaks to the value of early and ongoing evaluation of patients with extensive burns and those with facial burns by an ophthalmologist.

Role of the Rehabilitation Team

Rehabilitation was traditionally viewed as a separate "phase" in the care of injured patients, but today we recognize the long-term functional impact of interventions made by therapists during the immediate postburn hours. Accordingly, assessment by the rehabilitation team (occupational and/or physical therapists) should take place on the day of admission. A comprehensive burn evaluation should include the following elements [57, 58]:

- History of how injury occurred
- Patient's preinjury functional and activity level

- Location and depth of burn injury, to include TBSA burn and calculation of cutaneous functional units (CFUs)
- Associated injuries such as fractures, inhalation injury, exposed tendon/bone
- Edema, range of motion, strength, sensation measurements
- Activities of daily living assessment
- Functional mobility status
- Positioning needs
- Short-term and long-term goals
- Treatment plan

Since the hands are involved in more than 80% of patients with severe burns [59], monitoring hand edema is of significant importance during initial resuscitation. Use of a figure-of-eight hand edema measurement technique has been shown to be reliable and valid in the burn population [60]. This is a practical technique that can be performed rapidly and can be used to examine the efficacy of initial edema management techniques during resuscitation.

Positioning programs should be initiated immediately upon admission, as edema generally peaks within 12–48 h postburn [61]. The focus should be on reduction of edema, minimizing the risk of peripheral neuropathy, and promoting joint alignment [57]. This is especially prudent in burns of extremities that are deep-partial to full-thickness in depth, as well as in burns involving over 20% TBSA. In larger burns, edema formation is more severe and lasts longer, due to increased capillary permeability and the massive fluid volumes required for resuscitation [62].

Positioning programs should be individualized, closely monitored, and adjusted depending on the patient's medical status [57]. Generally speaking, elevation of the extremities includes placement of the involved hand or foot above the elbow or knee, which should in turn be at or above the level of the heart [63]. Caution is advised with hand orthosis use during initial resuscitation, due to the risk of causing external pressure and tissue ischemia [63].

Burn injury location is important in determining the functional impact of the injury and the resultant therapy workload. The CFU concept is a way of quantifying this relationship. It is based on how skin is recruited and how it moves during joint range of motion. Based on this analysis, grossly 100 major CFUs were identified, excluding the neck and face [64]. Therapists can utilize the completed Lund-Browder diagram to identify CFUs at that are at risk of contracture or deformity. For instance, a burn to a single hand (dorsal and volar surface) only represents 2% TBSA, but comprises at least 30 CFUs accounting for approximately 30% of all CFUs in the body. Thus, the hand is at very high risk for deformity and decreased function. We utilize the calculation of CFUs during the initial phases of burn injury to assist in determining therapy time and resource allocation [65, 66].

The rehabilitation team plays a vital role in the initial management and resuscitation of a burn injury. Therapists' unique skill set places them in an ideal position to assist the multidisciplinary team in the identification of key elements vital to preservation of limb and function:

- Extremity perfusion, through the careful assessment of edema and use of edema management techniques
- Neuromuscular status of the extremities, through assessment and identification of sensory and/or motor deficits
- Identification of tendon or bony anomalies such as exposed tendons and fractures

Teamwork

The care of patients with burn shock is complex and requires the coordinated efforts of a multidisciplinary team [67]. At the US Army Burn Center, we have devoted significant effort to improving communication among members of our team by means of processes such as the following:

TABLE 4.2 US Army Institute of Surgical Research Burn Resuscitation Checklist	
	Hour postburn
	Mean arterial blood pressure
	Lactate
	Base deficit
	PaO_2-to-FiO_2 ratio
	Bladder pressure
	Pulses
	Urine output
	Pressor doses
	Crystalloid rate
	Colloid rate
	Total volume received to date (mL/kg)

- Twice-daily multidisciplinary team rounds, starting with a briefing by the bedside ICU nurse
- Task lists ("to-do lists") managed by the charge nurse
- Custom (burn-specific) multivariable data display tools
- Three-way crisis communication techniques
- Focused after-action reviews

The first 48 hours is a time during which it is particularly important to employ all of these processes, and more. For example, we have found it helpful to schedule conference calls every 6 hours during the course of a difficult resuscitation among the various team members. During these calls, a standardized checklist of key variables can be used to guide the discussion (Table 4.2):

Final Thoughts

The successful initial evaluation and treatment of extensively burned casualties are challenging, but critical to both survival and optimal long-term outcomes. Early communication with a burn center and timely transport are keys to success. Under most circumstances, transport can and should be accomplished within hours of injury. In austere, mass-casualty, or military environments, this may not be possible—if so, postponing evacuation until after the resuscitation phase is complete, but before infection sets in, may be the best choice. Adherence to the principles described in this chapter will support the successful early care of burn patients.

Acknowledgments The opinions or assertions contained herein are the private views of the authors and are not to be construed as official or as representing the views of the Department of the Army or the Department of Defense.

L.C.C. is an inventor of Burn Navigator (Arcos Medical, Inc., Houston, TX). He has assigned his rights to the US Army. He is funded by the Department of Defense to conduct studies of plasma for burn shock resuscitation. The authors declare no other conflicts of interest.

The authors gratefully acknowledge Mr. W. Scott Dewey for helpful comments, and Ms. Susan Reyna, Library Assistant, US Army Institute of Surgical Research.

References

1. Hammond JS, Ward CG. Transfers from emergency room to burn center: errors in burn size estimate. J Trauma. 1987;27:1161–5.
2. Osler T, Glance LG, Hosmer DW. Simplified estimates of the probability of death after burn injuries: extending and updating the Baux score. J Trauma Acute Care Surg. 2010;68(3):690–7.
3. Anonymous. Burn Center Referral Criteria. Chicago, IL: American Burn Association; n.d.. http://ameriburn.org/public-resources/burn-center-referral-criteria/. Accessed 7 Oct 2020.
4. Cancio LC. Airway management and smoke inhalation injury in the burn patient. Clin Plast Surg. 2009;36(4):555–67.
5. Zak AL, Harrington DT, Barillo DJ, Lawlor DF, Shirani KZ, Goodwin CW. Acute respiratory failure that complicates the resuscitation of pediatric patients with scald injuries. J Burn Care Rehabil. 1999;20(5):391–9.
6. Ishimaru T, Goto T, Takahashi J, Okamoto H, Hagiwara Y, Watase H, et al. Association of ketamine use with lower risks of post-intubation hypotension in hemodynamically-unstable patients in the emergency department. Sci Rep. 2019;9(1):17,230.

7. Hampson NB, Piantadosi CA, Thom SR, Weaver LK. Practice recommendations in the diagnosis, management, and prevention of carbon monoxide poisoning. Am J Respir Crit Care Med. 2012;186(11):1095–101.

8. Chung KK, Wolf SE, Renz EM, Allan PF, Aden JK, Merrill GA, et al. High-frequency percussive ventilation and low tidal volume ventilation in burns: a randomized controlled trial. Crit Care Med. 2010;38(10):1970–7.

9. Arturson MG. The pathophysiology of severe thermal injury. J Burn Care Rehabil. 1985;6(2):129–46.

10. Shirani KZ, Vaughan GM, Mason AD Jr, Pruitt BA Jr. Update on current therapeutic approaches in burns. Shock. 1996;5(1):4–16.

11. Demling RH, Smith M, Bodai B, Harms B, Gunther R, Kramer G. Comparison of postburn capillary permeability in soft tissue and lung. J Burn Care Rehabil. 1981;2:86–92.

12. Lukewich MK, Rogers RC, Lomax AE. Divergent neuroendocrine responses to localized and systemic inflammation. Semin Immunol. 2014;26(5):402–8.

13. Carlson DL, Horton JW. Cardiac molecular signaling after burn trauma. J Burn Care Res. 2006;27(5):669–75.

14. Goodwin CW, Dorethy J, Lam V, Pruitt BA Jr. Randomized trial of efficacy of crystalloid and colloid resuscitation on hemodynamic response and lung water following thermal injury. Ann Surg. 1983;197(5):520–31.

15. Pruitt BA Jr, Mason AD Jr, Moncrief JA. Hemodynamic changes in the early postburn patient: the influence of fluid administration and of a vasodilator (hydralazine). J Trauma. 1971;11(1):36–46.

16. Cancio LC, Mozingo DW, Pruitt BA Jr. The technique of fluid resuscitation for patients with severe thermal injuries. J Crit Illn. 1997;12:183–90.

17. Lawrence A, Faraklas I, Watkins H, Allen A, Cochran A, Morris S, et al. Colloid administration normalizes resuscitation ratio and ameliorates "fluid creep". J Burn Care Res. 2010;31(1):40–7.

18. Cancio LC, Salinas J, Kramer GC. Protocolized resuscitation of burn patients. Crit Care Clin. 2016;32(4):599–610.

19. Gurney JM, Kozar RA, Cancio LC. Plasma for burn shock resuscitation: is it time to go back to the future? Transfusion. 2019;59(S2):1578–86.

20. Anonymous. Advanced burn life support course: provider manual 2018 update, Chicago, IL. American Burn Association.

p. 2018. http://ameriburn.org/wp-content/uploads/2019/08/2018-abls-providermanual.pdf. Accessed 7 Oct 2020.

21. Baxter CR. Fluid volume and electrolyte changes of the early postburn period. Clin Plast Surg. 1974;1:693–709.

22. Engrav LH, Colescott PL, Kemalyan N, Heimbach DM, Gibran NS, Solem LD, et al. A biopsy of the use of the Baxter formula to resuscitate burns or do we do it like Charlie did it? J Burn Care Rehabil. 2000;21(2):91–5.

23. Chung KK, Wolf SE, Cancio LC, Alvarado R, Jones JA, McCorcle J, et al. Resuscitation of severely burned military casualties: fluid begets more fluid. J Trauma. 2009;67(2):231–7.

24. Cancio LC, Chavez S, Alvarado-Ortega M, Barillo DJ, Walker SC, McManus AT, et al. Predicting increased fluid requirements during the resuscitation of thermally injured patients. J Trauma. 2004;56(2):404–13.

25. Chung KK, Salinas J, Renz EM, Alvarado RA, King BT, Barillo DJ, et al. Simple derivation of the initial fluid rate for the resuscitation of severely burned adult combat casualties: in silico validation of the rule of 10. J Trauma. 2010;69(Suppl 1):S49–54.

26. Graves TA, Cioffi WG, McManus WF, Mason AD Jr, Pruitt BA Jr. Fluid resuscitation of infants and children with massive thermal injury. J Trauma. 1988;28(12):1656–9.

27. Jeng JC, Lee K, Jablonski K, Jordan MH. Serum lactate and base deficit suggest inadequate resuscitation of patients with burn injuries: application of a point-of-care laboratory instrument. J Burn Care Rehabil. 1997;18(5):402–5.

28. Andel D, Kamolz L-P, Roka J, Schramm W, Zimpfer M, Frey M, et al. Base deficit and lactate: early predictors of morbidity and mortality in patients with burns. Burns. 2007;33(8):973–8.

29. Herrero De Lucas E, Sanchez-Sanchez M, Cachafeiro Fuciños L, Agrifoglio Rotaeche A, Martínez Mendez JR, Flores Cabeza E, et al. Lactate and lactate clearance in critically burned patients: usefulness and limitations as a resuscitation guide and as a prognostic factor. Burns. 2020;

30. Cancio LC, Galvez E Jr, Turner CE, Kypreos NG, Parker A, Holcomb JB. Base deficit and alveolar-arterial gradient during resuscitation contribute independently but modestly to the prediction of mortality after burn injury. J Burn Care Res. 2006;27(3):289–96.

31. Ivy ME, Atweh NA, Palmer J, Possenti PP, Pineau M, D'Aiuto M. Intra-abdominal hypertension and abdominal compartment syndrome in burn patients. J Trauma. 2000;49(3):387–91.

32. Holm C, Mayr M, Tegeler J, Horbrand F, Henckel von Donnersmarck G, Muhlbauer W, et al. A clinical randomized study on the effects of invasive monitoring on burn shock resuscitation. Burns. 2004;30(8):798–807.

33. Kulp GA, Herndon DN, Lee JO, Suman OE, Jeschke MG. Extent and magnitude of catecholamine surge in pediatric burned patients. Shock. 2010;33(4):369.

34. Soussi S, Berger MM, Colpaert K, Dünser MW, Guttormsen AB, Juffermans NP, et al. Hemodynamic management of critically ill burn patients: an international survey. Crit Care. 2018;22(1):194.

35. Ennis JL, Chung KK, Renz EM, Barillo DJ, Albrecht MC, Jones JA, et al. Joint Theater Trauma System implementation of burn resuscitation guidelines improves outcomes in severely burned military casualties. J Trauma. 2008;64(2 Suppl):S146–51.

36. Salinas J, Chung KK, Mann EA, Cancio LC, Kramer GC, Serio-Melvin ML, et al. Computerized decision support system improves fluid resuscitation following severe burns: an original study. Crit Care Med. 2011;39(9):2031–8.

37. Silversides JA, Major E, Ferguson AJ, Mann EE, McAuley DF, Marshall JC, et al. Conservative fluid management or deresuscitation for patients with sepsis or acute respiratory distress syndrome following the resuscitation phase of critical illness: a systematic review and meta-analysis. Intensive Care Med. 2017;43(2):155–70.

38. Wang YB, Ogawa Y, Kakudo N, Kusumoto K. Survival and wound contraction of full-thickness skin grafts are associated with the degree of tissue edema of the graft bed in immediate excision and early wound excision and grafting in a rabbit model. J Burn Care Res. 2007;28(1):182–6.

39. Cancio LC, Reifenberg L, Barillo DJ, Moreau A, Chavez S, Bird P, et al. Standard variables fail to identify patients who will not respond to fluid resuscitation following thermal injury: brief report. Burns. 2005;31(3):358–65.

40. Markell KW, Renz EM, White CE, Albrecht ME, Blackbourne LH, Park MS, et al. Abdominal complications after severe burns. J Am Coll Surg. 2009;208(5):940–7.

41. Hobson KG, Young KM, Ciraulo A, Palmieri TL, Greenhalgh DG. Release of abdominal compartment syndrome improves survival in patients with burn injury. J Trauma. 2002;53(6):1129–33; discussion 33-4.

42. De Laet IE, Malbrain ML, De Waele JJ. A clinician's guide to management of intra-abdominal hypertension and abdomi-

nal compartment syndrome in critically ill patients. Crit Care. 2020;24(1):97.

43. Parra MW, Al-Khayat H, Smith HG, Cheatham ML. Paracentesis for resuscitation-induced abdominal compartment syndrome: an alternative to decompressive laparotomy in the burn patient. J Trauma. 2006;60(5):1119–21.

44. Chung KK, Lundy JB, Matson JR, Renz EM, White CE, King BT, et al. Continuous venovenous hemofiltration in severely burned patients with acute kidney injury: a cohort study. Crit Care. 2009;13(3):R62.

45. Neff LP, Allman JM, Holmes JH. The use of therapeutic plasma exchange (TPE) in the setting of refractory burn shock. Burns. 2010;36(3):372–8.

46. Tanaka H, Matsuda T, Miyagantani Y, Yukioka T, Matsuda H, Shimazaki S. Reduction of resuscitation fluid volumes in severely burned patients using ascorbic acid administration: a randomized, prospective study. Arch Surg. 2000;135(3):326–31.

47. Abrams RA, Brown RA, Botte MJ. The superficial branch of the radial nerve: an anatomic study with surgical implications. J Hand Surg Am. 1992;17(6):1037–41.

48. Salisbury RE, McKeel DW. Ischemic necrosis of the intrinsic muscles of the hand after thermal injuries. J Bone Joint Surg Am. 1974;56-A:1701–7.

49. Smith MA, Munster AM, Spence RJ. Burns of the hand and upper limb—a review. Burns. 1998;24(6):493–505.

50. Sheridan RL, Hurley J, Smith MA, Ryan CM, Bondoc CC, Quinby WC Jr, et al. The acutely burned hand: management and outcome based on a ten-year experience with 1047 acute hand burns. J Trauma. 1995;38(3):406–11.

51. Sterling J, Gibran NS, Klein MB. Acute management of hand burns. Hand Clin. 2009;25(4):453–9.

52. Salisbury RE, Taylor JW, Levine NS. Evaluation of digital escharotomy in burned hands. Plast Reconstr Surg. 1976;58(4):440–3.

53. Hirche C, Almeland SK, Dheansa B, Fuchs P, Governa M, Hoeksema H, et al. Eschar removal by bromelain based enzymatic debridement (Nexobrid®) in burns: European consensus guidelines update. Burns. 2020;46:782–96.

54. Jandera V, Hudson DA, de Wet PM, Innes PM, Rode H. Cooling the burn wound: evaluation of different modalites. Burns. 2000;26(3):265–70.

55. Mosier MJ, Pham TN, Klein MB, Gibran NS, Arnoldo BD, Gamelli RL, et al. Early enteral nutrition in burns: compliance

with guidelines and associated outcomes in a multicenter study. J Burn Care Res. 2011;32(1):104–9.

56. Mai AP, Fortenbach CR, Wibbenmeyer LA, Wang K, Shriver EM. Preserving vision: rethinking burn patient monitoring to prevent orbital compartment syndrome. J Burn Care Res. 2020;41(5):1104–10.

57. Serghiou MA, Ott S, Cowan A, Kemp-Offenberg J, Suman OE. Burn rehabilitation along the continuum of care. In: Herndon DN, editor. Total burn care. 5th ed. Elsevier; 2018. p. 476–508.

58. Chapman T, Serghiou M, Niszczak J. Therapy management of the burned hand and upper extremity. In: Skirven TM, Osterman AL, Fedorczyk JM, Amadio PC, Feldscher SB, Shin EK, editors. Rehabilitation of the hand and upper extremity. 7th ed. Elsevier; 2021. p. 1154–86.

59. Germann G, Hrabowski H. Burned hand. In: Wolfe SW, Hotchkiss RN, Pederson WC, Kozin SH, Cohen MS, editors. Green's operative hand surgery. 7th ed. Philadelphia: Elsevier; 2017. p. 1926–57.

60. Dewey WS, Hedman TL, Chapman TT, Wolf SE, Holcomb JB. The reliability and concurrent validity of the figure-of-eight method of measuring hand edema in patients with burns. J Burn Care Res. 2007;28(1):157–62.

61. Hedman TL, Quick CD, Richard R, Renz EM, Fisher S, Rivers E, et al. Rehabilitation of burn casualties. In: Pasquina PF, Cooper RA, editors. Textbooks in military medicine: care of the combat amputee. Borden Institute, Department of the Army; 2009. p. 277–380.

62. Howell J. Management of the burned hand. In: Richard R, Staley M, editors. Burn care and rehabilitation: principles and practice. FA Davis Company; 1994. p. 531–75.

63. Richard R, Baryza MJ, Carr JA, Dewey WS, Dougherty ME, Forbes-Duchart L, et al. Burn rehabilitation and research: proceedings of a consensus summit. J Burn Care Res. 2009;30(4):543–73.

64. Richard RL, Lester ME, Miller SF, Bailey JK, Hedman TL, Dewey WS, et al. Identification of cutaneous functional units related to burn scar contracture development. J Burn Care Res. 2009;30(4):625–31.

65. Richard R, Jones J, Dewey W, Anyan W III, Faraklas I. Small and large burns alike benefit from lengthier rehabilitation time [abstract]. J Burn Care Res. 2015;36:S108.

66. Richard R, Santos-Lozada AR, Dewey WS, Chung KK. Profile of patients without burn scar contracture development. J Burn Care Res. 2017;38(1):e62–9.
67. Whipple AO. Basic principles in the treatment of thermal burns. Ann Surg. 1943;118:187–91.

Chapter 5
Inhalation Injury

Axel Rodriguez and Alexis McQuitty (iD)

Introduction

Inhalation injury is major cause of death for patients burned in structural fires, which often occur in enclosed spaces with inability to flee the incident [1]. Smoke inhalation may be present in up to 20% of reported burn cases and is identified in 60–70% of patients who die in burn centers. The degree of injury depends on many factors: gas components of fire accidents, presence of soot (particulate matter), and magnitude of exposure to flame or steam [2]. If inhalation injury is suspected in a patient with any burn size, a referral to a burn center should occur promptly. Early intervention, treatment, and monitoring in a burn ICU may improve patient outcome. In addition to extremes of age and the total body surface area (TBSA) burn, inhalation injury is an important predictor of mortality [3–5].

A. Rodriguez · A. McQuitty (✉)
Department of Anesthesiology, University of Texas Medical Branch, Galveston, TX, USA
e-mail: axrodrig@utmb.edu; almcquit@utmb.edu

© The Author(s), under exclusive license to Springer Nature 145
Switzerland AG 2023
J. O. Lee (ed.), *Essential Burn Care for Non-Burn Specialists*,
https://doi.org/10.1007/978-3-031-28898-2_5

Pathophysiology

Airway injury and respiratory complications may occur in patients with large TBSA burns, scald burns without head/neck involvement, prolonged intubation, and direct thermal inhalation of steam, chemicals, or hot gases [6]. Despite research gains in nutrition, the hypermetabolic response to burn injury, and novel skin grafting techniques, there is still much to be learned about the pathophysiology, inflammatory response, and long-term consequences of inhalation injury [7].

Inhalation injury may be divided into 3 classes: thermal injury (restricted to upper airway structures except in cases of blast injury or steam inhalation), local chemical irritation throughout the respiratory tract, and systemic toxicity (inhalation of toxins such as carbon monoxide or hydrogen cyanide). Airway compromise may occur within minutes to days from severe edema, bronchospasm, and mucous plugs or cast formation. The effects of fire and smoke exposure are pathologic at several distinct anatomic levels, from mild upper airway inflammation to severe systemic consequences (see Fig. 5.1 [8]).

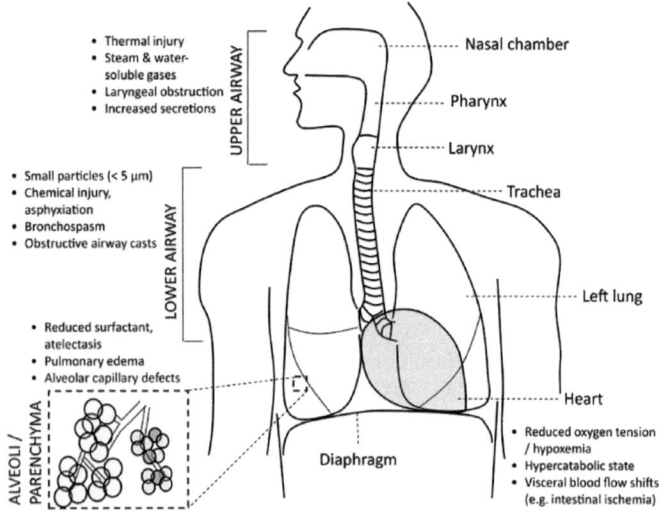

FIGURE 5.1 Respiratory and systemic effects of inhalation injury. Source: [8]

In the presence of steam, thermal injury to distal lung tissue occurs as steam has a higher heat capacity than air and will cause direct injury to the distal tracheobronchial tree [9]. Inhalation of hot dry air does not seem to have significant effects on the lower respiratory tract, as most of the heat is dissipated in the nasopharynx (but laryngospasm, supraglottic edema, and possible suffocation may occur). Profound distal lung injury and death may ensue in smoke inhalation patients who are entrapped in enclosed spaces with loss of consciousness. In conscious patients, subglottic injury rarely occurs, due to the reflex closure of the vocal cords. After exposure to smoke for an extended period, the following may occur in varying degrees: initial interstitial edema with decreased pulmonary compliance/bronchospasm, hypoxemia (with or without carbon monoxide), loss of hypoxic pulmonary vasoconstriction and resultant ventilation/perfusion mismatch, and late pneumonia or respiratory failure [9, 10].

Assessment and Grading

The initial assessment of the patient with suspected inhalation injury should include recognition and immediate treatment of limb or life-threatening injuries, as burn patients may also have associated trauma. Large cutaneous burns may distract physicians from other critical injuries; thus, providers should follow the guidelines outlined by the American College of Surgeons and the American Burn Association. Immediate priorities are outlined by the Advanced Trauma Life Support (ATLS) and Advanced Burn Life Support (ABLS) courses [11–13]. The initial focus is airway maintenance (recognition of current or impending obstruction), cervical spine protection, adequate ventilation, and maintenance of perfusion pressure. The presence of hypoxia or respiratory distress on arrival should alert the provider to rule out other immediate life-threatening pathology, such as tension pneumothorax. Oxygen should be initiated in patients with suspected inhalation injury, and continuous monitoring should occur, as airway edema will continue to increase over several hours, especially after fluid resuscitation [14, 15].

Although facial burns may be indicative of a possible inhalation injury, a history of a closed space flame burn should be a warning sign [16]. Predictors of inhalation injury with high sensitivity include a combination of several factors: large TBSA burn, flame burns in enclosed space, soot in mouth, and dyspnea [1, 17]. Facial burns, singed hair, and mild hoarseness are classic signs of probable inhalation injury but lack sensitivity and specificity [18]. Only completely asymptomatic patients without signs of inhalation injury (see Denver criteria below) may be discharged from the emergency department setting; otherwise, the patient should be stabilized and transferred to a burn center or admitted for close monitoring [19].

Multiple modalities may assist with the diagnosis of inhalation injury. The current standard for diagnosis of inhalation injury is bronchoscopy; initial chest radiographs or computed tomography (CT) scans often appear normal until secondary complications develop [15]. Inflammation is progressive, and patients should be assessed by bronchoscopy on arrival and repeated again within 48 h as needed. Chest radiographs or CT scans may be utilized to identify initial coexisting traumatic injuries. CT scans with a radiology score (RADS) to grade severity of inhalation injury may complement bronchoscopic findings within 24 h of injury and have the advantage of being noninvasive and allowing for evaluation of the lower airways [19]. Other clinical testing includes radionuclide studies with xenon-133, pulmonary function tests, carboxyhemoglobin levels (see Management section), and arterial blood gas analysis.

All symptomatic patients should have an evaluation by flexible bronchoscopy and/or nasopharyngoscopy [4, 20] to estimate the extent of injury and to evaluate the development of mucosal edema. If these scopes are not available, then guidelines for evaluation and intubation in a pre-burn center should be followed (see Management section). A complete diagnostic exam should be performed by experienced personnel, and care should be taken to avoid impairment of airway patency [21]. Nasopharyngoscopy is well-tolerated in non-intubated patients and should also be performed in intubated patients to assess pharyngeal edema. Sedation adjuncts and medications, if needed, include local anesthetic atomizers (lidocaine), dexmedetomidine, and ketamine. An antisialagogue/anticholinergic agent, such as glycopyrrolate, is often added to pediatric regimens. Narcotics and benzodiazepines should be used with caution as they may cause respiratory depression in a difficult airway patient. Children are at greater risk of airway obstruction (with relatively smaller airway diameters), as are patients with circumferential burns to the neck [1, 15]; these patients should be monitored in an acute care setting with a low threshold for intubation.

A key component of most studies is the importance of examining symptomatic patients, as many patients with inhalation injuries may not demonstrate the usual signs of facial burns [20]. Facial burns have a high correlation with true vocal cord edema, and body burns have a high correlation with both true and false vocal cord edema (we find this to be true in large scald burns at our institution). Diagnosis of inhalation injury by evaluation of the upper airway only (with laryngoscopy or nasopharyngoscopy) is not associated with poor outcomes or mortality [22]; however, the addition of bronchoscopic evidence of injury correlates well with mortality and ventilator/ICU days. It is necessary to confirm lower airway damage by bronchoscopy because physical findings, such as singed facial hair and carbonaceous sputum in the oropharynx, are indicators of thermal injury at the level of the pharynx and cannot predict lower airway damage [23].

The Abbreviated Injury Score (AIS, a bronchoscopic grading scale), shown in Table 5.1, correlates with subsequent clinical outcomes and may guide management [3, 24]. A complete diagnostic exam involves assessment of the supraglottic, glottis opening, and subglottic (tracheobronchial) areas [25]. Because airway edema may not occur immediately but may develop over a period of hours, a high index of suspicion and frequent reevaluations of the respiratory status are essential [15]. Patients

Table 5.1 Bronchoscopic criteria to grade inhalation injury (Abbreviated Injury Score)

Grade	Class	Description
0	No injury	Absence of carbonaceous deposits, erythema, edema, bronchorrhea, or obstruction
1	Mild injury	Minor or patchy areas of erythema, carbonaceous deposits in proximal or distal bronchi
2	Moderate injury	Moderate degree of erythema, carbonaceous deposits, bronchorrhea, with or without compromise of the bronchi
3	Severe injury	Severe inflammation with friability, copious carbonaceous deposits, bronchorrhea, bronchial obstruction
4	Massive injury	Evidence of mucosal sloughing, necrosis, endoluminal obliteration

Sources for this table [24, 29]

with moderate to severe injury by the AIS may worsen over the first few days; therefore, repeat bronchoscopy may be needed. In addition to age and TBSA, predictors of mortality and prolonged ICU care include severe injury by bronchoscopy, a decline in PaO_2/FiO_2 ratio at 48 h, decreased pulmonary compliance, pneumonia, and Acute Physiology and Chronic Health Evaluation II (APACHE II) scores on admission [3, 26–28].

Management

The treatment of inhalation injury, other than carbon monoxide and hydrogen cyanide, is supportive care after early recognition, lung protective ventilation strategies, inhaled/nebulized medications, and bronchoscopy to guide therapy [15, 25]. Immediate intubation, when indicated, and avoidance of prolonged mechanical ventilation may prevent acute and long-term complications.

Airway Management

Approximately 1/3 of admissions to burn centers with intuba-tion are extubated promptly, indicating an unnecessary intu-bation in the pre-burn center setting [18, 30]. The decision to intubate should be based on the current airway examination and not on presumed future sequelae. Routine prophylactic intubation may cause more harm. There are many risks of intubation: inability to intubate, unplanned extubation (inability to secure endotracheal tube [ETT] on burned face), tracheal trauma, suction-catheter trauma, poor pulmonary toilet, and ventilator-associated pneumonia [30]. Intubation-related complications are more common in those intubated in a pre-burn center setting [18]; however, in hospitals without burn physicians or those with airway expertise, early intuba-tion may be lifesaving. Stridor and laryngeal edema may progress rapidly during burn resuscitation in those with signs and symptoms of inhalation injury.

In patients without overt airway obstruction and difficult oxygenation/ventilation, supplemental humidified oxygen should be sufficient while the primary and secondary physical assessments are completed [1]. Impending loss of the airway is highly unlikely in those with adequate gas exchange at the time of initial examination [18]. Although multiple signs of inhalation injury may be present, the key to success is early identification of symptomatic patients. The decision to intu-bate a burn patient with severe stridor (indicating airway obstruction) is not difficult, but challenges occur in those with possible inhalation injury, minimal symptoms, and the need for transport [16].

While conservative management without intubation after immediate nasopharyngoscopy and bronchoscopy occurs at many burn centers with anesthesiologists on stand-by, pre-burn centers should follow guidelines for intubation [31, 32]. Many authors state that large TBSA burns should be intu-bated irrespective of where the burn occurred as the amount of resuscitation fluid that they require may lead to edema, which makes intubation impossible on arrival at the burn center [30]. In addition to the ATLS intubation guidelines [11], the Eastern Association for the Surgery of Trauma has guidelines for emergency intubation in smoke inhalation patients [33]:

– Airway obstruction
– Severe cognitive impairment (GCS score ≤8)
– Major cutaneous burn (≥40%)
– Major burns and/or smoke inhalation with an anticipated prolonged transport time
– Impending airway obstruction with moderate-to-severe facial or oropharyngeal burn or severe airway injury identified by nasopharyngoscopy and/or bronchoscopy.

Early studies showed that the classic signs of inhalation injury do not always predict the need for intubation; however, patients with soot in the oral cavity, facial burns, and large cutaneous burns should be monitored closely because these findings indicate a higher likelihood of laryngeal edema and the need for intubation [34]. Badulak et al. [35] noted that traditional American Burn Association criteria for intubation in patients with thermal burns are associated with long-term, unnecessary intubations; additional signs of injury were added to create the Denver criteria (Table 5.2), which serve as conservative intubation recommendations for pre-burn center providers while still reducing unnecessary intubations. Patients lacking these criteria should be closely monitored and may avoid intubation. In patients with a questionable

TABLE 5.2 Denver criteria

Indications for intubation with thermal burns	
• Full thickness facial burns	• Altered mentation
• Stridor	• Hypoxia/hypercarbia
• Respiratory distress	• Hemodynamic instability
• Swelling on laryngoscopy	• Suspected smoke inhalation
• Upper airway trauma	• Singed facial hair

Source for this table [35]

need for intubation, our center utilizes nasopharyngoscopy to examine upper airway edema and injury.

Although many patients may not require immediate intubation, it is recommended to contact a burn center in all patients with suspected inhalation injury. In patients without signs and symptoms of a compromised airway, burns with a lower need for pre-transfer intubation are the following [30]:

- Burns that occur from causes other than flame injury
- Burns that do not occur in enclosed spaces
- Burns that are less than 20% TBSA
- Burns that have no full-thickness (third degree) burns to the face
- Patient is within a reasonable distance to a burn center (less than 3 h).

Patients with severe burns should be presumed to have a difficult airway, and the medical personnel with the most airway experience should perform the intubation. In centers without airway expertise (experienced anesthesiologist and/or otolaryngologist), a multidisciplinary team approach may be successful; this pre-burn center team may consist of a general surgeon, emergency physician, anesthesiologist, respiratory therapist, and a pre-hospital emergency medical technician or paramedic. The intubation sequence should follow practice guidelines for management of the difficult airway by the American Society of Anesthesiology [36] (https://www.asahq.org) and the ATLS guidelines [11].

Nasotracheal intubation, secured by a septal tie (in those without facial trauma), is most common in our burn center, and it may be performed without paralysis and with minimal sedation [20]. For emergent oral intubation (usually with videolaryngoscopy assistance), it is crucial to maintain the ETT security; upper airway edema makes reintubation difficult [37]. Options to secure the ETT include the following: use of multiple umbilical cotton ties, around the head, above and below the ears, and tied around the ETT; use of dental wire around teeth or inserted between the maxilla and teeth, then the wire is secured around the ETT; placement of a red rubber catheter through the nose and out of the mouth to create a loop, and the ETT is tied to the loop with thin cotton umbilical tape [38]. Less ETT cuff pressure may be needed due to tracheal edema [39].

There is no evidence to support the routine use of tracheostomy in burn patients [1]. Tracheostomy should be avoided initially, as upper airway edema usually resolves in 3–6 days with treatment [15, 40]. With the exception of severe vocal cord injury, the indications for tracheostomy in this population are similar to non-burn patients: inability to intubate orally or nasally, adjunct to head or neck trauma management, airway protection in high spinal cord or traumatic brain injury, multiple failed weaning trials after prolonged intubation.

Extubation guidelines for burn patients follow conventional clinical criteria, including airway patency, neurological status, muscular weakness, pulmonary secretions, and chest compliance [41]. A positive ETT leak test should be documented prior to extubation. Additionally, our center utilizes nasopharyngoscopy to identify persistent upper airway edema, and we often extubate with direct fiberoptic visualization. This is useful in a small subset of patients with large ETT relative to body size (for example pediatric patients). Securing a face mask post-extubation for continuous positive airway pressure may not be possible with facial burns; high flow nasal cannula is a good alternative [41].

Carbon Monoxide and Hydrogen Cyanide

Carbon monoxide toxicity should be suspected in patients with inhalation injury, especially if the burn occurred in an enclosed space. Hemoglobin binds carbon monoxide (CO) with a much higher affinity than oxygen. The formation of carboxyhemoglobin (COHb) results in reduced oxygen delivery [37]. Patients may have normal pulse oximetry reading. Standard pulse oximeters use a wavelength also absorbed by COHb and may have normal to high readings with CO toxicity. For this reason, levels must be assessed by blood sample

CO-oximetry. A COHb level is abnormal if >3% in a non-smoker or >10% in a smoker [19]. Significant toxicity may still exist with near-normal levels, depending on the blood sample timing and oxygen administration.

Patients with low COHB toxicity (10–20%) may have headache, dizziness, abdominal pain, and nausea. With higher levels, dyspnea and syncope may occur. Hypotension, seizures, coma, and possibly irreversible neurologic injury are common with levels >50% [42]. Treatment for suspected or confirmed carbon monoxide poisoning is administration of high-flow supplemental oxygen for at least 6 h [1, 13]. The evidence for hyperbaric oxygen therapy is inconclusive, but it should be considered for those with persistent metabolic acidosis, loss of consciousness, myocardial ischemia, and pregnancy [19, 42].

Inhaled hydrogen cyanide (HCN), produced in many household fires, may have a synergistic effect with CO. Tissue hypoxia, lactic acidosis, dyspnea, hypotension, and seizures may occur [29]. Laboratory analysis is not readily available and may take hours to days to obtain a result. Levels >3 mg/L are potentially lethal, and a level <1 mg/L is considered mild. Patients with suspected HCN toxicity should be treated, and this often occurs in the pre-hospital setting. Hydroxocobalamin is the first-line therapy, given as a standard dose of 5 g IV over 15 min. Red discoloration of the skin and urine is common. Older combination therapy has many side effects but may be used if hydroxocobalamin is not available. If hydroxocobalamin (Cyanokit™) is not available, a combination of sodium nitrite (300 mg IV) and sodium thiosulfate (12.5 g IV) may be used as a second-line therapy. This combination (Nithiodote™) has the risks of hypotension and methemoglobinemia [2, 19].

Mechanical Ventilation

Mechanical ventilation (MV) is an additional risk factor for mortality, indicating severe injury diagnosed by bronchoscopy [23], and prolonged intubation is associated with tracheobronchial injury, compared to pure upper airway injury [25]. Several studies have shown that patients with inhalation injury require increased fluids during resuscitation [3, 24], and this correlates with a decreased PaO_2/FiO_2 ratio and longer MV times [25, 43]. Ventilation goals for inhalation injury are similar to lung-protective strategies derived from National Heart, Lung, and Blood Institute ARDS Network data (www.ardsnet.org). Most conventional ventilator modes may be used to achieve tidal volumes 6 mL/kg, plateau pressures <30 cm water, and initial higher positive end-expiratory pressure [8, 44].

Poor oxygenation and ventilation may occur in those with extensive cutaneous injuries, higher grades of inhalation injury, fibrin casts, and mucous plugs. Alternative or advanced ventilator modes may be required to optimize airway patency, reduce ventilation-perfusion mismatching, and prevent the development of pneumonia [45]. Higher tidal volumes can be considered transiently in the pediatric population [7, 46]. High-frequency percussive ventilation and airway [47] pressure release ventilation have both been used to enhance oxygenation in inhalation injury, but no mortality benefit has been noted. High-frequency oscillatory ventilation is not recommended [7, 45, 46].

Medical Therapy

Treatment for inhalation injury is currently supportive, although many pharmacologic agents and respiratory measures have been used extensively by burn centers with varying degrees of success. Therapeutic nebulized agents may be classified as mucolytic agents, bronchodilators, or anticoagulants. Respiratory management includes intensive bronchial hygiene, oral care, incentive spirometry, and early ambulation. The potential role of steroids and other inflammatory agents is an active area of research [8]. The empirical use of corticosteroids is not recommended [46, 48] in all patients; however, corticosteroid therapy may decrease post-extubation stridor (and possible need for reintubation) in patients with airway edema. In a subset of patients with upper airway edema, heliox (a mixture of helium and oxygen) has been used in our institution to avoid intubation or as adjunct for early extubation [49]. Personnel with burn airway expertise are present when we use this gas mixture to improve laminar flow in small airways. Evidence-based guidelines for treatment of inhalation injury are summarized in Table 5.3.

TABLE 5.3 Guidelines for treatment of inhalation injury

Respiratory care→	Humidified high-flow oxygen to maintain SpO_2 >90%
	Cough, deep breathing every 2 h, incentive spirometry exercises
	Turn patient side to side every 2 h
	Chest physiotherapy and nasotracheal suctioning
	Early ambulation
	Sputum cultures and antibiotics if indicated
	Repeat bronchoscopy for lavage and/or surveillance
Oxygenation→	Lung-protective mechanical ventilation
	Alternative: high-flow percussive ventilation
	Prone position, neuromuscular blockade
	Pulmonary vasodilators, extracorporeal membrane oxygenation
Medications→	Nebulized 20% N-acetylcysteine (3 mL) every 4 h
	Nebulized bronchodilator (albuterol) every 4 h (as needed for wheezing or scheduled)

(continued)

TABLE 5.3 (continued)

	Alternate aerosolized heparin 5000–10,000 units (in 3 mL normal saline) every 4 h
Airway edema→	Elevated head of bead
	Corticostcroids
	Heliox
Other→	Pulmonary function tests at hospital discharge
	Patient and family education
	Scheduled follow-up appointments

Sources for this table [1, 13, 15, 18, 37, 40, 45, 46, 50]

Mucolytic agents address the issue of inspissated mucus and hypersecretion after severe inhalation injuries [45]. N-acetylcysteine (NAC), commonly used, enhances airway clearance and possesses anti-inflammatory properties. It may act as an airway irritant and should be used with bronchodilators to reduce bronchospasm. Beta-2 agonists, such as albuterol or salbutamol, relax bronchiole smooth muscle, inhibit bronchospasm, and may improve PaO_2/FiO_2 ratio [7]. Some patients may also benefit from the muscarinic receptor antagonists, ipratropium or tiotropium; these inhaled anticholinergic medications function as bronchodilators. Nebulized heparin is added to aid the breakdown of fibrin casts. These nebulized medications can be continued for 7 days or until extubated [7, 45].

Complications

In addition to airway edema and obstruction, the most common early complication is respiratory tract infection [2]. Prophylactic antimicrobial therapy is not recommended in inhalation injury, but it should be initiated once the diagnosis of pneumonia occurs and sputum cultures are available [2, 46]. Bronchoscopy can be used for the initial diagnosis and for bronchoalveolar lavage (BAL); pneumonia is a complication of prolonged intubation, and sequential bronchoscopy may reduce intubation times and hospital stay [24, 51, 52].

The degree of injury diagnosed by bronchoscopy (AIS) correlates with oxygen perturbations, development of acute respiratory distress syndrome (ARDS), prolonged mechanical ventilation, and increased fluid resuscitation needs [24]. In severe burn patients, multiple mechanisms contribute to ARDS: severe inhalation injury, sepsis, ventilator-induced lung injury, systemic inflammatory response to the burn [53]. Patients with inhalation injury may develop poor oxygenation and ARDS earlier than cutaneous burn patients without inhalation injury [54]. The Berlin definition should be used to diagnosis ARDS in burn patients [44, 55] (see Table 5.4). Treatment for ARDS in the burn center is patient-dependent and involves lung-protective mechanical ventilation strategy, side or prone positioning, echocardiography to

TABLE 5.4 Berlin definition for Acute Respiratory Distress Syndrome[a]

Onset→	Within 7 days of a known risk factor (example: acute burn with inhalation injury)
Chest imaging→	Bilateral opacities consistent with pulmonary edema (chest radiograph or computed tomography)
Pulmonary edema→	Non-hydrostatic edema, not fully explained by heart failure or fluid overload; echocardiography may be required to clarify cardiogenic versus non-cardiogenic pulmonary edema
Classification→	Mild: 200 mmHg < PaO_2/FiO_2 ≤ 300 mmHg
	Moderate: 100 mmHg < PaO_2/FiO_2 ≤ 200 mmHg
	Severe: PaO_2/FiO_2 ≤ 100 mmHg

Sources for this table [44, 55]
[a] Based on oxygenation measured with a minimum of 5 cmH_2O PEEP; for mild classification, oxygenation may also be assessed with noninvasive ventilation; for moderate or severe classification, the patient must be mechanically ventilated

clarify cardiogenic versus non-cardiogenic pulmonary edema, nebulized medications for inhalation injury, neuromuscular blockade if needed, and the nutritional and antioxidant enteral support required for the cutaneous burn [46]. A small percentage of patients will not respond to these interventions to improve oxygenation and ventilation, and this population may require the use of pulmonary vasodilators and/or extra-corporeal membrane oxygenation [56]. Pulmonary vasodilators include inhaled therapies, such as epoprostenol (synthetic prostacyclin) and nitric oxide.

Long-term sequelae in inhalation injury may be avoided with early extubation and treatment. Mild complications include vocal cord dysfunction with voice changes, endo-bronchial or vocal cord polyps, and persistent symptoms consistent with asthma or obstructive lung disease [6, 39]. Severe complications are rare and can be diagnosed rapidly with bronchoscopy. These include tracheal stenosis (seen more commonly in children with prolonged intubation), tracheoesophageal fistula, and tracheal rupture. Other complications are bronchiectasis, bronchiolitis obliterans, and vocal cord fusion. Many of these complications may have a delayed presentation; therefore, long-term follow-up is necessary [2]. Delayed airway obstruction may also occur due to severe scar contracture in facial burns with or without inhalation injury.

Conclusion

It is recommended that both adults and children with inhalation injury be observed in the acute setting with continuous monitoring, allowing for prompt treatment of airway edema and intervention prior to airway obstruction [40]. Inhalation injury is a complex medical problem requiring a multidisciplinary team and preventative therapies. Optimal management may require the collaboration of several medical providers: emergency physicians, intensivists, anesthesiologists, burn surgeons, otolaryngologists, plastic surgeons, speech pathologists, and physiotherapists [6].

References

1. Ahuja RB, Gibran N, Greenhalgh D, et al. ISBI practice guidelines for burn care. Burns. 2016;42(5):953–1021. https://doi.org/10.1016/j.burns.2016.05.013.

2. Walker PF, Buehner MF, Wood LA, et al. Diagnosis and management of inhalation injury: an updated review. Crit Care. 2015;19(1) https://doi.org/10.1186/s13054-015-1077-4.

3. Endorf FW, Gamelli RL. Inhalation injury, pulmonary perturbations, and fluid resuscitation. J Burn Care Res. 2007;28(1):80–3. https://doi.org/10.1097/bcr.0b013e31802c889f.

4. Bai C, Huang H, Yao X, et al. Application of flexible bronchoscopy in inhalation lung injury. Diagn Pathol. 2013;8(174):1–5. https://doi.org/10.1186/1746-1596-8-174.

5. Foster KN, Holmes JH. Inhalation Injury. J Burn Care Res. 2017;38(3):137–41. https://doi.org/10.1097/bcr.0000000000000539.

6. Reid A, Ha JF. Inhalational injury and the larynx: a review. Burns. 2019;45(6):1266–74. https://doi.org/10.1016/j.burns.2018.10.025.

7. Jones SW, Williams FN, Cairns BA, Cartotto R. Inhalation injury. Clin Plast Surg. 2017;44(3):505–11. https://doi.org/10.1016/j.cps.2017.02.009.

8. Dyamenahalli K, Garg G, Shupp JW, Kuprys PV, Choudhry MA, Kovacs EJ. Inhalation injury: unmet clinical needs and future research. J Burn Care Res. 2019;40(5):570–84. https://doi.org/10.1093/jbcr/irz055.

9. Trunkey DD. Inhalation injury. Surg Clin N Am. 1978;58(6):1133–40. https://doi.org/10.1016/s0039-6109(16)41681-6.

10. Chao K, Lin Y, Chiang C, Tseng C. Respiratory management in smoke inhalation injury. J Burn Care Res. 2019;40(4):507–12. https://doi.org/10.1093/jbcr/irz043.

11. Galvagno SM, Nahmias JT, Young DA. Advanced trauma life Support® update 2019. Anesthesiol Clin. 2019;37(1):13–32. https://doi.org/10.1016/j.anclin.2018.09.009.

12. American College of Surgeons; 2021. https://www.facs.org.

13. Advanced Burn Life Support Course, Provider Manual by ABLS Advisory Committee. American Burn Association 2017–2018. https://ameriburn.org.

14. Orozco-Peláez YA. Airway burn or inhalation injury. Colombian J Anesthesiol. 2018;46:26–31. https://doi.org/10.1097/cj9.0000000000000042.

15. Bittner E, Shank E, Woodson L, Martyn J. Acute and peri-operative care of the burn-injured patient. Anesthesiology. 2015;122(2):448–64.
16. Costa Santos D, Barros F, Frazao M, Maia M. Pre-burn center management of the airway in patients with face burns. Ann Burns Fire Disasters. 2015;XXVII(4):259–63.
17. Dyson K, Baker P, Garcia N, et al. To intubate or not to intubate? Predictors of inhalation injury in burn-injured patients before arrival at the burn centre. Emerg Med Austr. 2020; https://doi.org/10.1111/1742-6723.13604.
18. Cai AR, Hodgman EI, Kumar PB, Sehat AJ, Eastman AL, Wolf SE. Evaluating pre burn center intubation practices. J Burn Care Res. 2017;38(1):e23–9. https://doi.org/10.1097/bcr.0000000000000457.
19. Otterness K, Ahn C. Emergency department management of smoke inhalation injury in adults. Emerg Med Pract. 2020;20(3):1–24.
20. Robinson L, Miller R. Smoke inhalation injuries. Am J Otolaryngol. 1986;7:375–80.
21. Gigengack RK, Cleffken BI, Loer SA. Advances in airway management and mechanical ventilation in inhalation injury. Curr Opin Anaesthesiol. 2020; Publish Ahead of Print.; https://doi.org/10.1097/aco.0000000000000929.
22. Ching JA, Ching Y-H, Shivers SC, Karlnoski RA, Payne WG, Smith DJ. An analysis of inhalation injury diagnostic methods and patient outcomes. J Burn Care Res. 2016;37(1):e27–32. https://doi.org/10.1097/bcr.0000000000000313.
23. Kim Y, Kym D, Hur J, et al. Does inhalation injury predict mortality in burns patients or require redefinition? PloS One. 2017;12(9):e0185195. https://doi.org/10.1371/journal.pone.0185195.
24. Mosier MJ, Pham TN, Park DR, Simmons J, Klein MB, Gibran NS. Predictive value of bronchoscopy in assessing the severity of inhalation injury. J Burn Care Res. 2012;33(1):65–73. https://doi.org/10.1097/BCR.0b013e318234d92f.
25. Ikonomidis C, Lang F, Radu A, Berger MM. Standardizing the diagnosis of inhalation injury using a descriptive score based on mucosal injury criteria. Burns. 2012;38(4):513–9. https://doi.org/10.1016/j.burns.2011.11.009.
26. Aung M, Garner D, Pacquola M, Rosenblum S, Cleland H, Pilcher D. The use of a simple three-level bronchoscopic assessment of inhalation injury to predict in-hospital mortality

and duration of mechanical ventilation in patients with burns. Anaesth Intensive Care. 2018;46(1):67–73.

27. Hassan Z, Wong J, Bush J, Bayat A, Dunn K. Assessing the severity of inhalation injuries in adults. Burns. 2010;36(2):212–6. https://doi.org/10.1016/j.burns.2009.06.205.

28. Shirani K, Pruitt B, Mason A. The influence of inhalation injury and pneumonia on burn mortality. Ann Surg. 1987;205:82–7.

29. Dries D, Endorf F. Inhalation injury: epidemiology, pathology, treatment strategies. Scand J Trauma Resusc Emerg Med. 2013;12(31)

30. Romanowski KS, Palmieri TL, Sen S, Greenhalgh DG. More than one third of intubations in patients transferred to burn centers are unnecessary. J Burn Care Res. 2016;37(5):e409–14. https://doi.org/10.1097/bcr.0000000000000288.

31. Hogg G, Goswamy J, Khwaja S, Khwaja N. Laryngeal trauma following an inhalation injury: a review and case report. J Voice. 2017;31(3):388.e27–31. https://doi.org/10.1016/j.jvoice.2016.09.017.

32. Dingle LA, Wain RAJ, Bishop S, Soueid A, Sheikh Z. Intubation in burns patients: a 5-year review of the Manchester regional burns centre experience. Burns. 2020; https://doi.org/10.1016/j.burns.2020.07.019.

33. Mayglothling J, Duane T, Gibbs M, et al. Emergency tracheal intubation immediately following traumatic injury: an Eastern Association for the Surgery of Trauma practice management guideline. J Trauma Acute Care Surg. 2012;5(Suppl 4):S333–40. https://doi.org/10.1097/TA.0b013e31827018a5.

34. Madnani D, Steele N, de Vries E. Factors that predict the need for intubation in patients with smoke inhalation injury. ENT-Ear Nose Throat J. 2006;85(4):278–80.

35. Badulak JH, Schurr M, Sauaia A, Ivashchenko A, Peltz E. Defining the criteria for intubation of the patient with thermal burns. Burns. 2018;44(3):531–8. https://doi.org/10.1016/j.burns.2018.02.016.

36. Apfelbaum JL, Hagberg CA, Connis RT, et al. 2022 American Society of Anesthesiologists practice guidelines for management of the difficult airway. Anesthesiology. 2022;136(1):31–81. https://doi.org/10.1097/ALN.0000000000004002.

37. Sheridan RL, Ingelfinger JR. Fire-related inhalation injury. N Engl J Med. 2016;375(5):464–9. https://doi.org/10.1056/NEJMra1601128.

38. Woodson L, Sherwood E, Kinsky M, Talon M, Martinello C, Woodson S. Anesthesia for burned patients. In: Herndon DN, editor. Total burn care. 5th ed. Elsevier Inc; 2018. p. 131–54.
39. Hemmes SN, Serpa Neto A, Schultz MJ. Intraoperative ventilatory strategies to prevent postoperative pulmonary complications: a meta-analysis. Curr Opin Anaesthesiol. 2013;26(2):126–33. https://doi.org/10.1097/ACO.0b013e32835e1242.
40. Sabri A, Dabbous H, Dowli A, Barazi R. The airway in inhalational injury: diagnosis and management. Ann Burns Fire Disasters. 2017;30(1):24–9.
41. Desai SR, Zeng D, Chong SJ. Airway management in inhalation injury: a case series. Singapore Med J. 2020;61(1):46–53. https://doi.org/10.11622/smedj.2019048.
42. Smollin C, Olson K. Carbon monoxide poisoning. In: Papadakis M, McPhee S, Rabow M, editors. Current medical diagnosis and treatment 2021. 60th ed. McGraw Hill; 2021.
43. Navar P, Saffle J, Warden G. Effect of inhalation injury on fluid resuscitation requirements after thermal injury. Am J Surg. 1985;150:716–20.
44. Patel B. Acute hypoxemic respiratory failure. Merck Manual Professional Version. Merck Sharp & Dohme Corp; 2020.
45. Enkhbaatar P, Pruitt BA, Suman O, et al. Pathophysiology, research challenges, and clinical management of smoke inhalation injury. Lancet. 2016;388(10052):1437–46. https://doi.org/10.1016/s0140-6736(16)31458-1.
46. Deutsch CJ, Tan A, Smailes S, Dziewulski P. The diagnosis and management of inhalation injury: An evidence based approach. Burns. 2018;44(5):1040–51. https://doi.org/10.1016/j.burns.2017.11.013.
47. Chung KK, Wolf SE, Renz EM, et al. High-frequency percussive ventilation and low tidal volume ventilation in burns: a randomized controlled trial. Crit Care Med. 2010;38(10):1970–7. https://doi.org/10.1097/CCM.0b013e3181eb9d0b.
48. Greenhalgh D. Steroids in the treatment of smoke inhalation injury. J Burn Care Res. 2009;30(1):165–9. https://doi.org/10.1097/BCR.0b013e3181923c08.
49. Herman J, Baram M. In the midst of turbulence, Heliox kept her alive. Ann Am Thorac Soc. 2017;14(3):452–5. https://doi.org/10.1513/AnnalsATS.201610-776CC.
50. Atkinson TM, Giraud GD, Togioka BM, Jones DB, Cigarroa JE. Cardiovascular and ventilatory consequences of laparoscopic

surgery. Circulation. 2017;135(7):700–10. https://doi.org/10.1161/CIRCULATIONAHA.116.023262.

51. Carr J, Phillips B, Bowling W. The utility of bronchoscopy after inhalation injury complicated by pneumonia in burn patients: results from the National Burn Repository. J Burn Care Res. 2009;30:967–74. https://doi.org/10.1097/BCR.0b013e3181bfb77b.

52. Ziegler B, Hundeshagen G, Uhlmann L, et al. Impact of diagnostic bronchoscopy in burned adults with suspected inhalation injury. Burns. 2019;45(6):1275–82. https://doi.org/10.1016/j.burns.2019.07.011.

53. Woodson L. Diagnosis and grading of inhalation injury. J Burn Care Res. 2009;30(1):143–5. https://doi.org/10.1097/BCR.0b013e3181923b71.

54. Lam N, Hung T. ARDS among cutaneous burn patients combined with inhalation injury: early onset and bad outcome. Ann Burns Fire Disasters. 2019;32(1):37–42.

55. Bersten A, Bihari S. Acute respiratory distress syndrome. In: Bersten A, Handy J, editors. Oh's intensive care manual. 8th ed. Elsevier Limited; 2019. p. 428–38.

56. Ainsworth CR, Dellavolpe J, Chung KK, Cancio LC, Mason P. Revisiting extracorporeal membrane oxygenation for ARDS in burns: a case series and review of the literature. Burns. 2018;44(6):1433–8. https://doi.org/10.1016/j.burns.2018.05.008.

Chapter 6
Burn Wound Management

Paige J. South, Deepak K. Ozhathil, Amina El Ayadi (ⓘ)**,
and Steven E. Wolf** (ⓘ)

Introduction

Burn care was first described 3500 years ago in ancient cave paintings. From topical therapies to wound dressings, burn care has since then significantly advanced. The Edwin Smith Papyrus from 1600 BC Egypt advocated the use of resin and honey salve for treating burns, and the ancient Chinese treated burn wounds with extracts from tea leaves in 600 BC [1]. In 400 BC, Hippocrates described the use of bulky dressings impregnated with rendered pig fat and resin with alternating warm vinegar soaks, augmented with tanning solutions made from oak bark [1]. The Arabian physician Muhammad ibn Zakariya al-Razi established the first description of first aid for burns in 854 AD, recommending cold water for pain relief from burns [2]. The treatment of topical ointment for burns was described as an old Calcarea blended with plant oil or pig fat cooked with willow bark by Hong Ge in 300 AD [1]. Ambroise Paré treated burns with onions in the middle of the sixteenth century and was the first to describe early burn

―――――
P. J. South · D. K. Ozhathil · A. El Ayadi · S. E. Wolf (✉)
Department of Surgery, University of Texas Medical Branch,
Galveston, TX, USA
e-mail: pjsouth@utmb.edu; amelayad@UTMB.EDU;
swolf@UTMB.EDU

wound excision. Through these discoveries and many more, burn care success rates have improved over the years. Between 1942 and 1952, shock, sepsis, and multiorgan failure with burns covering 50% of children's total body surface area (TBSA) caused a 50% mortality [3]. Currently, a burn covering more than 95% TBSA in children can survive in more than 50% of cases [4]. The initial care and management of burn injuries have a significant impact on the lasting outcomes, healing, appearance, and function. This chapter seeks to describe modern burn wound management for non-burn specialists.

Skin Anatomy

Understanding the basics of skin anatomy and physiology is necessary to recognize the effect and proper treatment of burn wounds. The skin is the largest organ of the body and serves to maintain nutrients, regulate water and temperature, and protect against pathogens, mechanical injuries, and ultraviolet light. This organ is composed of three layers: the epidermis, dermis, and hypodermis.

The epidermis maintains hydration and prevents entry of virulent microorganisms, consisting of five layers: stratum basale, stratum spinosum, stratum granulosum, stratum lucidum, and stratum corneum. The deepest portion of the epidermis, the stratum basale, is the proliferative portion producing keratinocytes and melanocytes. The dermis provides structural toughness to the skin; it consists of collagen and extracellular matrix, blood vessels, hair follicles, sensory neurons, arrector pili muscles, sweat glands, and lymphatic vessels. The dermis contains two layers, the papillary layer (upper, thinner layer) and the reticular layer (deeper, thicker layer). Also known as the subcutaneous fascia, the hypodermis is the deepest layer of the skin and serves to anchor the dermal and epidermal layers.

Burn wound management should be tailored to the type and severity of the burn. Partial-thickness burns are defined as skin loss involving the epidermis and part of the dermis. This may appear as a blister, abrasion, or a shallow crater [5]. Contrarily, full-thickness burns affect the epidermis, dermis, and sometimes, may extend to the subcutaneous tissue. The importance of proper burn classification is paramount to precise management and treatment of the wound.

During wound healing, four biological phases transpire: vasoconstriction and hemostasis phase, inflammatory phase, proliferative phase, and remodeling phase. The initial hemostasis phase occurs about 10 min after the introduction of thermal insult. Here, the outpouring of lymphatic fluid and blood activates the immune system [6]. Occurring 1–3 days after burn, the inflammatory phase usually lasts several days and can be divided into two stages [7]. The early stage is characterized by hemostasis and chemotaxis phase, triggering the release of cytokines and neutrophil infiltration into the wound bed. The late phase occurs as monocytes differentiate into macrophages, removing bacteria and pathogens from the wound site, resulting in erythema, swelling, and pain. The proliferation phase is characterized by two steps in wound repair: angiogenesis and re-epithelization. This phase occurs 3–10 days following the injury and results in granulation tissue if inadequate keratinocytes are present. The final phase of wound healing is the remodeling or maturation phase. This process begins 3 weeks after the injury and may continue for up to a year. Here, collagen is produced and remodeled while the excess collagen, inflammatory cells, and keratinocytes are removed by apoptosis, thus increasing the strength of the skin surrounding the wound.

Care Algorithm

The initial assessment and treatment of burn injuries are vital to the healing of the wound. According to the World Health Organization (WHO), "the first six hours following the injury are critical" [8]. Prior to the assessment, first aid should be considered by removing all burned clothing and irrigation of the wounds with room temperature water to cool the burn for up to 20 min.

Minor Burns Treatment

Although burns occur frequently, the majority of these injuries are minor, involving a small surface area. Therefore, successful burn management can result from an outpatient visit. A typical burn outpatient visit will include assessment for infection, cleaning the wound, providing wound care instructions, and consideration for systemic antibiotics.

During wound cleaning, every effort should be taken to cleanse the wound with soap and water. For any blisters that are present, these can be left intact to minimize pain, but can be unroofed if extensive. The burn is then further cleaned using a mild water-based antiseptic such as chlorhexidine solution [8]. A thin layer of antimicrobial agents such as silver sulfadiazine, bacitracin zinc, or polymyxin B sulfate/bacitracin zinc may be applied. An outer dressing should then be applied. Several other options are available for wrapping the burn wound such as dressing the burn with petroleum gauze with or without antibiotics and dry gauze [8] or using a simple gauze dressing impregnated with paraffin followed by a gauze pad over the dressing [9]. Depending on the type of topical agents used, frequency of dressing change may vary with different agents. Regardless, the dressing should be inspected and changed at least every 24 h or as necessary. Alternatively, one of the many silver-containing dressings may be applied. The benefit of these dressings is that these need to be changed only every 4–7 days in most cases.

Regardless of the initial dressing method, it is important to properly instruct patients on wound/dressing monitoring to have a successful healing process. During each dressing change, wounds should be inspected for any signs of infection such as discoloration or cellulitis. Patients may be referred for surgery if the burn has not healed in 2 weeks.

Hospital Admission for Minor Burns

Admission to the hospital due to a burn that involves less than 10% TBSA may result from three reasons: pain control, additional injuries that require transfer to a specialist, or consideration for excision and grafting. At times, patients with recently sustained burns experience significant pain. Intravenous or oral opioids will be beneficial for pain control in addition to mild analgesics [10].

Although the burn may involve less than 20% TBSA, deeper partial-thickness burns may benefit from excision and grafting. Topical antibiotic ointments such as bacitracin zinc or polysporin B sulfate/bacitracin zinc can be tried initially. This conservative treatment allows time for the wounds to heal on their own [11]. If the wounds are not healing appropriately in this manner, surgery may be the best option.

Although these burns may appear minor, it is best to take precautions as some may require transfer to a burn center. According to the American Burn Association (ABA), burns that involve any special region (face, hands, feet, genitalia, perineum, or major joints); electrical burns; chemical burns; burn injuries in patients with preexisting medical disorders; partial-thickness burns greater than 10% TBSA; full-thickness burns; inhalation injury; and any burn injury that contributes to higher risk of morbidity or mortality should be referred for transfer to a specialized burn center. A burn center will be able to ensure proper healing and provide necessary resources specialized for each patient.

Major Burns Treatment

Patients with burns involving more than 10% TBSA are at risk for hypovolemia associated with edema development and invasive burn wound infection and sepsis. Such persons should be hospitalized. Major burn significantly disrupts the skin barrier, which can result in an infection entering the bloodstream, and development of an overwhelming inflammatory response. Common indications that burn sepsis has occurred are high fever, low platelet count, decreased urine output, and hemodynamic instability [12].

When a patient with a major burn is admitted, treatment of shock, airway injuries, and additional trauma take precedence over management of the burn wound [13]. The first hours of treatment for the burn injury are the most critical for survival and proper healing. Any burn that is greater than 20% TBSA in adults and greater than 10% TBSA in children is considered serious and requires airway maintenance, cardiac monitoring, and fluid resuscitation as early as possible.

Escharotomy and Wound Care

Any patient with full-thickness and deep partial-thickness circumferential burns of the chest or limbs should be assessed for escharotomy prior to transfer to a burn center [14]. Circumferential burns and the resulting eschar of extremity and torso can create circulatory and pulmonary complications due to loss of normal elasticity of the skin and generalized edema formation that result in compression of the underlying tissues. Compartment syndromes may result in the extremities and abdomen from circumferential burns [15]. Escharotomy will relieve this eschar effect, prevent further injury, and restore proper circulation.

An escharotomy is performed by creating an incision through burned eschar and into subcutaneous tissues at lateral and medial aspects of extremities, and along axillary lines in the chest. Other signs that indicate a need for escharotomy are numbness and decreased oxygen saturation of digits. Due to the inflexibility of eschar, the abdominal wall and chest have movement restrictions [16, 17]. In fact, infants under 12 months experience a predominant abdominal breathing

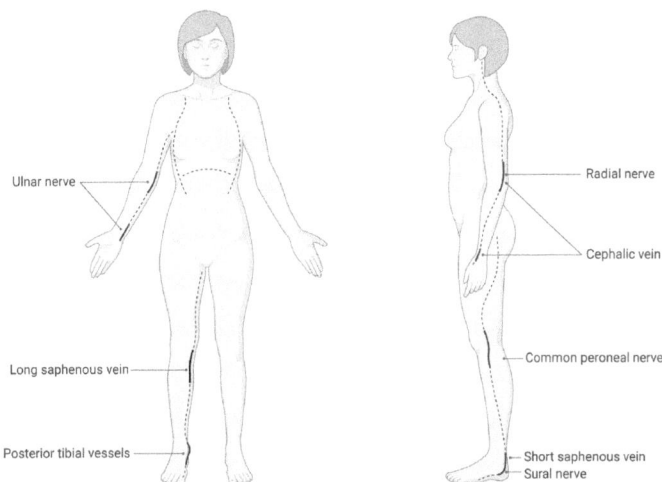

FIGURE 6.1 Escharotomy sites for incision. Incision location-specific to extremities and thorax [18]

pattern, leaving a splinting effect on the diaphragm. Therefore, any resulting compromised respiration benefits from escharotomy [14].

Escharotomy may be performed at the bedside. The upper limbs should be placed in a supine position and lower limbs in a neutral position. When making an incision in the limbs, electrocautery should be used along the medial and lateral mid-axial line bilaterally. In the chest wall and abdominal wall, incisions are made along the mid-axillary lines (Fig. 6.1). Across the abdomen and chest, these lines may be joined by a transverse elliptical incision. Residual restrictive areas may then be assessed by running a finger along the incision. The first 72 h following escharotomy are the most crucial due to possible risks of bleeding or incomplete releases [14]. For this reason, monitoring limb circulation and ventilator pressure are necessary.

174   P. J. South et al.

Major burn patients do not usually benefit from local wound treatment if they are in the process of transfer to a burn center where a more extensive assessment will take place. Therefore, dry dressing can be applied. In the case that transfer is not available within 12 h, the burn wound should be kept covered with application of antimicrobial ointment.

Burn Surgery

Burn Excision

Burn excision and grafting begin by removing all non-viable tissue. Blisters should be unroofed and any non-viable tissue excised. Early excision has proven beneficial in many aspects. Removing all damaged tissue has been shown to decrease the length of hospital stay, morbidity, mortality, bacterial colonization, and healing time [19–25].

Burn eschar can be surgically removed in three ways: tangential excision, fascial excision, or amputation. Regardless of the method used for burn excision, all excisions should begin after the patient is hemodynamically normal and has surpassed the acute stage. This is usually accomplished within the first 72 h of injury to prevent sepsis, bacterial contamination, and graft failure. Tangential excision is the most commonly used technique. Here, all burned tissue is removed while viable tissue is preserved. This technique produces better-preserved contours and reduces hospital length of stay. Although tangential excision generates significant blood loss, tourniquets and other techniques may be used to assist in the reduction of blood loss.

On the other hand, fascial excision is a more rapid method that results in less blood loss. This method is carried out for full-thickness burns, life-threatening burn wounds, and invasive burn wound sepsis. Unlike tangential excision, fascial excision often leads to significant contour defects and the development of lymphedema [26]. Lastly, amputation may be utilized for deep burns in unsalvageable limbs typically asso-

ciated with electrical injuries. Although many excisional techniques are available, special considerations and measures
should be taken into account for long-term function and
cosmesis.

Skin Grafting

Once necrotic tissue has been removed, a donor site is
selected for the procurement of normal skin that will be
transplanted to cover the prepared wound bed. Early grafting
may be practiced via several methods and is divided into two
main categories: skin replacements and skin substitutes. Skin
replacements, such as autografts, are the result of biological
skin application onto the burn wound. Skin substitutes, however, are temporary wound coverings made from a mixture of
biomaterial tissues. As an alternative for autograft skin, skin
substitutes include options such as allografts and xenografts.

Autograft Skin

An autograft skin is a permanent burn wound covering. This
ideal wound coverage is achieved by only using the epidermis and superficial layer of the dermis, minimizing the dermal component of donor skin. Autograft skin comes in two
forms: split-thickness skin graft or full-thickness skin graft.
Split-thickness skin grafts involve the epidermis and superficial layer of the dermis and are usually used to treat
extremity and torso burns. Because the epidermal appendages remain intact, donor site may be re-procured after
healing. To expand the donor skin, skin is often meshed to
increase coverage area by cutting slits into the skin graft
with a number of instruments available for meshing. On the
other hand, full-thickness skin grafts are procured from the
full layer of skin. Characterized with limited stretch, less
propensity for contracture and scarring, full-thickness skin
grafts tend to be associated with higher failure due to their
thicker dermis layer.

Skin Substitutes

Clean partial-thickness burn wounds are usually covered with skin substitutes such as an allograft, xenograft, or synthetic material. A variety of skin substitutes are available as each type of skin substitutes serves a different purpose.

Allograft Skin

Allograft skin is used as a temporary, biological dressing to cover the wound when autograft skin is not feasible or due to lack of available donor sites. While awaiting an autograft donor skin between procurement, allograft skin temporarily closes the wounds. Once donor sites are available for procurement, the temporary biological dressing is removed. This use of an allograft skin not only covers the wound, but also decreases wound size, decreases infection, and reduces pain. Allograft skin is more effective compared to other skin substitutes due to their versatility and immune characteristics as these become vascularized before ultimate rejection. On occasion, allograft skin is placed onto widely meshed autograft skin to protect and close the wound as the autograft skin underneath heals the interstices, known as the Alexander technique.

Other Skin Substitutes

A xenograft skin is a skin substitute where the skin is removed from another species. A xenograft skin is a cost-effective method for temporary wound coverage when compared to an allograft skin. Synthetic skin substitutes are made from a mixture of non-biological molecules such as bovine collagen, synthetic element, allograft, and porcine dermis [27]. Not present in normal skin, the non-biological components in synthetic skin substitutes are associated with a higher infection rate compared to autograft skin [27]. However, the materials used provide a stable, biodegradable temporary wound coverage that is mostly beneficial for major burns.

Other types of synthetic skin substitutes are AlloDerm®, Integra®, Biodegradable Temporizing Matrix (BTM®), and Matriderm®. These types of skin substitutes belong in the group of acellular skin substitutes which function as a dermal layer. These skin substitutes are made from natural biological materials and collagen. The silicone membranes of these dermal substitutes serve as the epidermis until removed and replaced with autograft skin.

It is important to recognize that several types of skin substitutes are available for use that cater to a variety of needs. Whereas some skin substitutes are more suitable for replacing solely the dermal layer, some are used to replace both the dermal and epidermal layers. Additionally, some skin substitutes are composed of different materials as they may help address other complications specific to the patient.

Conclusion

Acute management of a burn patient is most critical within the first 72 h of injury. It cannot be overemphasized that proper healing begins in the emergency department.

For each burn patient, the initial assessment is important since this process will indicate the magnitude and type of burn, additional injuries, approximate healing time, and length of hospital stay. All of these factors play a significant role in determining the most appropriate treatment needed for the patient. Usually, minor burns (generally less than 10% TBSA partial-thickness burns) may be treated as an outpatient unless otherwise stated by the ABA's Burn Criteria. Patients with burns involving more than 10% TBSA or those with full-thickness injuries, however, can experience infection, leading to hospitalization and surgery. Treatment of shock, pain relief, managing airway injuries, and addressing the care of additional trauma occur before management of the burn wound.

At times, certain injuries may benefit from escharotomy before transfer to a burn center to prevent circulatory and pulmonary complications from compression of the tissues.

Assessing for an escharotomy before transfer to a burn center is crucial. Additionally, early burn excision and grafting should begin promptly as it has proven to decrease the length of hospital stay, morbidity, mortality, and bacterial colonization [28]. When covering the wound, there are many dressing methods to choose from. Wound care should be tailored to individual patients as this care will significantly impact the wound-healing time.

References

1. Majno G. The healing hand : man and wound in the ancient world. Harvard University Press; 1975.
2. Gurlt EJ. Geschichte der Chirurgie und ihre Ausubung, Vol. 1. Berlin, Hirschwald; 1898.
3. Bull JP, Fisher AJ. A study of mortality in a burns unit: a revised estimate. Ann Surg. 1954;139(3):269–74. https://doi.org/10.1097/00000658-195403000-00002.
4. Wolf SE, Rose JK, Desai MH, Mileski JP, Barrow RE, Herndon DN. Mortality determinants in massive pediatric burns. An analysis of 103 children with > or = 80% TBSA burns (> or = 70% full-thickness). Ann Surg. 1997;225(5):554–65; discussion 565–559. https://doi.org/10.1097/00000658-199705000-00012.
5. Zulkowski K. Wound terms and definitions [Guide]. WCET J. 2015;35:22–7. https://www.colleaga.org/sites/default/files/attachments/wcet20wound20terms2020definitions201.pdf
6. Wallace HA, Basehore BM, Zito PM. Wound healing phases. In StatPearls; 2021. https://www.ncbi.nlm.nih.gov/pubmed/29262065
7. Coger V, Million N, Rehbock C, Sures B, Nachev M, Barcikowski S, Wistuba N, Strauss S, Vogt PM. Tissue concentrations of zinc, iron, copper, and magnesium during the phases of full thickness wound healing in a rodent model. Biol Trace Elem Res. 2019;191(1):167–76. https://doi.org/10.1007/s12011-018-1600-y.
8. World Health Organization. Management of burns; 2007. https://www.who.int/surgery/publications/Burns_management.pdf
9. Hudspith J, Rayatt S. First aid and treatment of minor burns. BMJ. 2004;328(7454):1487–9. https://doi.org/10.1136/bmj.328.7454.1487.

10. Tenenhaus M, Rennekampff H-O. Treatment of superficial burns requiring hospital admission; 2021. https://www.uptodate.com/contents/treatment-of-superficial-burns-requiring-hospital-admission#H2893372665

11. UC San Diego Health. About burns; 2022. https://health.ucsd.edu/specialties/burn-center/pages/about-burns.aspx

12. Greenhalgh DG. Sepsis in the burn patient: a different problem than sepsis in the general population. Burns Trauma. 2017;5:23. https://doi.org/10.1186/s41038-017-0089-5.

13. Baxter CR, Waeckerle JF. Emergency treatment of burn injury. Ann Emerg Med. 1988;17(12):1305–15. https://doi.org/10.1016/s0196-0644(88)80356-1.

14. Zhang L, Labib A, Hughes PG. Escharotomy. In: StatPearls; 2021. https://www.ncbi.nlm.nih.gov/pubmed/29489153

15. Schaefer TJ, Nunez Lopez O. Burn resuscitation and management. In: StatPearls; 2021. https://www.ncbi.nlm.nih.gov/pubmed/28613546

16. Pruitt BA Jr, Dowling JA, Moncrief JA. Escharotomy in early burn care. Arch Surg. 1968;96(4):502–7. https://doi.org/10.1001/archsurg.1968.01330220018003.

17. White CE, Renz EM. Advances in surgical care: management of severe burn injury. Crit Care Med. 2008;36(7 Suppl):S318–24. https://doi.org/10.1097/CCM.0b013e31817e2d64.

18. Tiong W. On scene first aid and emergency care for burn victims. Int Public Health J. 2012;4:3–24. https://www.researchgate.net/publication/269701993_On_Scene_First_Aid_and_Emergency_Care_for_Burn_Victims

19. Barret JP, Herndon DN. Effects of burn wound excision on bacterial colonization and invasion. Plast Reconstr Surg. 2003;111(2):744–50; discussion 751–742. https://doi.org/10.1097/01.PRS.0000041445.76730.23.

20. Chamania S, Patidar GP, Dembani B, Baxi M. A retrospective analysis of early excision and skin grafting from 1993-1995. Burns. 1998;24(2):177–80. https://doi.org/10.1016/s0305-4179(97)00117-4.

21. Committee IPG, Steering S, Advisory S. ISBI practice guidelines for burn care. Burns. 2016;42(5):953–1021. https://doi.org/10.1016/j.burns.2016.05.013.

22. Edmondson SJ, Ali Jumabhoy I, Murray A. Time to start putting down the knife: a systematic review of burns excision tools of randomised and non-randomised trials. Burns. 2018;44(7):1721–37. https://doi.org/10.1016/j.burns.2018.01.012.

23. Engrav LH, Heimbach DM, Reus JL, Harnar TJ, Marvin JA. Early excision and grafting vs. nonoperative treatment of burns of indeterminant depth: a randomized prospective study. J Trauma. 1983;23(11):1001–4. https://doi.org/10.1097/00005373-198311000-00007.

24. Israel JS, Greenhalgh DG, Gibson AL. Variations in Burn excision and grafting: a survey of the american burn association. J Burn Care Res. 2017;38(1):e125–32. https://doi.org/10.1097/BCR.0000000000000475.

25. Munster AM, Smith-Meek M, Sharkey P. The effect of early surgical intervention on mortality and cost-effectiveness in burn care, 1978-91. Burns. 1994;20(1):61–4. https://doi.org/10.1016/0305-4179(94)90109-0.

26. Nitescu C, Calota DR, Florescu IP, Lascar I. Surgical options in extensive burns management. J Med Life. 2012;5(Spec Issue):129–36. https://www.ncbi.nlm.nih.gov/pubmed/31803300

27. Browning JA, Cindass R. Burn debridement, grafting, and reconstruction. In: StatPearls; 2021. https://www.ncbi.nlm.nih.gov/pubmed/31869181

28. Goswami P, Sahu S, Singodia P, Kumar M, Tudu T, Kumar A, Sinha PK. Early excision and grafting in burns: an experience in a tertiary care industrial hospital of eastern India. Indian J Plast Surg. 2019;52(3):337–42. https://doi.org/10.1055/s-0039-3402707.

Chapter 7
Treatment of Facial Burns

Alen Palackic, Robert P. Duggan, Rahul Shah, Jong O. Lee, and Ludwik K. Branski

A. Palackic
Department of Surgery, University of Texas Medical Branch, Galveston, TX, USA

School of Medicine, University of Texas Medical Branch, Galveston, TX, USA
e-mail: alpalack@utmb.edu

R. P. Duggan
Division of Plastic, Aesthetic and Reconstructive Surgery, Department of Surgery, Medical University of Graz, Graz, Austria
e-mail: rpduggan@utmb.edu

R. Shah
School of Medicine, University of Texas Medical Branch, Galveston, TX, USA

Department of Medicine, Vanderbilt University Medical Center, Nashville, TN, USA
e-mail: rahul.shah@vumc.org

J. O. Lee
Department of Surgery, University of Texas Medical Branch, Galveston, TX, USA

Shriners Children's Texas, Galveston, TX, USA
e-mail: jolee@utmb.edu

© The Author(s), under exclusive license to Springer Nature Switzerland AG 2023
J. O. Lee (ed.), *Essential Burn Care for Non-Burn Specialists*, https://doi.org/10.1007/978-3-031-28898-2_7

181

L. K. Branski (✉)
Department of Surgery, University of Texas Medical Branch,
Galveston, TX, USA

Division of Plastic, Aesthetic and Reconstructive Surgery,
Department of Surgery, Medical University of Graz, Graz, Austria

Shriners Children's Texas, Galveston, TX, USA
e-mail: lubransk@utmb.edu

Introduction

The human face is vital for communication, allowing for the transmission of nonverbal information and subtle emotions. Furthermore, our faces process numerous sensory inputs, facilitating our perception of the outside world. The face has a unique and complex anatomy, consisting of skin, fat, muscle, and skeleton encasing and supporting sensory structures such as the eyes, the nose, and the ears. Facial burns can be truly devastating. Obliteration of facial landmarks, burn scar contractures, and loss of sensory structures may significantly impair how a patient interacts with the world. The resulting pain, edema, and scarring can lead to facial cosmetic and functional deformities and lasting physical and psychological impairment [1, 2].

Optimal care of the burned face is lifesaving and helps maximize future cosmetic and functional results. In general, care consists of the primary assessment, airway control, and wound care. Later, postburn management focuses on scar management, reconstruction, and rehabilitation. Because other vital structures such as the eyes, ears, and the upper and lower respiratory tracts are commonly involved, the initial management of the injury can become particularly challenging, requiring an intensive, multidisciplinary effort. The face is divided into distinct aesthetic units and subunits, first described by Gonzalez-Ulloa in 1987 [3]. These aesthetic units play a vital role in the surgical management of the burned face, in placement of skin grafts and other reconstructions [4, 5]. Facial burn management aims to restore the facial subunits, achieve a cosmetically satisfactory symmetric face, and maximize the function of dynamic facial expression [6].

This chapter aims to summarize and discuss the different approaches for the treatment of facial burns.

Anatomy and Pathophysiology of Facial Burns

Skin is vulnerable to numerous environmental insults. Injuries can be caused by exposure to heat, cold, radiation, chemical, or electrical sources. Most commonly, though, burns are caused by thermal insults from liquids or flames [7, 8]. The face is commonly uncovered, leaving it more vulnerable to injuries [9]. The skin acts as the primary barrier against ultraviolet radiation, temperature extremes, toxins, and mechanical trauma. Furthermore, it functions as a sensory organ, mediates immunologic surveillance, and aids in thermoregulation and fluid homeostasis [1, 10].

The skin consists of the epidermis and the dermis. The severity of a burn injury is classified by the depth of tissue involved. Accurate assessment of burn extent and depth is critical for determining the level of care required in the acute setting and the need for surgical intervention. Burn injuries that solely affect the epidermis are classified as superficial burns (first-degree). First-degree burns can be painful and cause the skin to become erythematous. While painful, these burns heal spontaneously without scarring. Partial-thickness burns involve injury down to the dermis. Superficial partial-thickness burns (second-degree) are painful, require topical wound care, typically do not scar, and do not require surgical procedures. Deep partial-thickness burns (second-degree) are less painful due to the destruction of pain receptors, drier than superficial partial-thickness burns, may require surgery, and are more prone to scarring. Full-thickness burns (third-degree) extend through the dermis, require skin grafting, and are at high risk for infections. Fourth-degree burns involve underlying structures such as muscle or bone [7].

Unique anatomical aspects at different depths of the facial skin are important in healing. Wound healing depends on several factors, including epithelial cell proliferation and migration of epidermal appendages. The face and the scalp contain a high concentration of these appendages, including sebaceous glands, apocrine glands, and hair follicles. In the face, these structures are usually localized in the deeper dermis and the underlying subcutaneous tissue. The high concentration and density of appendages in the deeper areas provide a great capacity to re-epithelialize spontaneously [1, 10].

When a thermal insult occurs, local blood supply influences the depth of the burn. The face is well vascularized. The greater the blood supply, the better an area can disperse heat, reducing burn depth and severity [9]. Due to the vascularity of the face, significant blood loss occurs with excision of burns, which has to be taken into consideration for surgical interventions [11].

The skin's thickness and flexibility affect overall burn depth and the development of complications such as contractures. Compared to the skin on the lips and eyelids, most facial skin is relatively thick. The skin on the forehead mostly sits on muscle and bone and is not very pliable, so it does not tend to contract after severe burn injuries. The skin on the face and the neck mostly overlies muscles and fat and is highly flexible. When burned, it tends to lead to contractures of the deeper layers of the skin [9]. The eyelids are often involved in severe facial burn injuries. The blink reflex protects the eye and the margin of the eyelid so that only the skin is exposed to the offending agent. Deep burns and scar contracture can result in ectropion, leading to incomplete eye closure. Ectropion increases the risk for desiccation and corneal ulceration leading to perforation and a threat to vision [4]. The nose and the ears consist of bony structures and cartilage, which are poorly vascularized with thin overlying skin. Deep burns in this area can expose the underlying structures and lead to vital tissue loss and deformity. Burn injuries to the nose, eyelids, and ears represent a significant challenge in the field of reconstructive burn surgery [1].

Inhalation Injury

Inhalation injury refers to tissue damage to the respiratory tract and the lungs following thermal or chemical insult. These types of injuries are common in severe facial burns [12]. The potential for concomitant inhalational injury in facial burn must be considered, and failure to identify inhalational injury expediently can be life threatening. Several studies have shown that patients with burn injuries experience more significant morbidity and mortality when there is concomitant inhalation injury [13–15]. Clinical suspicion of inhalation injury is suspected by certain risk factors, such as burns including the face and neck, singed facial or nasal hair, altered voice, stridor, oral or nasal soot deposits, and carbonaceous sputum. Due to edema, the most immediate threat from inhalation injury is upper airway obstruction [16]. Acute upper airway obstruction occurs in 20–33% of hospitalized burn patients with inhalation injury, which can rapidly progress from mild pharyngeal edema to complete upper airway obstruction [17]. Furthermore, patients without significant airway edema may rapidly decompensate when fluid resuscitation begins.

In general, there are three primary mechanisms and causes of inhalation injuries. First, direct thermal trauma can involve the upper respiratory tract and, rarely, subglottic structures [18]. The upper respiratory tract protects the structures distally from extreme heat or cold as it serves as a heat exchanger [12]. Second, smoke inhalation can pass the glottis. Chemical irritants are present in smoke, and the severity of the trauma is determined by the length of exposure, chemical composition, and the size of the particles. Third, systemic toxicity may occur when carbon monoxide or cyanide is present in the inhaled gases [12].

The diagnosis of inhalation injuries is challenging and is typically based on the physical examination, the patient history, and burn mechanism and bronchoscopy. Regarding the patient history, information about the mechanism of injury, the exposure, and the combustion source are crucial for diagnosis. For instance, blast injuries can indicate injuries distal to the larynx, and the source of combustion can identify particulate and chemical irritants. Tools other than physical examination and patient history are also often used to support the diagnosis of inhalation injury. Pulse oximetry, arterial blood gas analysis, and chest X-ray should be carried out as a baseline. However, they are insensitive tools for lung injuries in the initial phase of the trauma, as the inflammatory infiltrate occurring in response to injury may take one to two days to develop [12]. The flexible fiberoptic bronchoscopy directly visualizes the tissue damage and remains the "gold standard" to confirm inhalation injuries [19].

The treatment of inhalation injuries is not specific, depends on various factors, and primarily consists of supportive care. Initially, the focus is on airway management. There are multiple indications for prophylactic and early intubations. Intubation can be lifesaving for patients with burns to the face and inhalation injuries. Nasal intubation may be preferred in patients with partial-thickness burns. Patients with severe burn (≥30% total body surface area [TBSA] or full-thickness burns of the face) may require long-term ventilation, which may be managed by tracheostomy. This allows better access for treatment of the face and requires less sedation [1, 12, 20].

Management of Facial Burns

Facial burn can be devastating and may result in a change in appearance, scar formation, functional impairment, and psychiatric disability. Deep burns can require long-term rehabilitation and reconstructive procedures. With an accurate and swift treatment strategy, wound healing and scar prevention can be improved, and further follow-up procedures avoided.

The general approach for treating facial burns is similar to that of the rest of the body. The treatment strategy depends on the depth and size of the burn. Superficial partial-thickness burns are treated conservatively, as they heal spontaneously, re-epithelialize on their own within

14 days, and have a low risk of significant scarring. Conversely, full-thickness burns require excision and skin grafting. Wounds of undetermined depth pose a major challenge for the effective treatment of burns, as they may or may not heal within 21 days. Determining the exact burn depth is challenging upon the initial examination but is an integral component of initial management. A delay in re-epithelialization by 2–3 weeks dramatically increases the risk for hypertrophic scarring [21]. Decades ago, burn wounds were commonly treated conservatively with daily wound care because it was postulated that early excision and skin grafting of the face should be avoided [22–24]. Nowadays, most authors recommend early surgical intervention between 10 and 14 days to achieve the best cosmetic outcome in full-thickness facial burns [1, 25, 26]. In severe facial burn injuries, burn severity and depth are not uniform across the injured area. When to excise and graft a wound are crucial in the treatment regime and the patient's outcome.

In the acute setting, after admission to the hospital, patients undergo initial cleansing with an antiseptic prior to debridement of the necrotic tissue and blister. This facilitates the assessment of the depth of the burn wound [27]. Superficial partial-thickness burn wounds are treated with antimicrobial agents with the goal of re-epithelialization within 14 days. Antimicrobial agents play an essential role in the management of facial burns as they control microbial burden as well as superficial infections that may slow healing or give rise to systemic disease [27]. Ideally, the topical antimicrobial has broad-spectrum coverage, limited toxicity, and adequate local eschar penetration without systemic absorption. Products that are inexpensive and have a long shelf life are also desirable [27, 28]. Antimicrobials should be applied several times a day to keep the wound moist. The face should be cleaned at least once a day to reduce the risk of infection. There are many different topical antimicrobial agents used to treat facial burns. Topical antibiotic ointments such as bacitracin zinc and polymyxin B sulfate/bacitracin zinc are antimicrobial agents that are commonly used in partial-thickness burns. They are easy to apply and remove and lack in tissue and systemic toxicity [27]. Several antimicrobial, biologic dressings are available that aid epithelialization in partial-thickness burns and protect against desiccation and infection [29].

Management of Deep Facial Burns

Early excision and grafting are compulsory in full-thickness burns. Partial-thickness burns can be treated conservatively but must be assessed frequently. Several studies demonstrate the increasing prevalence of hypertrophic scarring in burns taking longer than 21 days to heal completely [30]. Therefore, delayed healing leads to the need for additional reconstructive procedures. If healing within 21 days can be anticipated, daily wound care should be continued until healing is complete. If it is clear the wound will not heal within 21 days, the patient should be considered for excision and grafting [31].

Several factors must be considered once the decision is made to excise and graft the wound. Procuring a graft from a donor site with similar color and quality as the face is crucial for long-term cosmesis. Skin from unburned areas of the scalp generally has the best color match but carries a risk of transferring unwanted hair to the face [4, 9]. As an alternative, one can procure a skin graft from the upper back. Skin grafts placed on the face must be unmeshed [4]. Skin grafting to the face also must take into consideration the aesthetic facial units and subunits. Scars at the junctions of these units are less noticeable; therefore, any surgery aims to place incisions, or skin graft seams, at the junctions [9]. The excision can be performed with various instruments, but a Goulian knife/Weck blade is used for the majority of the face. The excision should be at a uniform depth in mixed burn areas. Significant blood loss may occur with excision of the face. Therefore, it is vital to ensure that blood products are readily available [1, 9, 31]. To facilitate hemostasis, topical epinephrine can be helpful. Furthermore, hemostasis can be achieved by electrocautery [4]. Other studies have reported fibrin sealant as an adjuvant tool to control hematoma formation in facial burn surgeries [27, 32, 33]. Meticulous hemostasis of the recipient site is critical as hematoma is an important cause of graft failure, necessitating further operations and delaying wound closure [9]. After excision, it is crucial to decide whether the wound bed is ready for autografting or whether temporary wound coverage is more appropriate. When accurate excision and hemostasis can be ensured, immediate placement of autograft is feasible [31]. If not, the use of an allograft or dermal substitute can be indicated as the initial coverage.

When a patient experiences a full-thickness facial burn, the severity and extent of additional burns inform whether or not the face receives immediate coverage. Following excision of the face, allograft can be used as temporary coverage. After a few days, a second operation is performed to evaluate the allograft. If it is adherent and undergoing vascularization, the face can be covered with an autograft. The use of dermal substitutes as temporary coverage allows for the use of thinner donor skin and may reduce the scarring. We, at times, use dermal substitutes such as Biodegradable Temporizing Matrix (BTM) (Polynovo Biomaterials Pty. Ltd., Australia). BTM is a dermal matrix composed of three layers: a biodegrading foam, a bonding layer, and a sealing membrane. This matrix prevents wound contraction while promoting re-epithelialization [34, 35]. BTM requires a minimum of 2–3 weeks for vascularization before covering the face with autograft skin [9].

Scar Management of the Face

Conservative Approach

Facial burn injuries are devastating and can lead to a long-term physical and psychosocial disability. Implementing an early scar management regimen in the rehabilitation phase is crucial. The most commonly used noninvasive methods are massage therapy, pressure therapy, and the local application of silicone sheets. The application of silicone gel has been used since the 1980s and has become the standard of care in plastic surgery. In the early phase of healing, silicone gel application seems to positively impact the remodeling process [36]. It softens, improves elasticity, and decreases hypertrophy of the scars. Silicone sheets create a hydrated environment, which then decreases fibroblast activity and impair scar development. Furthermore, a hydrated environment may decrease nociceptor activity in the scar and decrease neurogenic inflammation driving hypertrophic scarring [37]. Face masks are used as pressure therapy, usually in deeper burn injuries. The benefits of the combination of pressure therapy and silicone gel have also been reported [38, 39].

Surgical Approach

Although there have been big advancements in the conservative approach, surgery still remains the most used treatment approach when dealing with facial burn scars. Each scar and each anatomical region have to be evaluated individually. In the acute phase (within first months), we focus on anatomical regions that may impair the function due to contractures, such as the mouth, the eyelid, and the neck. In the late stage (months to years postburn), we commonly follow the reconstructive ladder and also consider combining surgical techniques with laser therapy and corticosteroids if needed. Burn scar contractures of the face are commonly treated with tissue rearrangement techniques in combination with ablative carbon dioxide (CO_2) laser treatment.

Laser Therapy

The most applied laser in the main body of the literature is the fractional CO_2 laser (The UltraPulse® Lumenis). This is an ablative fractional resurfacing (AFR) laser with different setting options: ActiveFXTM (lowest energy and highest density) and DeepFXTM (balance between energy and density). These two settings are commonly applied for superficial and deep treatments, respectively. The ActiveFXTM and DeepFXTM fractional CO_2 lasers can also be combined in one single session, respectively. Several studies show that the ablative fractional laser improves the scar's height, volume, thickness, and overall texture [40, 41]. Hypertrophic scars with red or raised appearance are commonly treated with intense pulsed light (IPL). In our experience and intralesional corticosteroid injections, typically with triamcinolone (Kenalog 10 mg or 40 mg Bristol Myers Squibb, New York City, New York, USA) is beneficial. Scars with intense pruritus are also considered for IPL therapy or fat grafting. The surgeon should also consider applying these approaches in multiple sessions with a break of 6–8 weeks in between sessions. This allows the wound to heal and time for observation of the laser treatment benefits.

Burn Reconstruction of Anatomical Regions

As aforementioned, the treatment strongly depends on the anatomical region. The neck is the most challenging area to treat in terms of contractures. A simple, one-stage application of split-thickness skin graft (STSG) will most likely result in secondary contractures. Other common approaches involve bioartificial skin substitutes combined with STSG. The commonly applied Integra Dermal Regeneration Template offers great aesthetic result; however there are reports of contracture recurrence in 50% of cases [42]. The Biodegradable Temporizing Matrix (BTM) plus STSG is another bioartificial skin substitute that may potentially better prevent contracture recurrence. In our experience, a possible approach to prevent contractures is a two-stage approach with the French/McCauley technique with surgical release plus allograft skin grafting, followed by second-stage grafting with thick STSG from the back.

Scalp alopecia is also a very commonly treated condition postburn. Smaller defects can be treated with tissue rearrangement techniques. If the alopecia is too large, we use tissue expansion to increase the surface area of the hair-bearing scalp gradually. Later, the expander is removed, and scarred tissue is excised, with the area of alopecia now being covered by the expanded scalp.

Scarring and contractures in the perioral region can lead to long-term functional deficits with impairment of speech, eating, and facial expression. Local V-Y advancement flaps are applied to release the commissures around the mouth. Upper lip eversion is commonly treated with scar release, excision, and full-thickness skin grafting. Similarly, we treat lower lip eversion with excision and full-thickness skin grafting.

One of the most common early complications in the face postburn is keratopathy due to eyelid ectropion. The reconstruction should be an early priority as it reduces the risk for keratopathy. For the reconstruction of eyelids, we always use a full-thickness skin graft for the lower lid and thick STSG for the upper lids. Donor skin for the graft should match the color. The pre- and postauricular regions are preferred as donor sites; however, as they are often burned as well, other sites including the supraclavicular region and the groin are commonly used as grafts and match the color and texture.

The reconstruction of the nose represents a challenging area to treat. Local tissue rearrangement techniques are limited due to surrounding burns and grafts often do not match the color nor texture. The nasal inferiorly based turndown flap, consisting of the dorsal surface of the nose and covered with skin graft, has been established as useful surgical technique. The incision is carried through the scar contracture of the dorsum of the nose, folded down toward the tip to create an inferiorly based flap, and grafted with a split-thickness or thin full-thickness skin graft [43].

Summary

The treatment of facial burn is one of the most challenging aspects of burn surgery. Superficial burns are treated conservatively with antimicrobial agents. Full-thickness burns require excision and skin grafting for the best outcome. Indeterminate depth burns pose the most significant challenge. The timing and decision to excise the wound critically impact facial scarring and the ultimate aesthetic outcome. If a burn wound does not seem to heal in 2–3 weeks, then excision and skin grafting should be considered. Scars and contractures have to be evaluated individually and the anatomical regions considered carefully. Scar contractures are commonly released with tissue rearrangement techniques in combination with ablative CO_2 laser treatment.

References

1. Dziewulski P, Villapalos JL. Acute management of facial burns. In: Jeschke MG, Kamolz L.-P., Sjöberg F., Wolf SE, editors. Handbook of burns: acute burn care, Vol. 1. Wien: Springer-Verlag Wien, 2012. 291–302 p.
2. Ye EM. Psychological morbidity in patients with facial and neck burns. Burns. 1998;24:646–8.
3. González-Ulloa M. Regional aesthetic units of the face. Plast Reconstr Surg. 1987;79(3):489–90.
4. Aly MEI, Dannoun M, Jimenez CJ, Sheridan RL, Lee JO. Operative wound management. In: Herndon DN, editor. Total burn care. 5th ed. New York: Elsevier Inc.; 2018. p. 114–130.e2.
5. Cole JK, Engrav LH, Heimbach DM, Gibran NS, Costa BA, Nakamura DY, et al. Early excision and grafting of face and neck burns in patients over 20 years. Plast Reconstr Surg. 2002;109:1266–73.
6. Dougherty WR, Spence RJ. Reconstruction of the burned face/cheek: acute and delayed. In: Sood R, Achauer BM, editors. Achauer and Sood's burn surgery: reconstruction and rehabilitation. Elsevier/Saunders; 2006. p. 234–53.

7. Jeschke MG, van Baar ME, Choudhry MA, Chung KK, Gibran NS, Logsetty S. Burn injury. Nat Rev Dis Primers. 2020;6(1):11. Published 2020 Feb 13.

8. Burn incidence fact sheet. Chicago: American Burn Association (http://ameriburn.org/who-we-are/media/burn-incidence-fact-sheet/. opens in new tab).

9. Greenhalgh DG. Management of facial burns. Burn Trauma. 2020;25(9):1127–30.

10. Bagby SK. Acute management of facial burns. Oral Maxillofac Surg Clin North Am. 2005;17(3 Spec Iss):267–72.

11. Housinger TA, Lang D, Warden GD. A prospective study of blood loss with excisional therapy in pediatric burn patients. J Trauma. 1993;34(2):262–3.

12. Woodson LC, Branski LK, Enkhbaatar P, Talon M. Diagnosis and treatment of inhalation injury. In: Herndon DN, editor. Total burn care. 5th ed. New York: Elsevier Inc.; 2018. p. 184–194.e3.

13. Osler T, Glance LG, Hosmer DW. Simplified estimates of the probability of death after burn injuries: extending and updating the baux score. J Trauma. 2010;68:690–7.

14. Tian H, Wang L, Xie W, et al. Epidemiology and outcome analysis of facial burns: A retrospective multicentre study 2011-2015. Burns. 2020;46(3):718–726.15.

15. Darling GE, Keresteci MA, Ibanez D, Pugash RA, Peters WJ, Neligan PC. Pulmonary complications in inhalation injuries with associated cutaneous burn. J Trauma. 1996;40:83–9.

16. Woodson LC, Sherwood ER, Kinsky MP, Talon M, Martinello C, Woodson SM. Anesthesia for burned patients. In: Herndon DN, editor. Total burn care. 5th ed. New York: Elsevier Inc.; 2018. p. 131–157.e4.

17. Kobayashi K, Ikeda H, Higuchi R, Nozaki M, Yamamoto Y, Urabe M, et al. Epidemiological and outcome characteristics of major burns in Tokyo. Burns. 2005;31(Suppl. 1):S3–S11.

18. Moritz AR, Henriques FC, McLean R. The effects of inhaled heat on the air passages and lungs: an experimental investigation. Am J Pathol. 1945;21(2):311–31.

19. Cancio LC. Airway management and smoke inhalation injury in the burn patient. Clin Plast Surg. 2009;36(4):555–67.

20. Aggarwal S, Smailes S, Dziewulski P. Tracheostomy in burns patients revisited. Burns. 2009;35(7):962–6.

21. Deitch EA, Wheelahan TM, Rose MP, Clothier J, Cotter J. Hypertrophic burn scars: analysis of variables. J Trauma. 1983;23:895–8.

22. Bell JL. Treatment of acute thermal burns of the face. Am J Surg. 1959;98:923–9.
23. Boswick JA Jr. Burns of the head and neck. Surg Clin North Am. 1973;53:97–04.
24. McIndoe AH. Total reconstruction of the burned face. The Bradshaw Lecture 1958. Br J Plast Surg. 1983;36:410–20.
25. Cubison TC, Pape SA, Parkhouse N. Evidence for the link between healing time and the development of hypertrophic scars (HTS) in paediatric burns due to scald injury. Burns. 2006;32(8):992–9. Epub 2006 Aug 8.
26. McDonald WS, Deitch EA. Hypertrophic skin grafts in burned patients: a prospective analysis of variables. J Trauma. 1987;27(2):147–50.
27. Leon-Villapalos J, Jeschke MG, Herndon DN. Topical management of facial burns. Burns. 2008;34(7):903–11.
28. Monafo WW, West MA. Current treatment recommendations for total burn therapy. Drugs. 1990;40:364–73.
29. Chester DL, Papini R. Skin and skin substitutes in burn management. Trauma. 2004;6(2):87–99.
30. Fraulin FOG, Illmayer SJ, Tredget EE. Assessment of cosmetic and functional results of conservative versus surgical management of facial burns. J Burn Care Res. 1996;17:19–29.
31. Friedstat JS, Klein MB. Acute management of facial burns. Clin Plast Surg. 2009;36(4):653–60.
32. Gulati S. Use of fibrin glue in excision and grafting of facial burns. J Burns Surg Wound Care [Serial Online]. 2002;1(1):18.
33. Adant JP. Skin grafting with fibrin glue in burns. Eur J Plast Surg. 1996;16:292–7.
34. Greenwood JE, Dearman BL. Comparison of a sealed, polymer foam biodegradable temporizing matrix against Integra® dermal regeneration template in a porcine wound model. J Burn Care Res. 2012;33:163–73.
35. Li A, Dearman BL, Crompton KE, Moore TG, Greenwood JE. Evaluation of a novel biodegradable polymer for the generation of a dermal matrix. J Burn Care Res. 2009;30:717–28.
36. Parry I, Sen S, Palmieri T, Greenhalgh D. Nonsurgical scar management of the face: Does early versus late intervention affect outcome? J Burn Care Res. 2013;34(5):569–75.
37. Mustoe TA. Evolution of silicone therapy and mechanism of action in scar management. Aesthetic Plast Surg. 2008;32(1): 82–92. https://doi.org/10.1007/s00266-007-9030-9.

38. Li-Tsang CW, Zheng YP, Lau JC. A randomized clinical trial to study the effect of silicone gel dressing and pressure therapy on posttraumatic hypertrophic scars. J Burn Care Res. 2010;31:448–57.
39. Momeni M, Hafezi F, Rahbar H, Karimi H. Effects of silicone gel on burn scars. Burns. 2009;35:70–4.
40. Hultman CS, Friedstat JS, Edkins RE, Cairns BA, Meyer AA. Laser resurfacing and remodeling of hypertrophic burn scars: the results of a large, prospective, before-after cohort study, with long-term follow-up [published correction appears in Ann Surg. 2015 Apr;261(4):811]. Ann Surg. 2014;260(3):519–32.
41. Anderson RR, Donelan MB, Hivnor C, et al. Laser treatment of traumatic scars with an emphasis on ablative fractional laser resurfacing: consensus report. JAMA Dermatol. 2014;150(2):187–93.
42. Hunt JA, Moisidis E, Haertsch P. Initial experience of Integra in the treatment of post-burn anterior cervical neck contracture. Br J Plast Surg. 2000;53(8):652–8.
43. Taylor HO, Carty M, Driscoll D, Lewis M, Donelan MB. Nasal reconstruction after severe facial burns using a local turndown flap. Ann Plast Surg. 2009;62(2):175–9.

Chapter 8
Treatment of Hand Burns

Tina L. Palmieri

Introduction

The hands, although comprising <10% of overall body surface area, are involved in >90% of severe burns [1]. Because people interact with the environment predominantly via their hands, even a partial loss of hand function can result in difficulties in performing the simplest tasks. Hands are particularly important in completing activities of daily living; loss of hand use is associated with a 57% loss of total function for an individual [2]. Hands are also visible representations of our selves. We see our hands more often than our face, and hands are frequently what is noticed by others. Appearance has become the focus of outcome research after hand injury [3]. In children with large burns, the presence of a burn injury in a visible area, such as the hands, is more strongly associated with psychological consequences and worse health related quality of life outcomes than the overall severity of the burn [4, 5]. Hence, the appearance, as well as the function, of hands is important. The initial treatment of a hand burn sets the stage for future hand function; hence, it is important for non-

T. L. Palmieri (✉)
Shriners Children's Northern California, University of California Davis, Sacramento, CA, USA
e-mail: tlpalmieri@ucdavis.edu

© The Author(s), under exclusive license to Springer Nature Switzerland AG 2023
J. O. Lee (ed.), *Essential Burn Care for Non-Burn Specialists*,
https://doi.org/10.1007/978-3-031-28898-2_8

burn and non-plastic surgery practitioners to understand the basic principles of management of hand burns. Delayed treatment of a hand burn can result in lifelong disability. The purpose of this chapter is to provide the non-burn physician with the tools to appropriately evaluate and manage the acute presentation of a hand burn.

Anatomy of Hand Skin

Understanding skin anatomy is the cornerstone of accurate diagnosis and management of hand burns. The skin of the hand is unique anatomically compared to other body regions. The dorsal hand and palmar hand have different skin structure and function. While the dorsum of the hand has thin, flexible skin to facilitate movement and joint flexion, the palmar skin is thicker, attached to the palmar fascia, resistant to pressure, and contains essential sensory end organs [6]. As such, the dorsal surface is a motion facilitator, while the palm is designed structurally and biologically to facilitate grasping and holding objects. Injuries to the dorsal hand, due to the proximity of tendons to the skin surface, are prone to motion deficits, while palm injuries may have long-term impact on hand sensorium and grasp.

The etiology of burn injuries to the hand varies by anatomic region, as well as age. Dorsal hand burns are more commonly caused by scald or flame injuries, while palm burns, particularly in children, result from contact with a hot object, such as a curling iron or glass fireplace front [7, 8].Children explore their environment using their hands; hence, young children, especially toddlers, are at particular risk of palm injury. Due to the thickness of the palmar skin, third degree burns of the palm occur less frequently than dorsal hand burns. Other anatomic locations impose additional risks for long-term sequelae after burn injury. Nail bed burns can result in nail deviation, cleft, loss, or discoloration and adversely impact hand function [9]. The extensor tendons of the proximal interphalangeal joint (PIP) is another area of concern. The central slip of the extensor tendon inserts at the proximal interphalangeal joint (PIP), while 2 lateral bands continue distally to the base of the phalanx. Disruption of this mechanism causes the Boutonniere deformity. Finally, the fifth finger metacarpophalangeal joint, which is hypermobile, increases the likelihood for development of a boutonniere deformity months after excision and grafting [10].

Aim of Hand Burn Treatment

In general, tenets of hand burn care are to (1) promote a wound healing environment, (2) maintain circulation, (3) prevent infection, (4) obtain wound closure, and (5) maintain motion. Appropriate initial wound care relies on knowledge of the pathophysiology of burn wounds. Because definitive treatment of the hand burn is complex, requiring the input of surgeons, physiotherapists, occupational therapists, psychologists, and nursing, national burn treatment guidelines recommend that hand burns be treated in a burn center [11]. Due to the limited number of verified burn centers, most patients are initially evaluated in non-burn facilities. Timely referral of hand burns to a qualified burn provider is essential.

Initial Hand Burn Evaluation

The initial priority for burn injury treatment is to remove the patient from the heat source. This is generally accomplished at the injury scene. For small burns (less than 10%) immediate irrigation with cool tap water (NOT cold water and NOT ice) for 20–30 min may minimize the damage caused by heat exposure [12–14]. Initial medical evaluation focuses on assessment for life-threatening injuries following the guidelines set forth for initial trauma management. Injury history provides valuable insight into potential associated trauma (such as crush injury during a motor vehicle crash). The etiology of the burn injury (flame, scald, contact, chemical, electrical), duration of contact with the heat source, temperature of the heat source (if available), first aid applied at the scene, and prior hand injuries should be recorded. Hand radiographs are generally unnecessary unless there is associated crush or traumatic injury.

Determination of burn extent and depth is an essential element of the evaluation. Perhaps the most neglected yet essential step to enable accurate assessment of burn injury extent and depth is to wash the wound with soap and water to remove debris and soot that may obscure visualization of the wound beneath. Pain associated with the burn wound will need to be addressed prior to debridement. For initial burn treatment, patients frequently require intravenous narcotic administration to control pain. Low doses of short acting narcotics are recommended, as pain decreases precipitously after dressings are applied. Anxiolytic medications may be required, as well. Appropriate monitoring should be instituted. After pain is controlled, debridement can be accomplished by initially rinsing the wound with cool water, followed by utilization of wet wash rag saturated with room temperature water and soap (such as chlorhexidine). The rag can then be used to remove loose tissue and further clean the wound. At times scissors may be needed to remove adherent skin ends. The final step is to rinse off the soap and pat the wound dry. This allows for wound visualization and decreases infection risk.

Burn extent (i.e., how much of the body surface area is involved in the burn) is generally estimated by applying one of the three techniques: the palm rule, in which the patient's palm (including fingers) is 1% of the patient's body; the Rule of Nines, in which each body part is a multiple of 9; or employing the Lund-Browder chart, which adjusts body surface area estimates based on age. Upper extremity or hand burns that encompass the entire circumference of the arm or hand should be noted and extremity capillary refill assessed.

Burn depth determination can be particularly challenging for the hand due to the dynamic nature of the wound. The burn wound has three injury zones: coagulation, stasis, and hyperemia. The size of each zone over time is influenced by tissue perfusion and wound care. The tissue in the zone of coagulation is damaged beyond repair. The tissue in the zone of hyperemia, with minimal injury, will heal spontaneously within a week. The zone most influenced by initial treatment is the zone of stasis, in which there is significant, but not complete tissue injury. Appropriate wound management will allow healing of the zone of stasis, while inappropriate management or lack of perfusion will result in extension of the tissue injury. The goal of initial wound care is to minimize conversion of the zone of stasis to the zone of coagulation by optimizing the wound healing environment.

Burn injury depth is divided into three categories: first (superficial), second (partial-thickness), and third (full-thickness) degrees. First degree burns involve only the epidermis and do not blister but can be painful. A common first degree burn scenario is sunburn. A second degree burn traverses the epidermis and extends a variable distance into the dermis. Superficial second-degree burns are blistered, painful, moist, pink, and blanch on touch. These wounds should be managed in a moist environment to encourage epithelialization [15]. Deep second-degree burns are generally blistered, deeper red or mottled in color, have minimal blanching, and are usually somewhat less painful. These wounds should also initially be managed in a moist environment to encourage epithelialization, but the wounds should be closely monitored by a burn surgeon. Third-degree flame burns are white or leathery, generally have decreased sensation centrally, while third-degree scald burns are deep cherry red, dry, and mottled. Topical antimicrobials or silver dressings should be placed, and the patient referred to a burn surgeon for possible excision and grafting. Second and third-degree hand burns are best treated in a qualified burn center.

Most isolated hand burns can be referred for an outpatient clinic appointment within 1–3 days after injury. To date visual inspection of the wound for depth determination is commonplace, although advanced wound imaging modalities such as thermography and laser Doppler are gaining in popularity [16]. Presence of a blister makes determination of wound depth problematic, at best, because visualization of the skin beneath the blister is not possible.

Promote a Wound Healing Environment

Loose debris and broken blisters are removed from the wound, as they are a nidus for infection. Loose fingernails should be left in place (unless already gone). Loss of fingernails suggests the presence of a deep third-degree hand burn, and the patient should be immediately referred to a burn center. Palm blisters can be left intact; however, if the blister compromises circulation or impedes range of motion, they may require removal. Blisters contain inflammatory mediators [17]. Any blister ≤2 cm in height on the palm can usually be left intact without adverse outcomes. If the blister ruptures, however, the tissue pieces should be removed, and the skin beneath washed with soap and water as described above. Intact blisters should be wrapped in dry dressings, as topical antimicrobials such as silver sulfadiazine or bacitracin do not penetrate the blister and will result in skin maceration. Application of topical antimicrobials is appropriate after the blister has ruptured and the wound cleaned. The topical antimicrobial should be placed with a thickness of approximately 0.25″ and covered with loose dressings. Circumferential wrapping of hands should be monitored for impairment of perfusion. Elastic tube netting is the most efficacious method of holding dressings in place. Dressing changes depend on the dressing selected. Topical antimicrobials such as silver sulfadiazine and bacitracin should be changed daily, while silver dressings can be applied for 3−7 days. The patient should be referred to a burn center for outpatient management within the week.

Maintain Circulation

Maintaining circulation in the burned hand is essential to avoid extension of the zone of stasis to the zone of coagulation. This is particularly important in major burns (>20% total body surface area). Major burns should receive appropriate intravenous resuscitation. Hand and arm burns should be elevated above the level of the heart, and dressings placed loosely to avoid circulatory compromise of the extremity. Hand escharotomy for burn injury is rarely necessary and should be performed by a trained burn or hand surgeon, as they may cause blood loss or injury to underlying structures. After adequate intravenous sedation is assured, electrocautery is used to incise through burn eschar to pliable non-constricting tissue or fat. Arm escharotomies consist of incisions along the medial and lateral aspects of the extremity with the arm in supination. In the hand, the eschar is released with 2–3 longitudinal dorsal incisions between the tendons on the dorsal hand [18]. Digital escharotomies are rarely required on the lateral and medial aspects of the fingers and should be above the skin crease formed when the finger is bent at the DIP joint in order to avoid neurovascular injury. Circulation should be reassessed frequently after the performance of escharotomies, and fasciotomy in the operating room may be necessary if ischemia persists.

Prevent Infection

As emphasized above, burn hand infection is best prevented by early and complete wound debridement and cleaning with soap. A partial-thickness wound, which is classically pink, moist, and painful, will heal within 2 weeks and can be treated with topical bacitracin and Adaptic™ or petroleum gauze such as Xeroform™ once or twice daily. The advent of silver dressings, which can be applied and kept in place for 5–7 days, has facilitated management. However, proper application of silver dressings is important. The dressing needs to be secured to avoid dislodgement yet allow for movement. In general, tape should be avoided on burned skin, as it may denude the epithelial layer. Silver sulfadiazine should be reserved for third-degree burns. Although silver sulfadiazine has broad antimicrobial coverage, it leaves a thick residue on wounds that results in painful dressing changes, and it impedes wound healing [19]. Other topicals for third-degree wounds include mafenide acetate (reserved for ears, invasive infections), silver nitrate solution, and silver-containing dressings.

Obtain Wound Closure

Burn wound closure occurs either primarily through wound healing or secondarily via excision and grafting. The resultant healed skin or skin graft should be strong and pliable enough to allow maximal hand function while minimizing unsightly scar. Burns that heal within 2 weeks do not usually result in significant scarring or restriction in range of motion. Generally, all deep partial- or full-thickness burns that are not healing within 2–3 weeks should be considered for excision of the burn eschar with skin grafting [20, 21]. It is not necessary to wait 2 weeks prior to referral; the earlier the operative intervention, the less the scarring.

The foundation for surgical treatment of the burned hand is to perform the simplest technique that allows wound closure and optimized aesthetics without compromising function. Ideally, surgery should be performed as soon as possible after identification of grafting need to minimize scarring, but certainly within a week. Early excision decreases infection risk and facilitates wound excision, as the sub-eschar edema often separates the eschar from underlying tendons. The burn eschar is removed by tangentially excising (serial shaving) nonviable tissue using guarded blade (Goulian knife). Tourniquets can be employed to decrease blood loss and improve visualization of vital hand structures during excision. The wound is reexamined after tourniquet deflation, and hemostasis is obtained.

Skin grafts are generally either full-thickness or split-thickness. The size of full-thickness skin grafts is limited by the ability to close the donor site skin with sutures. Split-thickness skin grafts are thus used for larger grafts, such as grafts encompassing the entire dorsum of the hand and fingers. Because split-thickness skin grafts only contain a portion of the dermis, they may result in greater graft contraction, increased scarring, and less sensation than full thickness grafts. As such, the cosmetic outcomes can be compromised. Full-thickness skin grafts are reserved for smaller vital areas, such as the palm. In children, full-thickness grafting of the palm, using a full-thickness donor skin obtained from the child's inguinal crease, provides a durable graft that covers the entire surface of the palm [7]. However, full-thickness palm grafts will have darker pigmentation than the native palm skin, which has a paucity of melanocytes. Grafts can be inserted as sheets of skin (non-meshed) or meshed, in which holes are placed to extend the skin coverage. Meshed grafts are used in larger burns where donor sites are limited. Although meshed skin can cover more surface area, they heal by scarring of the interstices, resulting in a permanent meshed pattern that can increase contracture formation, compromising function, and aesthetics. Sheet split- or full-thickness skin grafts maximize cosmetic and functional outcomes, but the burn excision should include the dermal elements to prevent inclusion cyst development. Use of sheet grafts is contingent upon skin availability and adequacy of the wound bed. It may be impractical to use sheet grafts for major life-threatening burns. Allograft or skin substitutes may be used as temporary coverage when adequate donor site for hand grafts is not available.

Donor site location in split-thickness skin grafting is an important consideration for adults and children. In children, the back has decreased long-term donor site scarring and no difference in infection rate, pigmentation, or blistering compared to the thigh [22]. The back is our donor site of choice for split-thickness skin grafts in children. Sheet skin grafting, which maximizes both function and cosmesis, is advisable.

The six-inch dermatome can be used to obtain a graft of sufficient dimensions to completely cover the dorsum of the hand for most adults and all children without having seams. This dermatome is particularly suited to the wide flat surface of the back or transversely on the thigh. However, this dermatome requires additional expertise and should only be used by trained personnel.

Fourth degree burns (involving tendon, joint, muscle, bone), often from electrical injury or trauma, may compromise hand viability and function, and should be immediately referred to a burn center. Wounds are debrided and either autologous or cadaveric skin grafts or skin substitutes are used to determine tissue viability. In the event of joint instability, Kirschner wires can be inserted axially to immobilize the joint in a position of function until autografting is complete. Joint fixation may compromise movement: approximately 25% of patients treated with wire fixation have significant restriction in activities of daily living [23]. Free flaps may be required in the case of extensive fourth degree injury involving multiple fingers. Amputation is reserved for nonviable and non-salvageable situations.

Maintain Motion

Maintaining range of motion in the burned hand is imperative to prevent future contractures. Patients with partial-thickness burns should be instructed on exercises promoting extremity range of motion. This will both maintain motion and decrease edema. Splints may be needed to maintain the hand in a functional position in severe burns and postoperatively. Hand splints generally use 20 degrees of wrist extension, 70–90 degree metacarpophalangeal joint flexion, and extension of the interphalangeal joint. Passive range of motion should be initiated postoperatively as soon as grafts are stable. Involvement of an occupational therapist is essential to ensure compliance with strength, range of motion, and function of the hand. Although pressure garments can decrease edema and improve cosmesis, they should be closely monitored and modified. Silicone sheets may be helpful in decreasing scar prominence. Use of a moisturizer to facilitate scar massage usually helps to minimize itching and improve scar mobility.

Long-Term Issues in Hand Burns

With proper vigilance, patients with hand burns can regain full function. Burns that take longer than 10–14 days to heal are often subject to formation of significant scarring; however, thickening of the scar is gradual and not visible for 2–6 months after injury. As such, patients with second- and third-degree hand burns should be followed for at least a year to detect significant scar formation and contracture development. Evaluation of range of motion and strength, as mentioned above, is vital, and referral for hand therapy and/or to a burn or hand specialist is essential to assure maintenance of hand function. Pressure garments, specially fitting gloves that provide scar compression, are often prescribed to minimize hypertrophic scar formation in burned or grafted hands [24]. Pressure garments should be measured and fitted after burn wounds are healed and edema resolved. Despite appropriate therapy, patients can develop scar contractures due to delays in healing, genetic predisposition, or growth (in children). Contractures impeding hand function generally occur at joints, web spaces, and the palm in both ungrafted and grafted hand burns. Surgical contracture release is indicated for a hand burn scar that significantly impedes hand function despite appropriate splinting, stretching, and therapy. Timely release of hand burn scar contractures prevents loss of hand motion. Surgical burn scar contracture release, using the reconstructive ladder, is indicated for contractures that threaten joint function or hand growth. Waiting for a scar to "mature" (i.e., lose its pink color) for 6–12 months can result in permanent loss of function. However, early release should be reserved for fail-

ure of non-operative therapies, severe contractures impeding function, and in patients/families who are committed to
participating in post-operative hand therapy [25].

Another common long-term problem after hand burns is
pruritus, which can be debilitating. Although no single treatment modality successfully treats pruritus in all patients,
application of moisturizer combined with scar massage has
long been used to mitigate itch. Commonly used medications
include oral diphenhydramine, hydroxyzine, chlorphenira-
mine, gabapentin, and occasionally H2 blockers. Anecdotal
reports of laser use and reduction of pruritus have appeared
in the literature, but prospective trials are sparse [26].
Colloidal oatmeal baths have also been used effectively in the
treatment of burn pruritus [27].

Conclusion

Hand burns are frequent and morbid injuries that have significant long-term functional implications. Accurate assessment, treatment, and follow-up or referral are essential to
optimize patient health related quality of life. The anatomy of
the skin is a key factor determining the potential complications of hand burns. The basic tenets of hand burn care are to
(1) promote a wound healing environment, (2) maintain circulation, (3) prevent infection, (4) obtain wound closure, and
(5) maintain motion. All care of the burned hand is based on
these principles. Referral to a specialized burn center is warranted for any second- or third-degree hand burn; a hand
burn that does not heal within 2 weeks; or a hand burn that
impacts range of motion or function. Skin grafting is designed
to mitigate scar and prevent scar contracture and is generally
indicated for burns that do not heal within 2–3 weeks. Hand
therapy is essential to maintain function in delayed wound
healing situations or after surgery. In the long term, scarring,
itch, and contracture formation are the primary concerns.

Medications, therapy, and specialized pressure garments may be required. The overall care of the burned hand is founded in the application of basic principles and skill sets of multiple team members. With proper initial care, the patient with a hand burn can have a functional and cosmetically acceptable outcome.

References

1. Pan BS, Vu AT, Yakuboff KP. Management of the acutely burned hand. J Hand Surg Am. 2015;40:1477–84.
2. Keyerman PA, Andres LA, Lucas HD, et al. Reconstruction of the burned hand. Plast Reconstr Surg. 2011;127:752–9.
3. Johnson SP, Sebastin SJ, Rehim SA, Chung KC. The importance of hand appearance as a patient-reported outcome in hand surgery. Plast Reconstr Surg Glob Open. 2015;3(11):e552. https://doi.org/10.1097/GOX.0000000000000550.
4. Palmieri TL, Nelson-Mooney K, Kagan R, Stubbs T, et al. Impact of hand burns on health-related quality of life in children younger than 5 years. J Trauma. 2012;73(3):S197–204.
5. Maddern LH, Cadogan JC, Emerson MP. 'Outlook': a psychological service for children with a different appearance. Clinical child psychology and psychiatry. 2006;11(3):431–43.
6. Schmidt HM, Lanz U. Chirugische anatomie der hand 2, uberarb, und aktualisierte aufl. Ed. Stuttgart. G. Thieme; 2003.
7. Pham TN, Hanley C, Palmieri TL, Greenhalgh DG. Results of early excision and full-thickness grafting of deep palm burns in children. J Burn Care Rehabil. 2001;22:54–7.
8. Wibbenmeyer L, Gittelman MA, Kluesner K, Liao J, et al. A multicenter study of preventable contact burns from glass fronted gas fireplaces. J Burn Care Res. 2015;36(1):240–5.
9. Spauwen PH, Brown IF, Sauer EW, et al. Management of fingernail deformities after thermal injury. Scand J Plast Reconstr Surg Hand Surg. 1987;21:253–5.
10. Simpson RL, Flaherty ME. The burned small finger. Clin Plast Surg. 1992;19:673–82.

11. ACS Guidelines. Guidelines for trauma centers caring for burn patients. In: Resources for optimal care of the injured patient, Chapter 14; 2014, pp. 200–106.
12. Cuttle L, Kempf M, Liu PY, et al. The optimal duration and delay of first aid treatment for deep partial thickness burn injuries. Burns. 2010;36(5):673–9.
13. Venter TH, Karpelowsky JS, Rode H. Cooling of the burn wound: the ideal temperature of the coolant. Burns. 2007;33(7):917–22.
14. Cho YS, Choi YH. Comparison of three cooling methods for burn patients: a randomized clinical trial. Burns. 2017;43(3):502–8.
15. Rovee DT, Kurowsky CA, Labun J. Local wound environment and epidermal healing. Mitotic response. Arch Dermatol. 1972;106:330–4.
16. Jan SN, Khan FA, Bashir MM, et al. Comparison of laser doppler imaging (LDI) and clinical assessment in differentiating between superficial and deep partial thickness burn wounds. Burns. 2018;44:405–13.
17. Pan SC. Burn blister fluids in the neovascularization stage of burn wound healing: a comparison between superficial and deep partial-thickness burn wounds. Burn Trauma. 2013;1:27–31.
18. Smith MA, Munster AM, Spence RJ. Burns of the hand and upper limb-a review. Burns. 1998;24:493–505.
19. Palmieri TL, Greenhalgh DG. Topical treatment of pediatric patients with burns: a practical guide. Am J Clin Dermatol. 2002;3:529–34.
20. Sheridan, Salisbury RE, Wright P. Evaluation of early excision of dorsal burns of the hand. Plast Reconstr Surg. 1982;69:670.
21. Robson MC, Smith DJ Jr, VanderZee AJ, et al. Making the burned hand functional. Clin Plast Surg. 1992;19:663–71.
22. Greenhalgh DG, Barthel PP, Warden GD. Comparison of back versus thigh donor sites in pediatric patients with burns. J Burn Care Rehabil. 1993;14:21–5.
23. Sheridan RL, Baryza MJ, Pessina MA, et al. Acute hand burn in children: management and long-term outcome based on a 10-year experience with 698 injured hands. Ann Surg. 1999;229:558–64.
24. Atiyeh BS, El Khatib AM, Dibo SA. Pressure garment therapy (PGT) of burn scars: evidence-based efficacy. Ann Burns Fire Disasters. 2013;26(4):205–12.
25. Schwarz RJ. Management of postburn contractures of the upper extremity. J Burn Care Res. 2007;28:212–9.

26. Ebid AA, Ibrahim AR, Omar MT, El Baky AMA. Long-term effects of pulsed high-intensity laser therapy in the treatment of post-burn pruritus: a double-blind, placebo-controlled, randomized study. Lasers Med Sci. 2017;32(3):693–701. https://doi.org/10.1007/s10103-017-2172-3. Epub 2017 Feb 23.

27. Reynertson KA, Garay M, Nebus J, Chon S, Kaur S, Mahmood K, et al. Anti-inflammatory activities of colloidal oatmeal (Avena sativa) contribute to the effectiveness of oats in treatment of itch associated with dry, irritated skin. J Drugs Dermatol. 2015;14(1):43–8.

Chapter 9
Burn Wound Infection

Joseph E. Marcus, Kevin K. Chung, and Dana M. Blyth

Introduction

Burn wound infections are common complications after a burn injury. Depending on the burn center, they represent either the most common or second most common nosocomial infectious complication [1]. The two greatest risk factors for bacterial burn wound infection include delayed excision as well as increased total body surface area (TBSA) of burn injuries [2]. These skin and soft tissue infections tend to occur

J. E. Marcus
Department of Medicine, Infectious Diseases Service, Brooke Army Medical Center, Joint Base San Antonio, Fort Sam Houston, TX, USA
e-mail: Joseph.e.marcus3.mil@health.mil

K. K. Chung (✉)
Department of Medicine, Uniformed Services University, Bethesda, MD, USA

D. M. Blyth
Department of Medicine, Infectious Diseases Service, Walter Reed National Military Medical Center, Bethesda, MD, USA
e-mail: dana.m.blyth.mil@health.mil

© The Author(s), under exclusive license to Springer Nature Switzerland AG 2023
J. O. Lee (ed.), *Essential Burn Care for Non-Burn Specialists*, https://doi.org/10.1007/978-3-031-28898-2_9

early in the care of patients with burn injuries, with most infections occurring in the first week after burn [3]. While less prevalent, fungal wound infections are also seen, but later in hospitalizations and associated with older age, greater TBSA involvement, diabetes, use of total parenteral nutrition, and longer hospital stays [4]. Infections are not only associated with damage to the skin and underlying tissue, but can be associated with sepsis and development of multi-organ dysfunction and death [5].

Several factors work together to predispose a patient to burn wound infections. After a patient suffers a burn injury, there is compromise of the integrity of the protective epithelial layers and a devascularized, protein rich eschar is left behind that can harbor microorganisms. While the initial burn injury is associated with an immediate pro-inflammatory response, this response is quickly followed by immunosuppression that affects both the innate and adaptive immune system with macrophages, neutrophils, and Th-1 cells being primarily affected [6–8]. The combination of ease of pathogen entry from the loss of barrier as well as the decreased immunologic function leads to an increase in infectious potential for burn wounds.

Despite these risks, with modern burn management, wound infections are becoming less common and have less associated morbidity. Historically patients were managed with delayed debridement. After the injury, bacterial growth was tolerated to break down the eschar with additional passive debridement performed by immersion hydrotherapy and delaying grafting until there was separation of eschar and clear granulation tissue covering the wound [9]. Since the late 1980s when the benefits of early excision were shown, there has been increased use of early excision in the management of burns, and it is now considered the standard of care [10]. The use of early excision strategies resulted in a drop in burn wound sepsis from 6% to 1% [11]. With early debridement, there was a transition to early coverage of wounds which also reduced subsequent infection [12]. Definitive coverage is performed by application of autograft skin (taken from non-burned areas of the patient's own skin) or allograft skin (either fresh or frozen from cadavers). Temporary coverage can be performed with skin substitutes made from acellular animal collagen. Of note, with autograft skin, there is also risk of infection at site of procurement as well as site of engraftment [13]. Additional key advances in the treatment of burn patients include the use of topical antimicrobials, such as silver sulfadiazine, reducing the rates of burn wound infection by up to 50% [14, 15].

Diagnosis

The diagnosis of a burn wound infection starts with clinical suspicion. The most common changes associated with burn wound infection include erythema over the wound margin, edema, purulence, graft failure, and pain with systemic signs, such as fever [1]. These symptoms are generally associated with more invasive infections and are not sensitive or specific enough alone to make a diagnosis [16]. Therefore laboratory measures are usually needed to assist in the diagnosis.

The gold standard for diagnosis of a burn wound infection is histology demonstrating organism invasion into the dermis [17]. Compared to other methods, histology has the greatest specificity and is the most correlated with clinical outcome of any microbiological sampling technique [18]. Biopsy, however, is limited by the significant turn-around time in preparing and analyzing samples as well as the pathology expertise required to interpret the sample.

With biopsy, quantitative cultures can be performed to determine the causative organism, however, this is also a labor-intensive process. In quantitative cultures, a known weight of sample is collected, so that a determination of organisms per gram can be calculated. The number of organisms isolated by quantitative cultures is correlated with subsequent risk of sepsis [19]. Quantitative cultures have been used increasingly, but are generally restricted to large burn centers [20]. Systematic reviews have shown heterogeneity in

TABLE 9.1 Definitions of burn infections per American Burn Association

Wound colonization	$<10^5$ organisms/gram of tissue, no evidence of invasion on histology or biopsy. Asymptomatic
Wound infection	$>10^5$ organisms/gram of tissue, evidence of invasion on histology or biopsy. Symptomatic
Invasive wound infection	Wound infection + either separation of eschar, invasion into unburned tissue, or sepsis
Cellulitis	Wound infection + erythema, warmth or tenderness over wound
Necrotizing infections	Wound infection + deep wound necrosis

Adapted from Greenhalgh et al.

the different mechanisms of quantitative cultures from wounds and caution should be raised when interpreting cultures strictly by bacterial counts [21].

The American Burn Association developed a system to differentiate wound infection from colonization using quantitative cultures as well as histology. This schema is used in research and some larger burn centers (Table 9.1) [16]. As detailed earlier, both biopsy and quantitative culture require significant investment in clinicians and laboratory skills and are a challenge to perform even at large burn centers. Due to this significant investment, and conflicting techniques in the literature, there is great variability in the practice patterns of different institutions.

As most centers do not have the capability to perform biopsy (histopathology) and quantitative culture, the most widely used method is serial surveillance with superficial swabs. These swabs are collected after removal of all bandages and creams over a 1 cm area with enough force to cause minimal bleeding [22]. Other methods such as applying agar plates to wounds and using saline moistened gauze to collect samples are limited due to reliability and time required, respectively [23]. Superficial cultures may be used to make semi-quantitative classifications of bacterial inoculum with measurements such as "few organisms" to "many organisms." These semi-quantitative counts and the species of organisms recovered vary across different areas of the wound and therefore multiple samples from different locations of the wound should be taken at each collection to get a better representation of the biodiversity of flora and antimicrobial resistance to guide management [24]. The limitations of these cultures include sampling many organisms that are likely not pathogenic and the frequency of sampling to understand changes in flora.

In comparison to bacterial wound infections, fungal infections typically occur later in the course of a burn recovery. Fungal burn wound infection should be suspected when there is recurrent necrosis after serial debridements, decay seen on the wound edges, rapidly expanding caseating necrosis, or with graft failure especially in older patients with higher TBSA burn after spending several weeks in the hospital [1, 25]. Fungal infections typically are not diagnosed by quantitative cultures instead by clinical presentation, histology, and qualitative culture. On histopathology, fungal infections typically have at least 10^5 organisms per gram of tissues and have evidence of dermal invasion and is considered invasive when infection affects deeper tissue or blood vessels [18]. To accurately perform laboratory testing, two samples must be collected with each biopsy: one for histology and one for culture. Histology is used to determine the extent of infection, while culture is used to identify the causative fungus and to guide antifungals. Close coordination between the surgeon and the laboratory is essential to ensuring the appropriate tests on collected samples. Histology that shows fungal elements in non-viable tissue, such as eschar, is generally considered fungal wound colonization rather than infection [26]. Unfortunately, indirect markers of fungal invasion such as serum beta-D-glucan or galactomannan have poor predictive value for infections in patients with burn injuries [27].

There are research studies suggesting use of circulating fungal DNA to facilitate earlier diagnosis of fungal infections, but this is not yet available for clinical use [28].

Microbiology

After burn injuries, the initial sterilization of the burn site and eschar is rapidly followed by gram-positive colonization with a slow evolution to gram-negative bacteria and yeast, especially if there is antimicrobial pressure [29, 30]. Anaerobic bacteria are not thought to play a large role in burn wound infections [31]. This transition from early gram-positive colonization to gram-negatives and fungi has been shown repeatedly in single center studies. For example, one retrospective Dutch study looking at surveillance cultures on admission to a burn unit rarely showed drug-resistant or invasive species [32]. Within 24 h of admission, surveillance cultures showed pathologic species in up to a third of patients [33]. This was echoed in a different center where surveillance cultures had growth of gram-positive organisms on median day 4 versus median day 9 for gram-negative organisms [3].

Historically, one of the most concerning early gram-positive organisms was beta-hemolytic *Streptococcus* species, which can cause necrotizing infections [34]. Many burn centers would treat with five days of penicillin after admission to prevent this dreaded complication. However, with the modern strategy of early debridement, these infections became less common and penicillin prophylaxis appropriately has fallen out of favor [35]. Methicillin-resistant *Staphylococcus aureus* has become a more common pathogen in modern burn studies and many centers screen patients on admission and then weekly to facilitate early decolonization with appropriate topical agents [36].

Gram-negative organisms have also become more common causes of burn wound infections with Enterobacteriaceae such as *Escherichia coli* and *Klebsiella pneumoniae* are also commonly found throughout a patient's hospitalization, but generally are seen in the first several weeks of hospitalization [1, 3, 37]. *Pseudomonas aeruginosa* and other multidrug-resistant organisms appear after several weeks of hospitalization, causing 55% of bacterial infections after day 28 of hospitalization [1]. With improved early resuscitation of burn patients, associated hospitalizations have lengthened, which may be a contributor to the increased isolation of multidrug-resistant gram-negative organisms [38]. While one study has suggested that antibiotic resistance is uniform across many centers, the general consensus is that organisms are unique to each center requiring ongoing surveillance [39]. Furthermore, the Infectious Diseases Society of America recommends the creation of an antibiogram with stratification within institutions to reduce use of unnecessary or ineffective antibiotics [40].

Fungal pathogens are a less frequent cause of burn wound infections, but have significant associated mortality—equivalent to having an extra 33% TBSA burn in one study [26, 41]. Infections typically occur after the second week of hospitalization and are usually preceded by a period of colonization before development of infection [26]. *Candida* species tend to originate from the patient's own gastrointestinal tract and appear after broad-spectrum antibiotic use. Rates of *Candida* isolation appear lower with early use of autograft skin in burn injuries as compared to other means of skin coverage [42]. While *Candida* species are the most common fungal organism isolated, most are non-pathogenic, whereas molds are more pathogenic [26, 43]. Infections with molds are associated with a higher mortality than yeasts, with *Aspergillus* species being the most common, followed by members of Mucorales, including *Rhizopus* and *Mucor* [41]. Infections with Mucorales species are associated with significant mortality, even in the setting of rapid debridement and appropriate antifungal therapy [44].

While viral infections, specifically herpesviruses, may reactivate or cause primary infection during burn injuries, they normally are not the cause of burn wound infections. Varicella, in particular, is an important virus in children with burns, but is beyond the scope of this chapter [45].

Treatment

Topical

Topical antimicrobials represent an important component both for the prevention and treatment of burn wound infections (Table 9.2). While surgical debridement of infected tissue is fundamental, topical antibiotics are an adjuvant therapy that can improve outcomes [46]. Topical antimicrobials are administered over the entire burned surface at different intervals depending on the formulation. Each topical antimicrobial has its own spectrum of coverage and toxicity profile [37].

The distinguishing features of the most common topical antiseptics used for burn injuries are shown in the table. Some key points to note of individual therapies include:

Silver-based therapies: Silver may be applied topically as either a solution or through an impregnated-dressing. Both methods of delivery have the benefit of efficacy even against multidrug-resistant organisms. The main advantage of these therapies is their long record of use in many different burn centers with no documented evidence of resistance. However, unfortunately, silver solutions cannot penetrate eschar [47, 48]. While these antimicrobials are the most widely used, the largest systematic review to look at burn injuries found that there has not been definitive proof that using silver-based topical solutions reduced the number of burn wound infections [49]. Side effects of all silver containing therapies include toxicities to fibroblasts and thus should be used with caution [50, 51]. Small studies comparing nanocrystalline silver dressings to silver solutions have not found differences in wound healing [50]. The electrolyte abnormalities of silver nitrate are more prevalent with larger burn TBSA application, but are seen with as little as 15% TBSA [52, 53]. Silver nitrate may also cause skin discoloration, which makes it more difficult to monitor the wound over time.

Mafenide acetate: Mafenide acetate has the broadest gram-negative coverage of any topical antimicrobials used in burn

TABLE 9.2 Common topical antiseptics used in patients with burn injuries

Topical antiseptic	Application	Eschar penetration	Gram positive	Gram negative	Fungal	Notes
Sodium hypochlorite solution (Dakin's solution), 0.025–0.25% solution	2–4 times a day or continuous drip	Unknown	++	++	++	Side effects: Cytotoxicity to fibrocytes Unclear of duration of efficacy and stability of preparations
Mafenide acetate, 5% solution	2–4 times a day	Good	+	+++	−	Side effects: Acidosis (common), pain at application site Rarely used with concomitant inhalational injury due to acidosis
Mupirocin, 2% ointment	1–3 times a day	Unknown	+++	+	−	Side effects: Painful application
Nystatin, 6M units/gram	2–3 times a day	Good	−	−	+++	Minimal toxicity
Nanocrystalline silver dressings	Weekly	Moderate	++	++	+	Side effects: Fibroblast toxicity
Silver nitrate, 0.5% solution	2–4 times a day or continuous drip	Poor	++	++	+	Side effects: Hyponatremia, hypochloremia, skin discoloration (common), fibroblast toxicity Metabolic side effects frequency proportional to TBSA applied
Silver sulfadiazine, 1% cream	Daily	Poor	++	++	+	Side effects: Leukopenia (common), fibroblast toxicity

Adapted from Blyth et al, Cartotto et al, Stefanides et al.

care and has full penetration of the eschar [48, 54]. However, the associated risk of metabolic acidosis limits its use early in resuscitation and in those with concomitant inhalational injury. When used, monitoring for development of acidosis is recommended [55].

Mupirocin: This agent has been associated with the most gram-positive coverage in patients with burns when topically applied to the wound [54, 56, 57]. However, the use of nasal mupirocin has minimal effect in preventing *Staphylococcus aureus* burn wound colonization [58].

Other topical agents: Dakin's solution is notable for its broad spectrum of activity against bacteria as well as fungi, but its fibroblast toxicity limits its use [59]. The duration of efficacy is unclear and is a major challenge to the use of Dakin's solution. Nystatin is a potent antifungal that must be used in combination with an antibacterial topical treatment, as it has no antibacterial activity [60]

Systemic

Systemic antibiotics are often used in the treatment of burn wound infections but have no role as prophylaxis to prevent infections in patients with burns. The largest study using systemic antimicrobials in patients with burn injuries was performed in pediatric patients and resulted in no reduction in the development of wound infections and was associated with longer hospitalizations [61]. When infections develop, treatment should be guided by wound culture. Dosing of systemic antimicrobials in patients with burn injuries is complex due to a variety of factors including the significant fluids or blood products a patient receives, the hypermetabolic state associated with burns, and the common use of renal replacement therapy. Due to these factors, consideration should be made for a higher dose of systemic antibiotics than for patients without burn injuries [62, 63].

In general, systemic antibiotics should be targeted based on either burn center or patient specific resistance patterns and balance the benefits of therapy with the possible side effects. As described previously, systemic antibiotics are rarely the sole treatment for burn wound infections and should be used in conjunction with topical therapies and debridement. Close collaboration between experts in burn, critical care, infectious diseases, and pharmacology is needed to determine optimal dosing and duration, which is generally a short course once source control is achieved.

Invasive fungal infections are serious infections with a high associated mortality. The bedrock of therapy is surgical excision as an early study showed no surviving patients in groups treated with antifungals alone [64]. In conjunction with debridement, broad-spectrum antifungals are commonly used for empiric treatment of invasive fungal infections in addition to topical therapies. While voriconazole is commonly used for *Aspergillus* infections, mucormycosis has inherent resistance to this agent. As there is significant time required to identify the fungal pathogens, a combination of voriconazole and amphotericin is often used empirically while cultures are pending. Histology is generally not sufficient to make the correct identification of mold and clinicians should wait for cultures to return before narrowing antifungals. In a different population with significant risk of invasive fungal infections, the military's Clinical Practice Guidelines may provide a reference for therapy for invasive fungal infections, as they are commonly encountered in both populations [65]. Mold-active agents such as isavuconazole and posaconazole are being used more frequently in burn centers. With favorable safety profile, their use in the burn population compared to voriconazole and amphotericin is an area that warrants further investigation. Fungal infections generally receive at least two weeks of therapy after source control is achieved although it can be longer particularly if multiple body regions are affected [65].

Prevention

The incidence of burn wound infections has decreased significantly over the past several decades with early excision and skin grafting and the use of topical antimicrobials. However, despite these interventions, there are still outbreaks of burn wound infections [66].

Changes in the design of burn units have been shown to reduce the number of nosocomial infections. Patients should be consolidated to a single ward separated from other patients, with limits to the entry of people to the unit. All procedures, including surgical procedures would ideally occur in this unit to prevent transmission of bacteria from other parts of the hospital [1]. In general, patients with burns should be in individual rooms as they result in significantly less infections than when in open bays [67].

One area of the burn unit that has been tied to wound infection outbreaks in the past has been the Hubbard tanks for immersion hydrotherapy [68]. Even when the same water was not shared between patients, outbreaks occurred due to contamination of different components of the system [69]. Due to this risk, there has been a rapid transition to shower hydrotherapy. In 2010, only 10% of centers routinely performed immersion hydrotherapy [70]. Some centers have introduced chlorhexidine baths to reduce hospital acquired infections in patients with burns, where retrospective studies have shown to decrease wound colonization without delaying wound healing [71].

Providers, including physicians, nurses, therapists, and patient care technicians, should be rigorous about hand hygiene. It is standard practice in burn centers for all providers to wear new disposable gowns and gloves with each entry into a patient's room and to use individualized equipment for each patient rather than sharing equipment amongst different patients on a ward. In the burn intensive care unit, nurses should be assigned to patients on a 1:1 ratio to prevent transmission of infectious agents from one room to another [72].

Conclusion

Burn wound infections are decreasing in the setting of early debridement, topical antimicrobials, improved patient isolation, and decreased sharing of communal equipment in the care of burn patients. Diagnosis should be driven by changes in the wound appearance or patient hemodynamics. Gram-positive organisms predominate early in the patient's hospitalization with gram-negative bacterial and fungal infections appearing later in a patient's hospital course. Fungal infections are particularly concerning and have great morbidity associated with them. While there is variability in the treatment of patients with burn wounds, surgical debridement is the bedrock of therapy with addition of topical and systemic antimicrobials. Empiric antimicrobials should be guided by the unit antibiogram and/or patient's surveillance culture data, with subsequent narrowing based on cultures obtained at diagnosis. While more research is needed by multicenter trials to determine the optimal medication selection and treatment for burn wound infections, rigorous infection control practices must be upheld to continue to reduce the impact of these infections on patients with burn injuries.

References

1. Church D, Elsayed S, Reid O, Winston B, Lindsay R. Burn wound infections. Clin Microbiol Rev. 2006;19(2):403–34.
2. Alp E, Coruh A, Gunay GK, Yontar Y, Doganay M. Risk factors for nosocomial infection and mortality in burn patients: 10 years of experience at a university hospital. J Burn Care Res. 2012;33(3):379–85.
3. van Duin D, Strassle PD, DiBiase LM, Lachiewicz AM, Rutala WA, Eitas T, et al. Timeline of health care-associated infections and pathogens after burn injuries. Am J Infect Control. 2016;44(12):1511–6.
4. Blyth DM. Burns. In: Mandell Douglas and Bennett's principles and practice of infectious diseases, 9th ed. [Internet]. Elsevier; 2019.

5. Fitzwater J, Purdue GF, Hunt JL, O'Keefe GE. The risk factors and time course of sepsis and organ dysfunction after burn trauma. J Trauma. 2003;54(5):959–66.

6. Gamelli RL, He LK, Liu H. Marrow granulocyte-macrophage progenitor cell response to burn injury as modified by endotoxin and indomethacin. J Trauma. 1994;37(3):339–46.

7. Calum H, Moser C, Jensen P, Christophersen L, Maling DS, van Gennip M, et al. Thermal injury induces impaired function in polymorphonuclear neutrophil granulocytes and reduced control of burn wound infection. Clin Exp Immunol. 2009;156(1):102–10.

8. Lederer JA, Rodrick ML, Mannick JA. The effects of injury on the adaptive immune response. Shock (Augusta, GA). 1999;11(3):153–9.

9. Mayhall CG. The epidemiology of burn wound infections: then and now. Clin Infect Dis. 2003;37(4):543–50.

10. Herndon DN, Barrow RE, Rutan RL, Rutan TC, Desai MH, Abston S. A comparison of conservative versus early excision. Therapies in severely burned patients. Ann Surg. 1989;209(5):547–52; discussion 52-3.

11. Lloyd JR, Hight DW. Early laminar excision: improved control of burn wound sepsis by partial dermatome debridement. J Pediatr Surg. 1978;13(6d):698–706.

12. Jones I, Currie L, Martin R. A guide to biological skin substitutes. Br J Plast Surg. 2002;55(3):185–93.

13. Atiyeh BS, Hayek SN, Gunn SW. New technologies for burn wound closure and healing—review of the literature. Burns 2005;31(8):944-956.

14. Lindberg RB, Moncrief JA, Switzer WE, Order SE, Mills W Jr. The successful control of burn wound sepsis. J Trauma. 1965;5(5):601–16.

15. Fox CL Jr. Silver sulfadiazine—a new topical therapy for Pseudomonas in burns. Therapy of Pseudomonas infection in burns. Arch Surg (Chicago, Ill : 1960). 1968;96(2):184–8.

16. Greenhalgh DG, Saffle JR, Holmes JH, Gamelli RL, Palmieri TL, Horton JW, et al. American Burn Association consensus conference to define sepsis and infection in burns. J Burn Care Res. 2007;28(6):776–90.

17. Mitchell V, Galizia JP, Fournier L. Precise diagnosis of infection in burn wound biopsy specimens. Combination of histologic technique, acridine orange staining, and culture. The. J Burn Care Rehabil. 1989;10(3):195–202.

18. McManus AT, Kim SH, McManus WF, Mason AD Jr, Pruitt BA Jr. Comparison of quantitative microbiology and histopathology in divided burn-wound biopsy specimens. Arch Surg (Chicago, Ill : 1960). 1987;122(1):74–6.
19. Loebl EC, Marvin JA, Heck EL, Curreri PW, Baxter CR. The use of quantitative biopsy cultures in bacteriologic monitoring of burn patients. J Surg Res. 1974;16(1):1–5.
20. Kwei J, Halstead FD, Dretzke J, Oppenheim BA, Moiemen NS. Protocol for a systematic review of quantitative burn wound microbiology in the management of burns patients. Syst Rev. 2015;4:150.
21. Halstead FD, Lee KC, Kwei J, Dretzke J, Oppenheim BA, Moiemen NS. A systematic review of quantitative burn wound microbiology in the management of burns patients. Burns. 2018;44(1):39–56.
22. Levine NS, Lindberg RB, Mason AD Jr, Pruitt BA Jr. The quantitative swab culture and smear: a quick, simple method for determining the number of viable aerobic bacteria on open wounds. J Trauma. 1976;16(2):89–94.
23. Winkler M, Erbs G, König W, Müller FE. Comparison of 4 methods of bacterial count determination in burn wounds. Zentralblatt fur Bakteriologie, Mikrobiologie, und Hygiene Series A, Medical Microbiology, Infectious Diseases, Virology, Parasitology. 1987;265(1–2):82–98.
24. Steer JA, Papini RP, Wilson AP, McGrouther DA, Parkhouse N. Quantitative microbiology in the management of burn patients. I. Correlation between quantitative and qualitative burn wound biopsy culture and surface alginate swab culture. Burns. 1996;22(3):173–6.
25. Luo G, Tan J, Peng Y, Wu J, Huang Y, Peng D, et al. Guideline for diagnosis, prophylaxis and treatment of invasive fungal infection post burn injury in China 2013. Burns Trauma. 2014;2(2):45–52.
26. Horvath EE, Murray CK, Vaughan GM, Chung KK, Hospenthal DR, Wade CE, et al. Fungal wound infection (not colonization) is independently associated with mortality in burn patients. Ann Surg. 2007;245(6):978–85.
27. Blyth DM, Chung KK, Cancio LC, King BT, Murray CK. Clinical utility of fungal screening assays in adults with severe burns. Burns. 2013;39(3):413–9.
28. Legrand M, Gits-Muselli M, Boutin L, Garcia-Hermoso D, Maurel V, Soussi S, et al. Detection of circulating mucorales DNA in critically ill burn patients: preliminary report of a

screening strategy for early diagnosis and treatment. Clin Infect Dis. 2016;63(10):1312–7.

29. Erol S, Altoparlak U, Akcay MN, Celebi F, Parlak M. Changes of microbial flora and wound colonization in burned patients. Burns. 2004;30(4):357–61.

30. Manson WL, Pernot PC, Fidler V, Sauer EW, Klasen HJ. Colonization of burns and the duration of hospital stay of severely burned patients. J Hosp Infect. 1992;22(1):55–63.

31. Murray PM, Finegold SM. Anaerobes in burn-wound infections. Rev Infect Dis. 1984;6(Suppl 1):S184–6.

32. Dokter J, Brusselaers N, Hendriks WD, Boxma H. Bacteriological cultures on admission of the burn patient: to do or not to do, that's the question. Burns. 2016;42(2):421–7.

33. Park HS, Pham C, Paul E, Padiglione A, Lo C, Cleland H. Early pathogenic colonisers of acute burn wounds: a retrospective review. Burns. 2017;43(8):1757–65.

34. Lesseva M, Girgitzova BP, Bojadjiev C. Beta-haemolytic streptococcal infections in burned patients. Burns. 1994;20(5):422–5.

35. Sheridan RL, Weber JM, Pasternack MS, Tompkins RG. Antibiotic prophylaxis for group A streptococcal burn wound infection is not necessary. J Trauma. 2001;51(2):352–5.

36. Pangli H, Papp A. The relation between positive screening results and MRSA infections in burn patients. Burns. 2019;45(7):1585–92.

37. Altoparlak U, Erol S, Akcay MN, Celebi F, Kadanali A. The time-related changes of antimicrobial resistance patterns and predominant bacterial profiles of burn wounds and body flora of burned patients. Burns. 2004;30(7):660–4.

38. Keen EF 3rd, Robinson BJ, Hospenthal DR, Aldous WK, Wolf SE, Chung KK, et al. Prevalence of multidrug-resistant organisms recovered at a military burn center. Burns. 2010;36(6):819–25.

39. Azzopardi EA, Azzopardi E, Camilleri L, Villapalos J, Boyce DE, Dziewulski P, et al. Gram negative wound infection in hospitalised adult burn patients—systematic review and metanalysis. PloS One. 2014;9(4):e95042.

40. Barlam TF, Cosgrove SE, Abbo LM, MacDougall C, Schuetz AN, Septimus EJ, et al. Implementing an antibiotic stewardship program: guidelines by the Infectious Diseases Society of America and the Society for Healthcare Epidemiology of America. Clin Infect Dis. 2016;62(10):e51–77.

41. Maurel V, Denis B, Camby M, Jeanne M, Cornesse A, Glavnik B, et al. Outcome and characteristics of invasive fungal infections

in critically ill burn patients: A multicenter retrospective study. Mycoses. 2020;63(6):535–42.

42. Cochran A, Morris SE, Edelman LS, Saffle JR. Systemic Candida infection in burn patients: a case-control study of management patterns and outcomes. Surg Infect (Larchmt). 2002;3(4):367–74.

43. Ballard J, Edelman L, Saffle J, Sheridan R, Kagan R, Bracco D, et al. Positive fungal cultures in burn patients: a multicenter review. J Burn Care Res. 2008;29(1):213–21.

44. Devauchelle P, Jeanne M, Fréalle E. Mucormycosis in burn patients. J Fungi (Basel, Switzerland). 2019;5(1)

45. Kiley JL, Chung KK, Blyth DM. Viral infections in burns. Surg Infect (Larchmt). 2020;

46. Dai T, Huang YY, Sharma SK, Hashmi JT, Kurup DB, Hamblin MR. Topical antimicrobials for burn wound infections. Recent Pat Antiinfect Drug Discov. 2010;5(2):124–51.

47. Lansdown AB. Silver. I: its antibacterial properties and mechanism of action. J Wound Care. 2002;11(4):125–30.

48. Stefanides MM Sr, Copeland CE, Kominos SD, Yee RB. In vitro penetration of topical antiseptics through eschar of burn patients. Ann Surg. 1976;183(4):358–64.

49. Storm-Versloot MN, Vos CG, Ubbink DT, Vermeulen H. Topical silver for preventing wound infection. Cochrane Database Syst Rev. 2010;(3):Cd006478.

50. Wasiak J, Cleland H, Campbell F, Spinks A. Dressings for superficial and partial thickness burns. Cochrane Database Syst Rev. 2013;2013(3):Cd002106.

51. Cooper ML, Boyce ST, Hansbrough JF, Foreman TJ, Frank DH. Cytotoxicity to cultured human keratinocytes of topical antimicrobial agents. J Surg Res. 1990;48(3):190–5.

52. Cartotto R. Topical antimicrobial agents for pediatric burns. Burns Trauma. 2017;5:33.

53. Burke JF, Bondoc CC, Morris PJ. Metabolic effects of topical silver nitrate therapy in burns covering more than fifteen percent of the body surface. Ann N Y Acad Sci. 1968;150(3):674–80.

54. Glasser JS, Guymon CH, Mende K, Wolf SE, Hospenthal DR, Murray CK. Activity of topical antimicrobial agents against multidrug-resistant bacteria recovered from burn patients. Burns. 2010;36(8):1172–84.

55. White MG, Asch MJ. Acid-base effects of topical mafenide acetate in the burned patient. N Engl J Med. 1971;284(23):1281–6.

56. Rode H, Hanslo D, de Wet PM, Millar AJ, Cywes S. Efficacy of mupirocin in methicillin-resistant Staphylococcus aureus

burn wound infection. Antimicrob Agents Chemother. 1989;33(8):1358–61.

57. Strock LL, Lee MM, Rutan RL, Desai MH, Robson MC, Herndon DN, et al. Topical Bactroban (mupirocin): efficacy in treating burn wounds infected with methicillin-resistant staphylococci. J Burn Care Rehabil. 1990;11(5):454–9.

58. Jaspers ME, Breederveld RS, Tuinebreijer WE, Diederen BM. The evaluation of nasal mupirocin to prevent Staphylococcus aureus burn wound colonization in routine clinical practice. Burns. 2014;40(8):1570–4.

59. Barsoumian A, Sanchez CJ, Mende K, Tully CC, Beckius ML, Akers KS, et al. In vitro toxicity and activity of Dakin's solution, mafenide acetate, and amphotericin B on filamentous fungi and human cells. J Orthop Trauma. 2013;27(8):428–36.

60. Barret JP, Ramzy PI, Heggers JP, Villareal C, Herndon DN, Desai MH. Topical nystatin powder in severe burns: a new treatment for angioinvasive fungal infections refractory to other topical and systemic agents. Burns. 1999;25(6):505–8.

61. Ergün O, Celik A, Ergün G, Ozok G. Prophylactic antibiotic use in pediatric burn units. Eur J Pediatr Surg = Zeitschrift fur Kinderchirurgie. 2004;14(6):422–6.

62. Kiser TH, Hoody DW, Obritsch MD, Wegzyn CO, Bauling PC, Fish DN. Levofloxacin pharmacokinetics and pharmacodynamics in patients with severe burn injury. Antimicrob Agents Chemother. 2006;50(6):1937–45.

63. Conil JM, Georges B, Breden A, Segonds C, Lavit M, Seguin T, et al. Increased amikacin dosage requirements in burn patients receiving a once-daily regimen. Int J Antimicrob Agents. 2006;28(3):226–30.

64. Stone HH, Cuzzell JZ, Kolb LD, Moskowitz MS, McGowan JE Jr. Aspergillus infection of the burn wound. J Trauma. 1979;19(10):765–7.

65. Rodriguez CJ, Tribble DR, Murray CK, Jessie EM, Khan M et al. Invasive fungal infection in war wounds. Joint Trauma Service Clinical Practice Guidelines; 2016.

66. Lachiewicz AM, Hauck CG, Weber DJ, Cairns BA, van Duin D. Bacterial infections after burn injuries: impact of multidrug resistance. Clin Infect Dis. 2017;65(12):2130–6.

67. McManus AT, Mason AD Jr, McManus WF, Pruitt BA Jr. A decade of reduced gram-negative infections and mortality associated with improved isolation of burned patients. Arch Surg (Chicago, Ill : 1960, 1994;129(12):1306–9.

68. Mayhall CG, Lamb VA, Gayle WE Jr, Haynes BW Jr. Enterobacter cloacae septicemia in a burn center: epidemiology and control of an outbreak. J Infect Dis. 1979;139(2):166–71.
69. Embil JM, McLeod JA, Al-Barrak AM, Thompson GM, Aoki FY, Witwicki EJ, et al. An outbreak of methicillin resistant Staphylococcus aureus on a burn unit: potential role of contaminated hydrotherapy equipment. Burns. 2001;27(7):681–8.
70. Davison PG, Loiselle FB, Nickerson D. Survey on current hydrotherapy use among North American burn centers. J Burn Care Res. 2010;31(3):393–9.
71. Popp JA, Layon AJ, Nappo R, Richards WT, Mozingo DW. Hospital-acquired infections and thermally injured patients: chlorhexidine gluconate baths work. Am J Infect Control. 2014;42(2):129–32.
72. Thompson JT, Meredith JW, Molnar JA. The effect of burn nursing units on burn wound infections. J Burn Care Rehabil. 2002;23(4):281–6.

Chapter 10
Pediatric Burns

Eric S. Ruff, Nikhil R. Shah, Ramon L. Zapata-Sirvent, and Jong O. Lee

Introduction

Pediatric burns are a leading cause of injury and mortality both in the United States and abroad. Each day, over 300 children ages 0–19 are treated in emergency departments for burn-

E. S. Ruff (✉)
Department of Plastic and Reconstructive Surgery, University of Texas Medical Branch, Galveston, TX, USA
e-mail: esruff@utmb.edu; razapata@utmb.edu

N. R. Shah
Department of Surgery, University of Texas Medical Branch, Galveston, TX, USA
e-mail: nikshah@utmb.edu

R. L. Zapata-Sirvent
Department of Plastic and Reconstructive Surgery, University of Texas Medical Branch, Galveston, TX, USA

Shriners Children's Texas, Galveston, TX, USA
e-mail: esruff@utmb.edu; razapata@utmb.edu

J. O. Lee
Department of Surgery, University of Texas Medical Branch, Galveston, TX, USA

Shriners Children's Texas, Galveston, TX, USA
e-mail: jolee@utmb.edu

© The Author(s), under exclusive license to Springer Nature Switzerland AG 2023
J. O. Lee (ed.), *Essential Burn Care for Non-Burn Specialists*, https://doi.org/10.1007/978-3-031-28898-2_10

233

related injuries [1]. Recent studies, however, have shown that ED visits for pediatric burns have been decreasing, suggesting that care for less severe burns may be taking place in outpatient settings such as urgent care or primary care offices [2].

The type of burn injury is often related to the child's age and developmental stage. In the toddler age group, scald burns from hot liquids or grease predominate, as well as contact burns from stoves or grills. Younger children tend to suffer thermal burns from lighters or matches, while older children and teens are more likely to sustain flame burns from risk-taking activities such as use of flammable substances or fireworks [3]. Chemical burns and high-voltage (>1000 volts) electrical injuries may also be encountered in the pediatric population. Fire and flame-induced burns account for the majority of fatalities, whereas death due to scald burns are exceedingly rare. Risk factors for mortality in burned children are larger total body surface area (TBSA) burn, inhalation injury, multiorgan failure, age less than 4 years old, and non-accidental burn [4].

Notably, 16–20% of children admitted with burns are victims of abuse, which significantly increases mortality, though possibly due to concomitant injuries [3]. This should be considered when there is a delay in presentation or the history of the burn does not match the pattern of the injury. Anatomic location of the burn is an unreliable factor in differentiating non-accidental and accidental burns, however burns on both lower extremities convey a three times greater likelihood of being an abusive injury [5]. There are also patient- and parent-specific risk factors one should consider when there is suspicion of child abuse. Patient-specific risk factors include children with behavioral problems, chronic conditions, and disabilities. Parent-specific risk factors include unplanned pregnancies, single-parent household, mental illness, partner violence, and substance abuse. Obtaining collateral information from social workers can be beneficial; however, physicians do not need to definitively diagnose abuse but rather have reasonable cause to suspect it in order to report it to child protective services.

Emergency care of each pediatric burn patient requires an individualized care plan. Consideration must be given to the mechanism and size of the burn, age-specific relationship between body surface area and body weight when calculating fluid replacement, and physiological differences between children and adults. A critical understanding of these variables is essential to improving both short- and long-term outcomes in this population.

Pathophysiology

Patients suffering less than 15% TBSA burns generally have minimal systemic manifestations. Larger burns have the potential to cause overwhelming inflammatory states, especially in the pediatric patient [6]. Pathogenesis has been found to be largely multifactorial.

Breakdown of the integumentary barrier leads to large evaporative losses. This, in tandem with intravascular depletion from impaired function of capillary tight junctions, leads to devastating hypovolemic shock [4, 7]. The pediatric population has lower circulating volumes and can decompensate rapidly after such insults [8]. Burn injury also induces an overwhelming vasoplegic state. This is attributed to an array of endogenous substances, including nitric oxide, histamine, and reactive oxygen species [9]. The resulting distributive shock further reduces tissue perfusion.

Finally, the notion of post-burn cardiomyopathy has become increasingly prevalent, particularly in the initial 24–48 h period [10]. This is believed to be cytokine-mediated; interleukin-6, interleukin-8, and monocyte chemoattractant protein-1 have been found to be markedly elevated in children following thermal injury [11, 12]. Although reportedly reversible, cardiac depression poses diagnostic and resuscitative challenges [13]. Expeditious patient evaluation and intervention are crucial to systematically address all etiologies of burn shock.

Initial Evaluation

If feasible, a targeted history from a parent, caretaker, or witness should be taken to ascertain details about the burn occurrence, environment, and inciting events. Etiology of accidental versus non-accidental trauma should be further investigated as well. The time of presentation may be distant from the time of injury which should warrant alteration of resuscitation strategies. Patients presenting more than four hours after injury without appropriate explanation should raise concern for possible child abuse [14]. Nonetheless, all major burn patients are assumed to be trauma patients and must be evaluated in the same systematic approach.

As such, the airway and breathing take precedence. Supplemental oxygen should be applied if there is suspicion for inhalation injury, particularly after a house or building fire, during which prolonged smoke exposure is common. Physical examination may demonstrate significant facial burns, singed nasal hair or eyebrows, or carbonaceous soot in the oropharynx. Arterial blood gas and carboxyhemoglobin levels may assist in decision-making as pulse oximetry readings are typically normal in patients with carbon monoxide poisoning [15]. Warning signs that may indicate impending respiratory failure include tachypnea, stridor, and hoarseness, and should prompt emergent intubation [4].

Children with burns involving a large TBSA (>20%) or younger than two years old also necessitate a low threshold for intubation [3, 4, 16]. Younger children have considerably smaller airway diameters, thus even minimal edema from large volume fluid resuscitation may induce life-threatening obstruction. If ventilation becomes difficult or airway pressures increase in the setting of circumferential thorax burns, escharotomies may be indicated to restore adequate chest expansion.

Circulation is often challenging to assess in a severely burned patient. Palpation of distal pulses, assessment of capillary refill, and blood pressure monitoring should be attempted if possible; however, invasive monitoring may be necessary. In the infantile and younger pediatric population, a femoral arterial line is likely easier to secure. Of note, inability to appreciate extremity pulses in the setting of circumferential eschar may also indicate need for escharotomy.

Following evaluation of the trauma "ABCs," the secondary survey should ensue. Efficient "head to toe" evaluation is performed to identify additional traumatic injury. Those involved in explosive or electrical burns are at high risk for associated intracranial, intraabdominal, or orthopedic injuries. However, the inability of the neonatal or infant patient to convey and localize pain greatly limits early identification of these injuries. Thus it may be necessary to obtain full body radiographic and tomographic imaging following stabilization.

Clothing and coverings should be removed to expose all burn wounds. This step often occurs earlier during initial evaluation if the patient suffered chemical burns, as any residue retained on clothing could inflict further caustic injury [4]. The reflexive tendency to apply ice should be avoided. Clean sheets and blankets should be applied in order to maintain normothermia. External warming devices and room temperature manipulation may be required in the pediatric population, as they inherently have lower muscle and soft tissue mass. Desired ambient and core body temperatures range from 30 to 35 °C and 36 to 38 °C, respectively [17].

Extent of Injury

Only wounds that are partial- and full-thickness are accounted for when assessing extent of injury, especially if planning for surface area-based resuscitation. Clinical evaluation of wound depth is estimated to be accurate 60–75% of the time in the general population, however this may be even lower in children. Having thinner dermis, children's burn injury often requires 24–48 h to evolve; serial wound examinations may help delineate true depth [18, 19]. It is important to note that burns may often be mixed-thickness, however the deepest component is generally identified at the center. This is due to vessel thrombosis at the periphery, causing a centripetal pattern of injury.

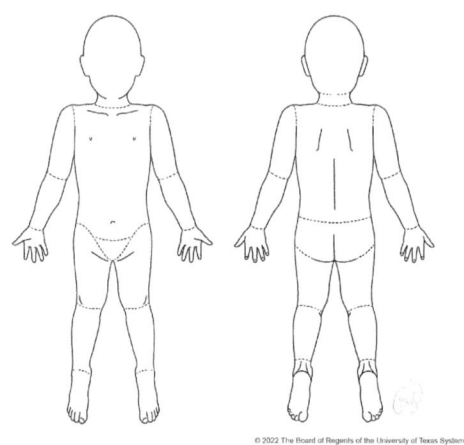

Area									
	0-1	1-4	5-9	10-14	15	Adult	%2°	%3°	%Total
Head	19	17	13	11	9	7			
Neck	2	2	2	2	2	2			
Anterior trunk	13	13	13	13	13	13			
Posterior trunk	13	13	13	13	13	13			
R buttock	2.5	2.5	2.5	2.5	2.5	2.5			
L buttock	2.5	2.5	2.5	2.5	2.5	2.5			
Genitalia	1	1	1	1	1	1			
R upper arm	4	4	4	4	4	4			
L upper arm	4	4	4	4	4	4			
R lower arm	3	3	3	3	3	3			
L lower arm	3	3	3	3	3	3			
R hand	2.5	2.5	2.5	2.5	2.5	2.5			
L hand	2.5	2.5	2.5	2.5	2.5	2.5			
R thigh	5.5	6.5	8	8.5	9	9.5			
L thigh	5.5	6.5	8	8.5	9	9.5			
R leg	5	5	5.5	6	6.5	7			
L leg	5	5	5.5	6	6.5	7			
R foot	3.5	3.5	3.5	3.5	3.5	3.5			
L foot	3.5	3.5	3.5	3.5	3.5	3.5			

Total _____

Lund and Browder Extent of Burn Chart

FIGURE 10.1 Lund and Browder chart for estimation of burn size in pediatric patient

The standard "Rule of Nines" cannot be readily applied to patients younger than 15 years of age due to a significantly higher surface area to body weight ratio. This skewed ratio manifests because of children's large cranial surface area compared to extremities [18, 19]. As such, Lund and Browder chart can be used, in order to rapidly assess extent of injury [20] (Fig. 10.1). For non-confluent regions, the patient's palmar surface with fingers adducted may approximate 1% of body surface area [21].

As discussed earlier, presence of facial burns suggests a likelihood of inhalation injury; however, definitive diagnosis is obtained with bronchoscopy. Ocular involvement, particularly corneal epithelial injury, is assessed with fluorescein test. Evidence of severe retrobulbar edema in the setting of inelastic periorbital eschar should prompt swift lateral canthotomy to avoid devastating effects of retinal ischemia due to increased ocular pressures [22].

The possibility of non-accidental trauma must always be considered in young children. Patterns of injury that raise suspicion include spared upper extremities, "stocking and glove" lower extremity symmetry, or clearly demarcated cigarette or iron shaped wounds. Burns appearing older than reported, wounds inconsistent with given history, or identification of concurrent fractures are also concerning for abuse [14, 23].

Perhaps the most important step after quantifying burn injury is to assess whether the evaluating center has appropriate medical and surgical capabilities to fully care for the burned pediatric patient in question. The American Burn Association has documented well-defined criteria to warrant transfer to a burn center—factors pertinent to pediatric patients include partial-thickness burns greater than 10% TBSA, burns involving face, genitalia, or perineum, inhalation injury, and burns in the setting of concomitant trauma.

Resuscitation

To prepare for forthcoming resuscitation, obtaining reliable intravenous (IV) access is paramount. Bilateral large bore peripheral IVs are preferred, even if inserted through burned skin. Should edema preclude peripheral IV access, a central vein can be cannulated [7, 21]. If all attempts fail, intraosseous access can be obtained; volumes upwards of 100 mL per hour can be infused into the bone marrow. Additionally, a Foley catheter is inserted to accurately measure urine output throughout the resuscitative process.

The ideal resuscitation fluid is isotonic and adequately replaces deficient electrolytes. In all ages, lactated Ringer's solution is most commonly used within the first 24 h [6]. Infants are prone to hypoglycemia due to their limited glycogen stores. Thus, strict blood glucose monitoring is imperative in children less than 1 year old and dextrose-containing maintenance fluids should be added as supplementation [21].

For burns less than 15–20% TBSA, large volume resuscitation is not indicated. Instead, maintenance fluid via IV or oral routes will suffice, with close clinical monitoring of volume status [24]. For larger burns, the Advanced Trauma Life Support (ATLS) 10th edition recommends a pediatric derivation of the Parkland formula, 3 mL/kg/% burn. Other commonly used pediatric resuscitation formulas are the Galveston and Cincinnati formulas which are based on body surface area (Table 10.1). Compared to the Parkland formula, the latter two include provisions for a maintenance rate as well as administration of 25% albumin to combat loss of oncotic gradient [11]. Colloid infusion, as early as 8–12 h after injury, has shown to decrease total crystalloid requirement during resuscitation [25, 26].

These formulas offer guidance for resuscitation, but require continuous adjustments as clinical and laboratory parameters change. Patients' hourly urine output is the most frequently relied upon set point, aiming to achieve a goal of 1 mL/kg/h in children less than 30 kg and 0.5 mL/kg/h in children greater than 30 kg [27]. Additional endpoints include base deficit <3 mEq/L, lactate <2 mmol/L, patient arousability, and warm extremities with full pulses [24, 28].

Close bedside monitoring is pivotal, as under- and overresuscitation both pose significant morbidity. Insufficient fluid volumes result in inadequate tissue perfusion and subsequent end-organ failure, whereas excessive volumes induce "fluid creep" and its devastating sequelae: pulmonary edema, pleural effusion, extremity or abdominal compartment syndromes, and acute respiratory distress syndrome [6, 27, 29]. Albumin infusion has been shown to help mitigate such complications [30].

TABLE 10.1 Pediatric formulas for burn fluid resuscitation

Formula	Calculation	Crystalloid	Colloid	Glucose	Administration
Parkland	3 mL/kg/%TBSA	Ringers lactate	None	None	½ over first 8 h ½ over next 16 h
Cincinnati	4 mL/kg/%TBSA + 1500 mL/m² total BSA	Ringers lactate	12.5 g of 25% albumin per liter of crystalloid in last 8 h of the first 24 h	5% dextrose as needed	½ over first 8 h ½ over next 16 h
Galveston	5000 mL/m² BSA burned + 2000 mL/m² total BSA	Ringers lactate	12.5 g of 25% albumin per liter of crystalloid	5% dextrose as needed	½ over first 8 h ½ over next 16 h

Patients with persistent hemodynamic instability receiving fluids at or exceeding calculated rates should prompt suspicion of other etiologies, including cardiogenic in nature. Hemodynamic monitoring in tandem with echocardiography may be implemented, with possible consideration of vasopressor support [10]. Real-time clinical interpretation is essential as resuscitation is a dynamic process.

Analgesia and Sedation

Pain management and sedation are important aspects of pediatric burn care. Aside from pain caused by the acute burn itself, the patients' subsequent hospital course and recovery will consist of innumerable dressing changes, operative procedures, and physical therapy. If undertreated, pain from these interventions can lead to feelings of depression, insomnia, fear, and helplessness even long after the injury [31]. Thus, analgesic and anxiolytic regimens must be implemented early and effectively.

Opioid medications are heavily utilized for pain management following burn injury [39]. Despite the current paradigm shift away from opioid administration in the field of medicine, burn pain is very challenging to treat. With frequent dressing changes and procedural interventions, patients suffer multiple bouts of acute pain superimposed with baseline pain from the initial injury. For rapid and effective analgesia, morphine sulfate and fentanyl are most commonly used via intermittent intravenous push [32].

Additionally, given the complex nature of burn pain, physicians should strive to incorporate multimodal therapy with the ultimate goal to reduce opioid requirement as time from injury lengthens. Scheduled acetaminophen and nonsteroidal anti-inflammatory drugs are often implemented as background pain control [33]. Gabapentin and pregabalin are important adjuncts known to address neuropathic pain [34, 35].

Sedation may be procedural or continuous. Many medications are used for both, but with varying doses and routes of administration depending on the indication. Continuous sedation is generally implemented in patients requiring intubation. Particularly in children intubated for inhalation injury, maintenance of adequate sedation is crucial to ensure security of the endotracheal tube. Commonly, benzodiazepines are co-administered with opioids due to their synergistic interaction. Dexmedetomidine has gained increasing popularity due to its partial analgesic effects, preservation of respiratory drive, and less hypotensive events [32, 36, 37]. Perhaps most relevant to the pediatric population is its ability to induce sedation that closely parallels natural sleep [31]. Propofol is another widely used agent, generally for short-term sedation. Benefits include its rapid clearance and recovery; conversely, it is known to cause hypotension due to global vasodilation and cardiac depression. Burn injury greatly impacts pharmacokinetics, thus it is important to monitor clinical response and titrate dosing accordingly [31, 32].

Procedural sedation must be tailored specifically to each patient, based on extent of wounds, pain tolerance, and dressings required. Intravenous benzodiazepines, such as midazolam and lorazepam, are most commonly selected as they produce rapid-onset effects with high potency. Particularly important in the pediatric population, these achieve anterograde and retrograde amnesia, anxiolysis, and muscle relaxation. Midazolam has the benefit of shorter duration of action (30–120 min) thus is the mainstay of procedural sedatives, especially if administered via the oral route [31]. Ketamine is a dissociative agent that produces sedation, analgesia, and amnesia. Having minimal effects on cardiopulmonary function, both IV and intramuscular ketamine are widely implemented as safe and effective therapy [38, 39]. Although not yet widely instituted, intranasal dexmedetomidine is a recently emerging agent for procedural premedication in children, demonstrating efficacy similar to that of benzodiazepines [40].

Aside from the aforementioned medications, many non-pharmacologic interventions can help diminish fear and anxiety. These include maintaining a sleep-wake cycle, intrusive noise reduction, ensuring comfortable positioning, and maximizing the presence of family members at the bedside [41]. Play therapy is an essential component of daily stress relief and social development; incorporating child life specialists into the care plan has shown to further alleviate periprocedural anxiety [32]. Fostering a sense of familiarity and normalcy for pediatric patients is crucial to facilitate convalescence.

Wound Management

Burn wound management principles are covered elsewhere in this textbook, however there are some important points to emphasize when managing pediatric burn patients. The current burn center protocol is to debride partial-thickness burns and apply a durable burn dressing, which has been shown to reduce pain [42, 43]. Nonetheless, the optimal dressing selection should provide a moist, protective wound healing environment.

Topical antimicrobials such as bacitracin, polymyxin, or silver sulfadiazine can be used on burns of limited extent to help minimize the risk of infection. Silver sulfadiazine (Silvadene), while bactericidal and relatively painless upon application, can promote accumulation of proteinaceous exudate on the wound surface and retard epithelialization. Prolonged use of silver sulfadiazine uncommonly causes a reversible leukopenia, thus monitoring may be indicated. Mafenide acetate (Sulfamylon) offers gram negative coverage, including *Pseudomonas* and has excellent penetration into eschar and cartilage. Thus it remains the drug of choice for extensive full-thickness burns involving the ear and nose, as exposed cartilage increases the risk of developing chondritis. Disadvantages include pain on application, lack of antifungal activity, and development of metabolic acidosis if applied to large surface areas due to inhibition of renal carbonic anhydrase after systemic absorption. Due to these potential adverse effects, its use should be limited to burns less than 20% TBSA.

Silver-impregnated fabric and foam dressings have largely replaced silver sulfadiazine and mafenide acetate. They contain biologically active silver ions, which provide antibacterial properties as well as facilitate absorption of excess wound exudate. These dressings can be changed every 7 days or until reepithelialization of the burn occurs with the additional benefit of less pain with less frequent dressing change, thus mitigating parental concern about dressing changes at home [44].

Other biologic options include allografts, xenograft, and amniotic membrane. Dermal substitutes such as acellular human dermal substitute, bovine collagen and shark cartilage glycosaminoglycan, and biodegradable temporizing matrix may also be utilized as a temporary wound covering to prepare a wound bed prior to grafting. These latter products may be best suited for use at burn centers with more extensive experience and training.

Surgical Treatment

It is widely recognized that early surgical excision and skin grafting have decreased morbidity and improved survival and cosmesis following burn injury in the pediatric population [27, 45]. Early excision decreases progression of the hypermetabolic burn state and reduces risk of subsequent wound infection [46]. As previously discussed, it is imperative for the evaluating physician to determine whether the center has appropriate medical and surgical capabilities to fully care for the burned pediatric patient.

Partial-thickness burns often present with loose, sloughing tissue and blisters that can be adequately managed in an outpatient setting or by an emergency physician. Management of blisters is a source of controversy in the burn community; however, the collective goals remain constant: preventing infection, reducing time to epithelialization, improving functional and aesthetic outcome, and optimization of patient comfort [47]. Sloughed tissue and broken blisters can be debrided with coarse gauze, soap, and warm water. Intact blisters may be broken to promote patient comfort or left in place to act as a biological dressing against infection. Some authors recommend blister debridement for lesions greater than 2 cm [43].

For large surface area partial- or full-thickness burns, surgical treatment is best undertaken at a burn center. Initial surgical management involves cleaning the wound and debridement of necrotic tissue. Typically, tangential excision of full-thickness burns is performed using Weck blade, or dermatome until healthy, viable tissue is encountered.

In some cases, serial debridements may be required as the wounds continue to declare their true depth during 24–48 h after burn, especially in cases of electrical injury. Skin grafting can often be performed at the time of excision, however in patients with massive (>40% TBSA) burns, the pace of definitive wound closure is limited by the availability of viable donor skin sites and hemodynamic status of the patient. In these situations, excision and grafting have to be completed in stages over a period of weeks. If there is concern regarding quality of the wound bed, final extent of burn depth or a patient's physiologic status, temporizing measures such as allografts, dermal substitutes, or negative pressure wound therapy devices may be utilized for short-term wound coverage [8]. These alternatives are left in place, for a period of days to weeks, to provide wound coverage, promote early mobilization, and minimize risk of infection [48–50].

Reconstruction

With improved resuscitative and surgical techniques, large burns in children once thought to be fatal are now successfully managed [6, 12, 51]. Due to improved survival rates, burn reconstruction has emerged as a major aspect of long-term pediatric burn care. While the technical components are beyond the scope of this text, knowledge of available resources and options for reconstruction allows the non-burn specialist to communicate effectively with reconstructive colleagues and provide appropriate counseling to patients and their families.

The basic concerns in pediatric burn reconstruction are function, comfort, and appearance. In addition to the physical wound or tissue defect, surgical planning should also account for overall social, emotional, and neurocognitive development of the child. Hypertrophic scarring, scar contractures, loss of form and function, and changes in color and texture of injured skin are common concerns among pediatric burn patients and their caretakers. To address these problems, understanding the principle of the reconstructive ladder is paramount. In short, one should employ the most simple technique if possible and progress to more complex techniques when necessary.

If there is minimal deficiency and surrounding tissues are easily mobilized, direct closure or local tissue rearrangement with Z-plasties can be performed to address hypertrophic scars or contractures. For larger or more complex defects, reconstruction with split or full-thickness skin grafts or locoregional flaps may be required. For select anatomic regions with a paucity of soft tissue, advancements in tissue expansion and free tissue transfer utilizing microsurgical techniques have made coverage of large wounds possible even in very young infants and children [52–54].

Finally, laser scar modulation has revolutionized burn reconstructive algorithms for children, often preceding other reconstructive efforts regardless of anatomic location [55, 56]. It is important to note that children may outgrow an initial adequate result and could require multiple reconstructive operations as they continue to grow and develop. Physicians should manage both patient and family expectations appropriately while providing them with the necessary tools for long-term follow-up, thus ensuring optimal reconstructive results.

Conclusion

Pediatric burn care has evolved substantially in recent decades, largely due to implementation of a holistic approach with collaboration from community physicians, nurses, dietitians, therapists, and surgeons [57]. The challenge remains in ensuring that providers account for anatomic and physiologic differences in children throughout the initial evaluation, acute resuscitation, and surgical management. Prompt referral to a multidisciplinary burn center is of utmost importance for major pediatric burns. Fortunately in this population, most burns are minor and can often be managed in the primary care setting with excellent long-term outcomes by utilizing the strategies presented in this chapter.

References

1. Burn Prevention. Centers for disease control and prevention. Centers for Disease Control and Prevention; 2019 [cited 2021Feb21]. https://www.cdc.gov/safechild/burns/index.html
2. Armstrong M, Wheeler KK, Shi J, et al. Epidemiology and trend of US pediatric burn hospitalizations, 2003-2016. Burns. 2020; https://doi.org/10.1016/j.burns.2020.05.021.
3. Reed JL, Pomerantz WJ. Emergency management of pediatric burns. Pediatr Emerg Care. 2005;21(2):118–29.
4. Strobel AM, Fey R. Emergency care of pediatric burns. Emerg Med Clin North Am. 2018;36(2):441–58. https://doi.org/10.1016/j.emc.2017.12.011.
5. Thombs BD. Patient and injury characteristics, mortality risk, and length of stay related to child abuse by burning. Ann Surg. 2008;247(3):519–23.
6. Romanowski KS, Palmieri TL. Pediatric burn resuscitation: past, present, and future. Burns Trauma. 2017;5:26. https://doi.org/10.1186/s41038-017-0091-y.
7. Gonzalez R, Shanti CM. Overview of current pediatric burn care. Semin Pediatr Surg. 2015;24(1):47–9. https://doi.org/10.1053/j.sempedsurg.2014.11.008.
8. Arbuthnot MK, Garcia AV. Early resuscitation and management of severe pediatric burns. Semin Pediatr Surg. 2019;28(1):73–8. https://doi.org/10.1053/j.sempedsurg.2019.01.013. Epub 2019 Jan 18.

9. Lambden S, Creagh-Brown BC, Hunt J, Summers C, Forni LG. Definitions and pathophysiology of vasoplegic shock. Crit Care. 2018;22(1):174. https://doi.org/10.1186/s13054-018-2102-1.

10. Howard TS, Hermann DG, McQuitty AL, Woodson LC, Kramer GC, Herndon DN, Ford PM, Kinsky MP. Burn-induced cardiac dysfunction increases length of stay in pediatric burn patients. J Burn Care Res. 2013;34(4):413–9. https://doi.org/10.1097/BCR.0b013e3182685e11.

11. Rae L, Fidler P, Gibran N. The physiologic basis of burn shock and the need for aggressive fluid resuscitation. Crit Care Clin. 2016;32(4):491–505. https://doi.org/10.1016/j.ccc.2016.06.001.

12. Kraft R, Herndon DN, Al-Mousawi AM, Williams FN, Finnerty CC, Jeschke MG. Burn size and survival probability in paediatric patients in modern burn care: a prospective observational cohort study. Lancet. 2012;379(9820):1013–21. https://doi.org/10.1016/S0140-6736(11)61345-7.

13. Jeschke MG, van Baar ME, Choudhry MA, Chung KK, Gibran NS, Logsetty S. Burn injury. Nat Rev Dis Primers. 2020;6(1):11. https://doi.org/10.1038/s41572-020-0145-5.

14. Rosado N, Charleston E, Gregg M, Lorenz D. Characteristics of accidental versus abusive pediatric burn injuries in an urban burn center over a 14-year period. J Burn Care Res. 2019;40(4):437–43. https://doi.org/10.1093/jbcr/irz032.

15. Macnow TE, Waltzman ML. Carbon monoxide poisoning in children: diagnosis and management in the emergency department. Pediatr Emerg Med Pract. 2016;13(9):1–24.

16. Mosier MJ, Peter T, Gamelli RL. Need for mechanical ventilation in pediatric scald burns: why it happens and why it matters. J Burn Care Res. 2016;37:e1–6.

17. Pruskowski KA, Rizzo JA, Shields BA, Chan RK, Driscoll IR, Rowan MP, Chung KK. A survey of temperature management practices among burn centers in North America. J Burn Care Res. 2018;39(4):612–7. https://doi.org/10.1093/jbcr/irx034.

18. Shah AR, Liao LF. Pediatric burn care: unique considerations in management. Clin Plast Surg. 2017;44(3):603–10. https://doi.org/10.1016/j.cps.2017.02.017.

19. Monstrey S, Hoeksema H, Verbelen J, Pirayesh A, Blondeel P. Assessment of burn depth and burn wound healing potential. Burns. 2008;34(6):761–9. https://doi.org/10.1016/j.burns.2008.01.009.

20. Lund CC, Browder NC. The estimation of areas of burns. Surg Gynecol Obstet. 1944;79:352–8.

21. Palmieri TL. Pediatric burn resuscitation. Crit Care Clin. 2016;32(4):547–59. https://doi.org/10.1016/j.ccc.2016.06.004.
22. Hurst J, Johnson D, Campbell R, Baxter S, Kratky V. Orbital compartment syndrome in a burn patient without aggressive fluid resuscitation. Orbit. 2014;33(5):375–7.
23. Campos JK, Wong YM, Hasty BN, et al. The effect of socioeconomic status and parental demographics on activation of department of child and family services in pediatric burn injury. J Burn Care Res. 2017;38:e722–33.
24. Sheridan RL. Burns in children. J Burn Care Res. 2017;38(3):e618–24. https://doi.org/10.1097/BCR.0000000000000536.
25. Müller Dittrich MH, Brunow de Carvalho W, Lopes LE. Evaluation of the "Early" use of albumin in children with extensive burns: a randomized controlled trial. Pediatr Crit Care Med. 2016;17(6):e280–6. https://doi.org/10.1097/PCC.0000000000000728.
26. Eljaiek R, Heylbroeck C, Dubois MJ. Albumin administration for fluid resuscitation in burn patients: a systematic review and meta-analysis. Burns. 2017;43(1):17–24. https://doi.org/10.1016/j.burns.2016.08.001.
27. Jeschke MG, Herndon DN. Burns in children: standard and new treatments. Lancet. 2014;383(9923):1168–78. https://doi.org/10.1016/S0140-6736(13)61093-4.
28. Peeters Y, Vandervelden S, Wise R, et al. An overview on fluid resuscitation and resuscitation endpoints in burns: Past, present and future. Part 1—Historical background, resuscitation fluid and adjunctive treatment. Anaesthesiol Intensive Ther. 2015;47:6–14.
29. Sheridan R. Less is more-revisiting burn resuscitation. Pediatr Crit Care Med. 2016;17(6):578–9. https://doi.org/10.1097/PCC.0000000000000747.
30. Navickis RJ, Greenhalgh DG, Wilkes MM. Albumin in burn shock resuscitation: a meta-analysis of controlled clinical studies. J Burn Care Res. 2016;37(3):e268–78. https://doi.org/10.1097/BCR.0000000000000201.
31. Fagin A, Palmieri TL. Considerations for pediatric burn sedation and analgesia. Burns Trauma. 2017;5:28. https://doi.org/10.1186/s41038-017-0094-8.
32. Pardesi O, Fuzaylov G. Pain management in pediatric burn patients: review of recent literature and future directions. J Burn Care Res. 2017;38(6):335–47. https://doi.org/10.1097/BCR.0000000000000470.

33. de Jong AE, Bremer M, van Komen R, et al. Pain in young children with burns: extent, course and influencing factors. Burns. 2014;40:38–47.
34. Cuignet O, Pirson J, Soudon O, Zizi M. Effects of gabapentin on morphine consumption and pain in severely burned patients. Burns. 2007;33:81–6.
35. Jones LM, Uribe AA, Coffey R, Puente EG, Abdel-Rasoul M, Murphy CV, Bergese SD. Pregabalin in the reduction of pain and opioid consumption after burn injuries: a preliminary, randomized, double-blind, placebo-controlled study. Medicine (Baltimore). 2019;98(18):e15343. https://doi.org/10.1097/MD.0000000000015343.
36. Shank ES, Sheridan RL, Ryan CM, Keaney TJ, Martyn JA. Hemodynamic responses to dexmedetomidine in critically injured intubated pediatric burned patients: a preliminary study. J Burn Care Res. 2013;34(3):311–7. https://doi.org/10.1097/BCR.0b013e318257d94a.
37. Fagin A, Palmieri T, Greenhalgh D, Sen S. A comparison of dexmedetomidine and midazolam for sedation in severe pediatric burn injury. J Burn Care Res. 2012;33(6):759–63. https://doi.org/10.1097/BCR.0b013e318254d48e.
38. Owens VF, Palmieri TL, Comroe CM, Conroy JM, Scavone JA, Greenhalgh DG. Ketamine: a safe and effective agent for painful procedures in the pediatric burn patient. J Burn Care Res. 2006;27(2):211–6; discussion 217. https://doi.org/10.1097/01.BCR.0000204310.67594.A1.
39. Hansen JK, Voss J, Ganatra H, Langner T, Chalise P, Stokes S, Bhavsar D, Kovac AL. Sedation and analgesia during pediatric burn dressing change: a survey of American Burn Association Centers. J Burn Care Res. 2019;40(3):287–93. https://doi.org/10.1093/jbcr/irz023.
40. Poonai N, Spohn J, Vandermeer B, Ali S, Bhatt M, Hendrikx S, Trottier ED, Sabhaney V, Shah A, Joubert G, Hartling L. Intranasal dexmedetomidine for procedural distress in children: a systematic review. Pediatrics. 2020;145(1):e20191623. https://doi.org/10.1542/peds.2019-1623.
41. Baarslag MA, Allegaert K, Knibbe CAJ, van Dijk M, Tibboel. Pharmacological sedation management in the paediatric intensive care unit. J Pharm Pharmacol. 2017;69(5):498–513.
42. Paddock HN, Fabia R, Giles S, et al. A silver-impregnated antimicrobial dressing reduces hospital costs for pediatric burn patients. J Pediatr Surg. 2007;42:211–3.

43. Hartstein B. Burn injuries in children and the use of biological dressings. Pediatr Emerg Care. 2013;29:939–45.
44. Gotschall CS, Morrison MIS, Eichelberger MR. Prospective, randomized study of the efficacy of mepitel on children with partial thickness scalds. J Burn Care Rehabil. 1998;19:279–83.
45. Israel JS, Greenhalgh DG, Gibson AL. Variations in burn excision and grafting: a survey of the American Burn Association. J Burn Care Res. 2017;38(1):e125–32. https://doi.org/10.1097/BCR.0000000000000475.
46. Gray DT, Pine RW, Harnar TJ, Marvin JA, Engrav LH, Heimbach DM. Early surgical excision versus conventional therapy in patients with 20 to 40 percent burns. A comparative study. Am J Surg. 1982;144:76–80.
47. Sargent RL. Management of blisters in the partial-thickness burn: an integrative research review. J Burn Care Res. 2006;27(1):66–81. https://doi.org/10.1097/01.bcr.0000191961.95907.b1.
48. Wang C, Zhang F, Lineaweaver WC. Clinical applications of allograft skin in burn care. Ann Plast Surg. 2020;84(3S Suppl 2):S158–60. https://doi.org/10.1097/SAP.0000000000002282.
49. Choi YH, Cho YS, Lee JH, Choi Y, Noh SY, Park S, Sung C, Lim JK, Kim J, Shin JJ, Yang B, Jeong J, Chun H, Kim KJ. Cadaver skin allograft may improve mortality rate for burns involving over 30% of total body surface area: a propensity score analysis of data from four burn centers. Cell Tissue Bank. 2018;19(4):645–51. https://doi.org/10.1007/s10561-018-9715-0.
50. Diegidio P, Hermiz SJ, Ortiz-Pujols S, Jones SW, van Duin D, Weber DJ, Cairns BA, Hultman CS. Even better than the real thing? Xenografting in pediatric patients with scald injury. Clin Plast Surg. 2017;44(3):651–6. https://doi.org/10.1016/j.cps.2017.02.001.
51. Palmieri TL, Taylor S, Lawless M, Curri T, Sen S, Greenhalgh DG. Burn center volume makes a difference for burned children. Pediatr Crit Care Med. 2015;16(4):319–24. https://doi.org/10.1097/PCC.0000000000000366.
52. De La Cruz Monroy MFI, Kalaskar DM, Rauf KG. Tissue expansion reconstruction of head and neck burn injuries in paediatric patients—a systematic review. JPRAS Open. 2018;18:78–97. https://doi.org/10.1016/j.jpra.2018.10.004.
53. Abellan Lopez M, Serror K, Chaouat M, Mimoun M, Boccara D. Tissue expansion of the lower limb: Retrospective study of 141 procedures in burn sequelae. Burns. 2018;44(7):1851–7. https://doi.org/10.1016/j.burns.2018.03.021.

54. Ziegler B, Hundeshagen G, Will PA, Bickert B, Kneser U, Hirche C. Role, management, and outcome of free flap reconstruction for acute full-thickness burns in hands. Ann Plast Surg. 2020;85(2):115–21. https://doi.org/10.1097/SAP.0000000000002412.

55. Patel SP, Nguyen HV, Mannschreck D, Redett RJ, Puttgen KB, Stewart FD. Fractional CO2 laser treatment outcomes for pediatric hypertrophic burn scars. J Burn Care Res. 2019;40(4):386–91. https://doi.org/10.1093/jbcr/irz046.

56. Zuccaro J, Muser I, Singh M, Yu J, Kelly C, Fish J. Laser therapy for pediatric burn scars: focusing on a combined treatment approach. J Burn Care Res. 2018;39(3):457–62. https://doi.org/10.1093/jbcr/irx008.

57. D'Cruz R, Martin HC, Holland AJ. Medical management of paediatric burn injuries: best practice part 2. J Paediatr Child Health. 2013;49(9):E397–404. https://doi.org/10.1111/jpc.12179.

Chapter 11
Elderly Burns

Robyn Richmond and Sharmila Dissanaike

Introduction

The 2010 United States Census shows that the fastest growing demographic is people over the age of 65 years [1]. A similar pattern is seen across the globe, and this trend is expected to continue over the coming decade. With an increasing elderly population nationwide and worldwide, all healthcare providers need to understand the influence of age on various medical conditions; burns are no exception.

The elderly sustain burns more commonly than younger adults, and their burns mostly occur at home [2, 3]. Because of decreased alertness, impaired cognition, and slower reaction time, their ability to escape from harm is diminished [4, 5]. Impaired mobility can lead to greater contact time with the thermal agent, resulting in larger total body surface area (TBSA) affected, deeper burns, and an increase in inhalational injury [6, 7].

R. Richmond (✉) · S. Dissanaike
Department of Surgery, Texas Tech University Health Sciences Center, Lubbock, TX, USA
e-mail: robyn.richmond@ttuhsc.edu; sharmila.dissanaike@ttuhsc.edu

© The Author(s), under exclusive license to Springer Nature Switzerland AG 2023
J. O. Lee (ed.), *Essential Burn Care for Non-Burn Specialists*,
https://doi.org/10.1007/978-3-031-28898-2_11

255

Initial Assessment and Resuscitation

The Advanced Burn Life Support course recommends a standardized approach to the burned patient, starting with initial assessment [8]. The primary survey follows a systematic assessment of life and/or limb-threatening injuries [8]. Although the primary survey remains the same in the elderly patient, there are several anatomic and physiologic changes that impact initial assessment that should be considered.

When assessing the airway in elderly burn patients, it is important to recognize that they are more likely to have loss of protective airway reflexes, making aspiration more likely [9]. Dentition can also affect the airway; poor dentition as well as dentures can affect the ability to bag-valve-mask and result in ineffective ventilation. Dentures may also become dislodged and occlude the airway [9]. One tip is to keep dentures in place during bag-valve-mask ventilation to improve the mask seal, but to remove dentures for intubation. Checking for loose teeth prior to intubation is another important step to guard against dislodgement and aspiration. Range of mouth opening may be decreased, which can affect the ability to open the mouth using standard "scissor" manual technique during endotracheal intubation. Cervical immobility secondary to age and/or arthritis can impede neck extension making intubation more difficult [9]. Proper positioning with support under the shoulders can improve visualization during intubation, as can video laryngoscopes if available.

Elderly patients have decreased lung and chest wall compliance, which can impair their ability to maintain normal oxygenation and ventilation at baseline [10]. This places them at high risk for respiratory failure [10]. Because of a limited ability to increase their heart rate, they typically are less likely to manifest tachycardia associated with hypoxia, which can make respiratory failure more insidious and difficult to diagnose [9]. Early recognition of impending respiratory failure is critical to prevent patients from emergent intubation with possible cardiovascular collapse.

The circulatory system in the elderly has significant changes compared to younger counterparts. The heart rate and cardiac output are more likely to be fixed for a number of reasons, including a blunted response to catecholamines [11]. In addition to a blunted response to catecholamines, myocyte mass decreases and afterload increases with age which can contribute to a depressed cardiac function. A fixed heart rate may also be a manifestation of a prescribed antihypertensive or antiarrhythmic medication. In the setting of shock, a decrease in the ability to increase heart rate and cardiac output results in significant vasoconstriction to maintain perfusion [12]. This response, in addition to hypertension in many elderly patients, results in relative normotension masking hypotension and hypoperfusion [12]. Because of this, a systolic blood pressure of 110 mmHg can be considered hypotensive in some elderly [12].

Burn resuscitation in the elderly should look similar to younger patients, and use of defined end points such as lactate, base deficit, and other organ system perfusion indicators are important. It should be noted, however, that use of advanced monitoring may be necessary in the elderly due to their physiologic differences and possible pre-existing conditions [9, 12].

Physiologic changes to the renal system with age include a decreased glomerular filtration rate and a decreased sensitivity to antidiuretic hormone [13]. This will affect the body's ability to concentrate urine, making urine output as a marker of tissue perfusion potentially unreliable [13]. The elderly are also at an increased risk for acute kidney injury, making resuscitation and maintenance of renal perfusion critical in these patients [13]. In addition, avoidance of nephrotoxic agents is important to prevent acute kidney injury.

The endocrine system is also affected by the aging process, with occult hypothyroidism and adrenal insufficiency being common [14]. These should be screened for and treated accordingly.

Loss of subcutaneous fat will affect depth of burn in the elderly, with similar burns resulting in a deeper burn in an older compared to a younger patient [15]. Thinner atrophic skin also puts the elderly at an increased risk for hypothermia following a large burn [16]. Avoidance and active treatment of hypothermia are critical in any burn patient. Ensuring warm rooms, warm blankets, and warmed intravenous fluids are easy first steps in caring for burn patients. More aggressive central warming measures with central venous devices, gastric tubes, urinary catheters, thoracostomy, or intra-abdominal devices should be considered in severely hypothermic patients if initial rewarming attempts are ineffective. In addition to loss of subcutaneous fat, reduced microcirculation and reduced turnover rate of the epidermis lead to prolonged wound healing in the elderly [16, 17].

Pre-existing Conditions and Medications

Knowledge of a patient's history, including pre-existing conditions (PECs) and home medications, is critical for care following burn injury. Elderly patients are more likely to suffer from PECs which can affect their response to injury, their response to resuscitation, and increase the likelihood of complications including mortality.

PECs that are associated with an increased mortality in trauma patients from one statewide database include liver disease, renal disease, cancer, and congestive heart failure [18]. Another large study identified five PECs that influence outcome in trauma: cirrhosis, congenital coagulopathy, chronic obstructive pulmonary disease (COPD), ischemic heart disease, and diabetes [19]. In addition, one quarter of all patients in that study greater than 65 years carried the diagnosis of at least one of the above listed PECs [19]. The burn literature also suggests that PECs increase the likelihood of complications following burns [20].

In addition to PECs, elderly patients are more likely to take daily, scheduled medications, both prescription and over the counter. One important consideration is beta blockers. Beta blockers are used in approximately 20% of elderly patients with coronary artery disease and 10% of patients with hypertension [21]. Consumption of beta blockers can impair interpretation of the physiologic response to a burn.

Anticoagulants and antiplatelets are also frequently taken by the elderly. Since these agents impair blood clotting, their effects must be considered when planning surgical treatment of burns. When present, it is important to weigh the consequences of stopping these agents, which may vary from a minor risk of stroke in a patient with atrial fibrillation and a low CHA_2DS_2-VASc score to a major risk of in-stent thrombosis and death, in a patient who has recently received drug-eluting stents for critical coronary stenosis. A thoughtful plan to manage these competing risks, balance them against the need for surgery, and prevent bleeding both intra-operatively and in the immediate post-operative period, must be developed.

Since COPD is a common disease in the elderly, most commonly from emphysema after a lifetime of smoking, it is not unusual to see burn injuries sustained while smoking on oxygen; in fact, this is an injury pattern unique to this demographic. Smoking related burn injuries involving home oxygen can carry a significant morbidity and mortality, most notably when inhalational injury is present and intubation is required [22, 23]. One series cites a relatively high mortality rate of over 14% despite most patients having a relatively low TBSA burn (less than 5%) [22]. In another review of the American Burn Association (ABA)'s National Burn Repository, inhalational injury was found to be the strongest predictor of mortality [23]. This is likely due to the baseline disease state in these patients, and if inhalational injury exists and intubation is required in these already pulmonary compromised patients, they are more likely to have prolonged intubation, possible tracheostomy, and a discharge destination other than home [23]. Inhalation injuries derived from smoking on oxygen are a phenomenon seen in patients with end-stage COPD. These patients almost always have other medical comorbidities that can complicate their medical course. The outcome in these cases is primarily dependent on involvement of the lower airways; in these cases, prolonged mechanical ventilation and a poor outcome are not unusual. Fortunately, most cases are a simple flash burn to the face, without significant consequence. While it is impossible to conduct a randomized controlled trial on this subject, there is evidence from surrogate markers that patients who continue to smoke on oxygen likely do not derive a survival benefit from long-term oxygen therapy, although they will symptomatically feel better [24].

Pain Control, Nutrition, and Surgical Treatment

Providing good pain control with a regimen that covers both baseline and procedural pain is an essential part of managing any burn patient. A misconception that there is a decrease in pain with increasing age is challenged by literature that suggests that there is reduced pain tolerance to stimuli in the elderly [25]. Assessment of pain may be more difficult because of concomitant dementia and communication disorders. Despite these challenges, it is essential that care and attention are paid to appropriately assessing and treating pain in elderly burn patients. Lack of adequate pain control also increases the risk of delirium in the elderly, which in turn worsens outcomes including mortality.

Nutritional supplementation is essential to meet the increased energy needs caused by the hypermetabolic state that ensues after a large burn; in addition, good nutrition is critical to healing of burn wounds, both with and without surgery. Elderly patients are at an increased risk for pre-existing nutritional deficiencies, therefore their nutritional needs must account for their deficits in addition to the requirements from their injury [20]. Dieticians should be consulted for all elderly burn patients, and formal assessment of nutritional status following current guidelines, including metabolic calorimetry for larger burns, should be undertaken.

It is critical that not only total caloric and fluid needs are met, but that additionally, the correct amount of protein and micronutrients is provided [26].

Surgical treatment of burns in the elderly is another special consideration. While early excision and grafting of full-thickness burns are the standard of care to reduce hospital length of stay (LOS) and mortality [27], some debate that a more conservative approach should be applied to the elderly because undergoing additional physiologic stress of early excision and grafting so soon after the burn injury does not shorten LOS and may actually increase mortality [28, 29].

Other authors report improved outcomes with an early excision and grafting approach with a decreased LOS and fewer episodes of sepsis and pneumonia [30]. There is evidence of a decrease in mortality with early excision and grafting in the elderly [31, 32]. As a general principle, it is recommended that when burn excision is needed in elderly patients, it is performed as soon as possible after completion of resuscitation and optimization of any medical conditions, including correction of anticoagulation.

Non-Accidental Injury

At the extremes of age, humans are especially vulnerable to trauma inflicted by others; therefore, a small proportion of burns in the elderly will result from abuse and neglect. While physicians are taught to look for signs of non-accidental trauma in children, this aspect is often overlooked in the frail, elderly patient. Patients who depend on others for help with activities of daily living have impaired mobility and cognitive decline, this possibility should be considered. Signs of general neglect such as untreated bedsores and poor hygiene, burn injury patterns that conflict with the account of injury given by caregivers, and delay in seeking medical care should all be considered red flags that may warrant reporting to adult protective services for further investigation.

Outcomes

The strong relationship between age and mortality in burns has been recognized for many years, as evidenced by the classic Baux score calculation of age + percent burn = % mortality. While improvements in burn care and resuscitation have fortunately superseded the grim expectations of this equation, it is still true that large burns, inhalation injury, and age over 60 remain the strongest predictors of poor outcome, with mortality in elderly increasing with age by approximately 1% per year [33].

Advances in critical care and surgical treatment of burns have improved survival over the last several decades [7]. A recent 20-year retrospective review showed an overall elderly mortality rate of 22.7% with a large increase in mortality after TBSA surpasses 20% [34]. Encouragingly, the mortality decreased by a rate of 2.9% for every 5 years of the study with an overall decrease in mortality by 11.6% over the 20-year study period [34].

Worse prognosis in elderly patients is one reason why transfer to an ABA verified burn center is recommended; however, even with state-of-the-art care, a significant proportion of elderly patients, especially those with larger burns and/or inhalation injury, will not survive. Another cohort will survive with disability and requirements for skilled nursing or long-term care. In order to provide optimal, individualized care tailored to a patient's wishes and long-term goals, it is important that discussions on their goals of care, expectations of treatment, and anticipated prognosis are started as early in the course as feasible. Early involvement of palliative care consultative services may assist in identifying cases where standard surgical treatment, intensive care, and a prolonged hospital course may not result in the patient's desired outcome, or is not compatible with patient wishes and goals of care. Recognition of this divergence in goals may help avoid subjecting patients to treatments that will not be beneficial in the long term; therefore, these resources should be utilized where available.

References

1. U.S. Census Bureau. 2010 Census shows 65 and older population growing faster than total U.S. population. 2011. https://www.census.gov/newsroom/releases/archives/2010_census/cb11-cn192.html#:~:text=According%20to%20the%202010%20Census,this%20population%20numbered%2035.0%20million.&text=In%202010%2C%20the%20older%20population,from%2012.4%20percent%20in%202000.

2. Petro JA, Belger D, Salzberg CA, Salisbury RE. Burn accidents and the elderly: what is happening and how to prevent it. Geriatrics. 1989;44(3):26–7.

3. Baux S, Mimoun M, Saade H. Burns in the elderly. Burns. 1989;15:239.

4. Barillo DJ, Goode R. Fire fatality study: demographics of fire victims. Burns. 1996;22:85–8.

5. Anous MM, Heimbach DM. Causes of death and predictors in burns patients more than 60 years of age. J Trauma. 1986;25:135–9.

6. Bessey PQ, Arons RR, Dimaggio CJ, Yurt RW. The vulnerabilities of age: burns in children and older adults. Surgery. 2006;140(4):705–15.

7. Lionelli GT, Pickus EJ, Beckum OK, DeCoursey RL, Korentager RA. A three decade analysis of factors affecting burn mortality in the elderly. Burns. 2005;31:958–63.

8. Advanced burn life support course provider manual 2018 update. http://ameriburn.org/wp-content/uploads/2019/08/2018-abls-providermanual.pdf.

9. Milzman DJ, Rothenhaus TC. Resuscitation of the geriatric patient. Emerg Med Clin N Am. 1996;14(1):233–44.

10. Sharma G, Goodwin J. Effect of aging on respiratory system physiology and immunology. Clin Interv Aging. 2006;1(3):253–60.

11. Barontini M, Lazzari JO, Levin G, Armando I, Basso S. Age-related changes in sympathetic activity: biochemical measurements and target organ responses. J Arch Gerontol Geriatr. 1997;25(2):175–86.

12. Oyetunji TA, Chang DC, Crompton JG, Greene WR, Efron DT, Haut ER, et al. Redefining hypotension in the elderly: normotension is not reassuring. Arch Surg. 2011;146(7):865–9.

13. Meyer BR, Bellucci A. Renal function in the elderly. Cardiol Clin. 1986;4(2):227–34.

14. Lewis MC, Abouelenin K, Paniagua M. Geriatric trauma: special considerations in the anesthetic management of the injured elderly patient. Anesthesiol Clin. 2007;25(1):75–90.

15. West MD. The cellular and molecular biology of skin aging. Arch Dermatol. 1994;130:87–95.

16. Hunt JL, Purdue GF. The elderly burn patient. Am J Surg. 1992;164:472–6.

17. Kurban RS, Bhawan J. Histologic changes in skin associated with aging. J Dermatol Surg Oncol. 1990;16(10):908–14.

18. Grossman MD, Miller D, Scaff DW, Arcona S. When is an elder old? Effect of preexisting conditions on mortality in geriatric trauma. J Trauma. 2002;52(2):242–6.

19. Morris JA, MacKenzie EJ, Edelstein SL. The effect of pre-existing conditions on mortality in trauma patients. JAMA. 1990;263(14):1942–6.

20. Keck M, Lumenta DB, Andel H, Kamolz LP, Frey M. Burn treatment in the elderly. Burns. 2009;35(8):1071–9.

21. Yelon JA. Geriatric trauma. In: Moore EE, Feliciano DV, Mattox K, editors. Trauma. 7th ed. New York: McGraw Hill; 2012.

22. Carlos WG, Baker MS, McPherson KA, Bosslet GT, Sood R, Torke AM. Smoking-related home oxygen burn injuries: continued cause for alarm. Respiration. 2016;91(2):151–5.

23. Assimacopoulos EM, Liao J, Heard JP, Kluesner KM, Wilson J, Wibbenmeyer LA. The national incidence and resource utilization of burn injuries sustained while smoking on home oxygen therapy. J Burn Care Res. 2016;37(1):25–31.

24. Lacasse Y, LaForge J, Maltais F. Got a match? Home oxygen therapy in current smokers. Thorax. 2006;61(5):374–5.

25. Gibson S, Helme R. Age-related differences in pain perception and report. Clin Geriatr Med. 2001;17:433–56.

26. Rollins C, Huettner F, Neumeister MW. Clinician's guide to nutritional therapy following major burn injury. Clin Plast Surg. 2017;44(3):555–66.

27. Janzekovic Z. A new concept in the early excision and immediate grafting of burns. J Trauma. 1970;10:1103–9.

28. Herd BM, Herd AN, Tanner NSB. Burns to the elderly: a reappraisal. Br J Plast Surg. 1987;40:278–82.

29. Kirn DS, Luce EA. Early excision and grafting versus conservative management of burns in the elderly. Plast Reconstr Surg. 1998;102:1013–7.

30. Kara M, Peters WJ, Douglas LG, Morris SF. An early surgical approach to burns in the elderly. J Trauma. 1990;30(4):430–2.

31. Burdge JJ, Katz B, Edwards R, Ruberg R. Surgical treatment of burns in elderly patients. J Trauma. 1988;28:214–7.
32. Deitch EA. A policy of early excision and grafting in elderly burn patients shortens the hospital stay and improves survival. Burns. 1985;12:109–14.
33. Taylor SL, Lawless M, Curri T, Sen S, Greenhalgh DG, Palmieri TL. Predicting mortality from burns: the need for age-group specific models. Burns. 2014;40(6):1106–15.
34. Harats M, Ofir H, Segalovich M, Visentin D, Givon A, Peleg K, et al. Trends and risk factors for mortality in elderly burns patients: a retrospective review. Burns. 2019;45(6):1342–9.

Chapter 12
Electrical Injuries

Manrique Guerrero, Casey Kohler, and Brett Arnoldo

Introduction

Electricity gives us the chance to run our technology from lights and personal computers to cars, space shuttles, and power plants, but it also comes with the chance of injury or death. The American Burn Association (ABA) Burn Incidence Fact Sheet from 2016 demonstrated that 4% of 30,000 burn admissions to burn centers were electrical in origin [1]. Electrical injuries are the most common causes of amputations related to burns [2]. There is a bimodal distribution of injury with most adults undergoing high-voltage injuries at work and children under six experiencing low-voltage injuries from electrical outlets and power cords [3–7].

M. Guerrero (✉)
Department of Surgery, University of South Florida Morsani School of Medicine, Tampa, FL, USA
e-mail: guerrerom@usf.edu

C. Kohler · B. Arnoldo
Department of Surgery, Case Western Reserve University School of Medicine, Cleveland, OH, USA
e-mail: Ckohler@metrohealth.org;
Brett.arnoldo@utsouthwestern.edu

267
J. O. Lee (ed.), *Essential Burn Care for Non-Burn Specialists*,
https://doi.org/10.1007/978-3-031-28898-2_12

Electrical injuries are unique and require early, aggressive management. Quick decisions regarding diagnosis and treatment of cardiac injuries or compartment syndrome must be made while appropriately resuscitating a patient to protect their kidneys from the devastating effects of myoglobinuria. These patients often need to be transferred to a specialized burn center to receive advanced wound care and reconstruction, as well as extensive physical and occupational therapy. However, important steps in care and survival start as soon as they land on your doorstep and whether you are a specialized center or not, early actions in the correct direction can make a big difference in survival.

Pathophysiology

Clinically electrical injuries can be classified into four types of injury: (1) True electrical injury by current flow; (2) arc injury from the electrical arc as it passes from the source to an object; (3) flame injury from ignition of clothing or surroundings, and (4) lighting strikes [8]. The mechanism by which these types of electrical injuries cause tissue damage is multifactorial with both thermal and nonthermal causes. The direct electrical forces can damage cell proteins, membranes, and other cellular structures. Just as devastating is the damage caused by heat generated from the electrical injuries [9]. How severe the injury depends on voltage, current, type of current, path of current flow, duration of contact, and the resistance at the point of contact.

Voltage can be categorized arbitrarily into low voltage (<1000 V) and high voltage (>1000 V). Low-voltage injuries will localize to the area of the contact point. Conversely, high-voltage injuries are characterized by extension into deep tissues and by spreading out to the surrounding structures. High-voltage insults tend to demonstrate a "tip of the iceberg" phenomenon affecting deep tissues at the contact point and tissues distally [10]. Thus, high-voltage injuries are often higher acuity and require urgent medical intervention.

It is important to note that domestic wiring in the United States operates on alternating current (AC) at 120 V. This allows the clinician to characterize indoor electrical injuries into a low-voltage type. However, at the industrial level, high-voltage injuries are more commonly seen. Industrial settings, computers, light emitting diodes (LED), solar cells, and electrical vehicles utilize direct current (DC) [11]. Furthermore, while the voltage during the electrical injury can be identified, the current cannot and is dependent on voltage and resistance as demonstrated by Ohm's law (Current = Voltage/Resistance). The resistance during an electrical injury varies with time. Initially it decreases slowly and then more rapidly until arcing occurs. The resistance will then rapidly rise to infinity and the current flow will cease. Interestingly, temperature at the contact site is directly proportional with the current flow. However, it will not increase distally and cause most of its thermal damage at the contact point. This phenomenon can commonly be seen in wrist and ankle injuries where distal digits can remain unharmed [10].

The path the current takes during the electrical injury can alter the clinical management of the patient. Heart conduction abnormalities and central nervous system deficits are seen when current traverses through these vital structures. Tetanic muscle contractions also commonly occur. The contractions are exhibited by either throwing the individual back or "pulling them into" continuous contact [12].

At 4000 °C, electricity arcs causing flash like injuries without actual current flow through the tissue. This is commonly seen in electricians and industrial workers as they labor near metallic objects within short distances of electrical power sources [8]. The same arcing of electricity may also throw the patient, causing additional trauma.

Finally, a thermal burn due to an electrical injury is the result of high temperatures caused by the power (heat) of a current [13]. The human body serves as a volume conductor; thus, the severity of the injury is inversely proportional to the cross-sectional area of the body part [11]. The most severe injuries with the highest heat are seen in the wrist and ankle.

More proximal regions such as the thighs and torso experience less heat. Deeper tissues and regions between 2 bones (tibia and fibula; ulna and radius) also retain heat to a greater degree. Furthermore, excessive heat production is associated with immediate and non-reversible macroscopic and microscopic vascular injury [14]. The injury pattern can progress for more than a week, thus outlining the importance of serial surgical debridements.

Types of Injuries

Low-Voltage Injuries

The most common type of electrical injury is low-voltage (<1000 V) alternating current. These are usually the injuries that occur around the house and are often localized to the points of contact. However, tissue damage can be deeper and more extensive if prolonged contact has occurred. Arrhythmias directly following the electrical injury are possible in low-voltage injuries but not as common as high voltage and do not require 24-h monitoring if initial EKG is normal [15]. The oral cavity is one the most common places for young children to experience an electrical burn, usually from chewing on an electrical cord [16]. It is important to note that the most serious complication of this injury is bleeding from the labial artery which usually happens 10–14 days after the original injury. The labial artery should be compressed digitally until it can be definitively controlled. If this complication occurs, there is a high chance that the child will require further treatment in the future including reconstructive surgery [17, 18].

High-Voltage Injuries

Injuries are considered high voltage if it is >1000 V and oftentimes are occupational exposures. Patients or witnesses usually know the exact amount of current that was being used during the injury. Most of the further treatments and complications discussed in this chapter relate to high-voltage injuries. These injuries are often devastating.

Lightning Strikes

In the United States, lightning kills more people than any other weather phenomenon with the most deaths occurring in Texas and Florida [19–21]. Although lightning strikes are millions of volts of electricity, injury severity varies greatly depending on distance from strike (closer the more severe) or if a nearby object has become incandescent causing a flash or flame burn, in addition to an electrical injury. The pathognomonic sign of lightning strikes is a Lichtenburg figure or keraunographic markings which are a dendritic, arborescent, or fernlike erythematous cutaneous branching pattern due to the extravasation of blood in the subcutaneous tissue. It will often fade within an hour of injury [22, 23]. Isolated burns to the tips of the toes can also be characteristic of a lightning injury [24]. When a lightning strike causes a cardiac or respiratory arrest, CPR is effective if initiated early, however, 10% will still die [25, 26]. Patients can still successfully be resuscitated even if the person appears dead or there is a delay in starting resuscitation. Glasgow Coma Scale or pupillary exam will be unreliable and is a poor predictor of outcome [27–29]. Patients will often develop ophthalmic injuries ranging from cataracts and uveitis to vitreous hemorrhage, retinal detachment, and optic neuropathy [28, 30, 31]. An ophthalmology consultation should be obtained when the patient arrives and follow-up should be arranged to monitor for any long-term complications. The ears also need to be examined because injuries are common with the most frequent being ruptured tympanic membranes [32]. Long term, it can cause sensorineural hearing loss and increase the risk of vertigo [33]. Neurologic complications are common with patients often presenting unconscious or with seizures. Paralysis and paresthesias may develop over the next several days after the injury. Keraunoparalysis, a complete tetraplegia and a loss of sensory awareness of the limbs and trunk, can occur but is usually transient [34]. It is important to have physical and occupational therapy involved early. If patients present with altered level of consciousness, intracranial pathology such as subdural hematoma, epidural hematoma, or intraparenchymal hemorrhages must be ruled out with a CT scan [21]. Lightning strike patients with neurologic injuries tend to recover better than other traumatic brain injuries, and a study of 10 patients over a 12.3 year period demonstrated no long-term neurologic or psychologic deficits [35]. However, 30% of lightning strike patients have been found to suffer from posttraumatic stress disorder [36].

Acute Management

Management of electric injuries should always start with the basics of Advanced Trauma Life Support (ATLS) and focus on airway, breathing, and circulation. Many of these patients may have a fall from height as injuries often occur on a ladder or working on power lines and should undergo a full trauma work-up to identify any concomitant injuries. There are unique challenges that present in injuries due to electric current that are not seen in other trauma patients or those who were thermally injured. These include:

1. Who needs electrocardiographic monitoring and for how long.
2. How to proceed with fluid resuscitation in patients with deep tissue injury or myoglobinuria.
3. Who is at risk for compartment syndrome and may need emergent surgical intervention.
4. Who is at high risk of respiratory failure secondary to pulmonary parenchymal injury.

Electrocardiographic Monitoring

Cardiac abnormalities can occur after low or high-voltage injury and are the most frequent cause of death [10, 37]. For this reason, it is imperative to obtain an EKG during the initial evaluation. The most common abnormality is non-specific ST changes, and sinus bradycardia or tachycardia is often seen [15, 38]. Atrial fibrillation is the most common dysrhythmia [38, 39], but ventricular fibrillation is the most common cause of on scene death [40]. EKG changes are usually present shortly after injury and a recent paper studying 490 low-voltage electrical injury patients demonstrated that there were no late onset malignant arrythmias. All arrythmias or abnormalities had been present on admission EKG [15].

A direct myocardial injury similar to a traumatic contusion may also occur in these patients but they do not have the same hemodynamic compromise as most myocardial infarctions. Many etiologies have been proposed, such as direct electrical current to the heart, coronary spasm and thrombus, and inadequate perfusion secondary to hypotension, however none has been definitely proven. There has been conflicting data using cardiac markers in electrical injury but no biomarker has proven to be consistently accurate. For instance, CK and CK-MB both can be elevated secondary to severe muscle injury [15, 41–46].

Therefore the question becomes, how to identify who needs cardiac monitoring. There are 5 indications for admission for cardiac monitoring:

1. Loss of consciousness at time of injury.
2. EKG abnormality or concern for ischemia.
3. Dysrhythmia either prior to or after ED admission.
4. Pre-hospital CPR.
5. Any patient with a standard indication for cardiac monitoring.

Asymptomatic patients with no cardiac risk factors and a normal EKG do not need inpatient monitoring. For those that need to stay for observation, the optimal length of monitoring is unknown, although most publications have used 24–48 h [47–49]. In our institution, we monitor at risk patients for approximately 24 h. If they have a low-voltage injury with no criteria for monitoring and no other indication for admission, they will be discharged home from the emergency department. Most high-voltage injuries will be admitted for observation, however, if they are going to have dysrhythmias, they tend to occur early in the hospital course [45]. Currently, we are looking into targeted temperature management for patients who present to the emergency department in a coma after cardiac arrest due to electrical injuries. Other than the mechanism of cardiac arrest, these patients fulfill the requirements put forth by the International Liaison Committee on Resuscitation, and we are hopeful that targeted temperature management will prove to be neurologically protective as it has in other populations [50].

Fluid Resuscitation and Rhabdomyolysis

Per consensus protocol, resuscitation for an electrical injury with a cutaneous burn greater than or equal to 20% total body surface area would be 4 mL/kg/% burn with the first half of the resuscitation volume given over the first 8 h. This is twice the recommended amount for cutaneous burns alone as electrical injuries often have extensive internal injuries which are underestimated. However, when large cutaneous burns are not associated with the electrical injury, there is no accepted formula to determine the starting fluid rate, although high-voltage injuries can require almost double the amount of fluid as a low-voltage injury [51].

In our institution, one of the first steps in evaluating an electrical injury is to look for pigmented urine. Visible myoglobinuria is a sign of rhabdomyolysis and ongoing ischemia which needs to be cleared promptly to avoid tubular obstruction and acute renal failure [52, 53]. This is achieved by starting the patient on 1.5–2 times the maintenance fluid rate of lactated Ringer's with a Foley catheter in place to maintain urine output at 100 mL/h. or twice the standard urine output in a burn patient. Aggressive resuscitation continues until the urine appears clear. Some burn centers have adopted the use of osmotic diuretics (mannitol) and alkalinization of the urine to help protect renal function during rhabdomyolysis, however, there is no level I evidence to support these measures [54]. If myoglobinuria has failed to improve after a few hours of aggressive resuscitation, it is a sign of ongoing muscle ischemia and the patient should be re-examined for a missed compartment syndrome or may require debridement of necrotic tissue. If there is no visible myoglobinuria, then the patient is started on a normal maintenance fluid rate and titrated to a goal urine output of 30–50 mL/h.

Compartment Syndrome

Electrical injuries and their sequalae place patients at risk for compartment syndrome. However, not all electrical injuries carry the same risk and patients with high-voltage electrical injuries are at highest risk for developing deep tissue damage and compartment syndrome.

Electrical injury results in an immediate inflammatory response, however, tense compartments and muscle necrosis may develop during the first 48 h after injury. Damaged muscle and edema within the investing fascia of the extremity may increase pressure to the point at which muscle blood flow is compromised. Venous blood flow obstruction is compromised first followed by arteriolar collapse [55, 56]. The actual absence of pulses is one of the last signs of compartment syndrome. A high index of suspicion is paramount for this early diagnosis, and adjunct tests such as serial CK's and compartment pressures are most often not needed. Treating compartment syndrome in electrical burn patients has changed in recent years. In the past, a very aggressive early approach of debridement and exploration was recommended, however, this approach led to amputation rates in the

35–40% range [57]. Newer indications for operation are evidence based and highlighted in the ABA guidelines. Indications include: (1) progressive neurologic dysfunction, (2) vascular compromise, (3) increased compartment pressure, and (4) systemic clinical deterioration from suspected ongoing myonecrosis. Patients not meeting these indications may be debrided on the third to fifth postinjury day [10].

If a patient develops compartment syndrome, four compartment fasciotomies of the lower leg are the standard of care. For forearm fasciotomies, the surgeon must decompress the flexor (volar) compartment, the mobile wad (brachioradialis, extensor carpi radialis longus, and extensor carpi radialis brevis), and the extensor (dorsal) compartment. The extensor compartment is simpler and requires a straight longitudinal incision over the dorsal surface of the forearm [40].

Debridement of clearly nonviable muscle is recommended at initial operation. A conservative approach is taken with tissue of questionable viability. Amputation at initial operation is done mostly for mummified or contracted nonviable extremities. After the initial operation, a second look at 24–48 h with debridement or amputation is usually performed. Skin coverage of the ensuing wound is temporarily achieved with a biological dressings such as allograft or xenograft [40]. Wounds with associated skin and muscle loss often require skin grafting; however, closure can sometimes be facilitated with negative pressure wound therapy (NPWT).

Wound Care

High-voltage injuries require a thorough evaluation to rule out urgent surgical intervention. If urgent surgical intervention is not required, initial wound care and observation are suitable. Low-voltage injuries affecting small areas that do not meet criteria for cardiac monitoring and have adequate pain control can be discharged home. For those injuries requiring local wound care, mafenide acetate cream works well for contact point with deep tissue injury. Mafenide acetate has great eschar penetration and broad antimicrobial coverage. Other topical antibiotics can be used alternatively or for more superficial injuries. These include silver sulfadiazine, bacitracin, and silver containing dressings [58].

Surgical excision of electrical burns is delayed for 48–72 h if patient does not require an urgent fasciotomy or debridement. This allows for revaluation of tissue with questionable viability which should be retained and reassessed every day. If necrotic tissue is present at revaluation, it should be removed. This pattern is repeated until all nonviable tissue is ultimately removed [59]. Some authors believe that a conservative course of tissue removal and wound closure using either or both skin grafts and flaps allow for the best functional outcome [60]. NPWT assisted closure devices can also help with these wounds. They can safely be placed over questionable tissue and later be removed for assessment every third to fifth day. If the hand is involved the consultation of a plastic surgeon with burn reconstruction experience can result in improved functionality of the extremity [40]. Daily physical therapy and functional splinting are vital to decrease contractures and round out the complete care of the patient.

Complications

Early complications of electrical injuries can be similar to other burn and ICU patients, including septic, cardiac, pulmonary, and renal complications. They have unique ocular and neurologic complications that can develop. Ocular issues can affect all aspects of the eye with cataracts being the most frequent ocular manifestation [61, 62]. Between 5 and 20% of patients will develop some degree of ocular changes; therefore, all electrical burn patients should have follow-up with an ophthalmologist [63]. Injuries can appear as early as 3 weeks or as delayed as 11 years with 77% of patients who develop cataracts eventually requiring surgery [64].

Neurologic complications are extremely variable and may present early directly after the injury or not manifest for years. Approximately 82% of patients will have some kind of neurologic complication. Defects include paresis, paralysis, Guillain–Barre Syndrome, amyotrophic lateral sclerosis, and transverse myelitis [65] with the most common reported symptoms being numbness (42%), weakness (32%), memory problems (32%), paresthesias (24%), and chronic pain (24%) [66]. Grube et al. found that 67% of high-voltage electrical injuries develop immediate central or peripheral neuropathies. It was also noted that there was no delayed onset of central neuropathies but one-third of peripheral neuropathies were persistent [12]. Neurologic complications are not limited to high-voltage injuries. Low-voltage injuries had similar neuropsychological symptoms, limited return to work (only 30% return), or delayed return to work [67, 68]. Early lesions are more likely to resolve than late lesions. Weakness is the most common clinical finding with function more affected than sensation, and spasticity is more common than flaccidity. It is important to get a complete baseline neurologic exam in these patients so they can be followed long term for complications. Patients also experience a range of psychological symptoms including anxiety (50%), nightmares (45%), insomnia (37%), and flashbacks (37%) [66]. Studies focused on neuropsychological testing have discovered that PTSD is a significant problem in this population leading to difficultly with cognition and decreased ability to return to work [69]. It has also been noted that there was a correlation with the no-let-go phenomenon seen in low-voltage injuries and higher rates of depression and PTSD [70]. Electrical burn patients who undergo long bone amputations have an 80% chance to develop heterotopic ossification at the cut ends of the amputation site with 28% requiring surgical revision. This does not occur in small bone amputations or in disarticulations [71]. While electrical burns only make up a fraction of burns seen in the hospital, they require tremendous resources both in terms of the acute and chronic care of these patients and the complications associated with electrical injury.

References

1. http://www.ameriburn.org/resources_factsheet.php. Accessed 21 Oct 2021.
2. Arnoldo BD, Purdue GF, Kowalske K, et al. Electrical injuries: a 20-year review. J Burn Care Rehabil. 2004;25(6):479–84.
3. Baxter CR, Waeckerle JF. Emergency treatment of burn injury. Ann Emerg Med. 1988;17(12):1305–15.
4. Skoog T. Electrical injuries. J Trauma. 1970;10(10):816–30.
5. Cawley JC, Homce GT. Occupational electrical injuries in the United States, 1992–1998, and recommendations for safety research. J Saf Res. 2003;34(3):241–8.
6. Taylor AJ, McGwin G Jr, Davis GG, Brissie RM, Rue LW 3rd. Occupational electrocutions in Jefferson County, Alabama. Occup Med (Lond). 2002;52(2):102–6.
7. Wick R, Gilbert JD, Simpson E, Byard RW. Fatal electrocution in adults—a 30-year study. Med Sci Law. 2006;46(2):166–72.
8. Nichter LS, Braynt CA, Kenney JG, et al. Injuries due to commercial electric current. J Burn Care Rehabil. 1984;5:124–37.
9. Lee RC. Cell injury by electric forces. Ann N Y Acad Sci. 2005;1066:85–91.
10. Arnoldo B, Klein M, Gibran NS. Practice guidelines for the management of electrical injuries. J Burn Care Res. 2006;27(4):439–47.
11. Hunt JL, Mason AD Jr, Masterson TS, Pruitt BA Jr. The pathophysiology of acute electric injuries. J Trauma. 1976;16(5):335–40.
12. Grube BJ, Heimbach DM, Engrav LH, Copass MK. Neurologic consequences of electrical burns. J Trauma. 1990;30(3):254–8.
13. Lee RC, Zhang D, Hannig J. Biophysical injury mechanisms in electrical shock trauma. Annu Rev Biomed Eng. 2000;2:477–509.
14. Hunt JL, McManus WF, Haney WP, Pruitt BA Jr. Vascular lesions in acute electric injuries. J Trauma. 1974;14(6):461–73.
15. Pilecky D, Vamos M, Bogyi P, et al. Risk of cardiac arrhythmias after electrical accident: a single-center study of 480 patients. Clin Res Cardiol. 2019;108:901–8.
16. Rai J, Jeschke MG, Barrow RE, Herndon DN. Electrical injuries: a 30-year review. J Trauma. 1999;46(5):933–6.
17. Pensler JM, Rosenthal A. Reconstruction of the oral commissure after an electrical burn. J Burn Care Rehabil. 1990;11(1):50–3.
18. Sadove AM, Jones JE, Lynch TR, Sheets PW. Appliance therapy for perioral electrical burns: a conservative approach. J Burn Care Rehabil. 1988;9(4):391–5.

19. Centers for Disease Control and Prevention. Lightning-associated deaths—United States, 1980–1995. MMWR Morb Moral Wkly Rep. 1998;47(19):391–4.
20. Tribble CG, Pershing JA, Morgan RF, Kenney JG, Edlich RF. Lightning injuries. Compr Ther. 1985;11(2):32–40.
21. Hiestand DGC. Lightning-strike injury. J Intensive Care Med. 1988;3:303–14.
22. Cherington M. James Parkinson: links to Charcot, Lichtenbergh, and lightning. Arch Neurol. 2004;61(6):977.
23. ten Duis HJ, Klasen HJ, Nijsten MW, Pietronero L. Superficial lightning injuries—their "fractal" shape and origin. Burns Incl Therm Inj. 1987;13(2):141–6.
24. Fahmy FS, Brinsden MD, Smith J, Frame JD. Lightning: the multisystem group injuries. J Trauma. 1999;46(5):937–40.
25. Moran KT, Thupari JN, Munster AM. Electric and lightning-induced cardiac arrest reversed by cardiopulmonary resuscitation. JAMA. 1986;255(16):2157.
26. Rahmani SH, Faridaalaee G, Jahangard S. Acute transient hemiparesis induced by lightning strike. Am J Emerg Med. 2015;33(7):984.e981–3.
27. Lee MS, Gunton KB, Fischer DH, Brucker AJ. Ocular manifestations of remote lightning strike. Retina. 2002;22(6):808–10.
28. Norman ME, Albertson D, Younge BR. Ophthalmic manifestations of lightning strike. Surv Ophthalmol. 2001;46(1):19–24.
29. Yi C, Liang Y, Jiexiong O, Yan H. Lightning-induced cataract and neuroretinopathy. Retina. 2001;21(5):526–8.
30. Handa JT, Jaffe GJ. Lightning maculopathy. A case report. Retina. 1994;14(2):169–72.
31. Dhillon PS, Gupta M. Ophthalmic manifestations postlightning strike. BMJ Case Rep. 2015;2015:bcr2014207594.
32. Bergstrom L, Neblett LW, Sando I, Hemenway WG, Harrison GD. The lightning-damaged ear. Arch Otolaryngol. 1974;100(2):117–21.
33. Modayil PC, Lloyd GW, Mallik A, Bowdler DA. Inner ear damage following electric current and lightning injury: a literature review. Eur Arch Otorhinolaryngol. 2014;271(5):855–61.
34. Charcot JM. Des accidents nerveux provoque' par la fondre. Bull Med. 1889;3:1323–6.
35. Muehlberger T, Vogt PM, Munster AM. The long-term consequences of lightning injuries. Burns. 2001;27(8):829–33.

36. Primeau M. Neurorehabilitation of behavioral disorders following lightning and electrical trauma. NeuroRehabilitation. 2005;20(1):25–33.
37. Orak M, Ustundag M, Guloglu C, Gokhan S, Alyan O. Relation between serum pro-brain natriuretic peptide, myoglobin, CK levels, and morbidity and mortality in high voltage electrical injuries. Intern Med. 2010;49(22):2439–43.
38. Chandra NC, Siu CO, Munster AM. Clinical predictors of myocardial damage after high voltage electrical injury. Crit Care Med. 1990;18(3):293–7.
39. Das KM. Electrocardiographic changes following electric shock. Indian J Pediatr. 1974;41(316):192–4.
40. Arnoldo BD, Purdue GF. The diagnosis and management of electrical injuries. Hand Clin. 2009;25(4):469–79.
41. Housinger TA, Green L, Shahangian S, Saffle JR, Warden GD. A prospective study of myocardial damage in electrical injuries. J Trauma. 1985;25(2):122–4.
42. McBride JW, Labrosse KR, McCoy HG, et al. Is serum creatinine kinase-MB in electrically injured patients predictive of myocardial injury? JAMA. 1986;255(6):764–8.
43. Dilworth DHD, Alford P. Evaluation of myocardial injury in electrical burn injuries. J Burn Care Rehabil. 1998;10:S239.
44. Saracoglu A, Kuzucuoglu T, Yakupoglu S, et al. Prognostic factors in electrical burns: a review of 101 patients. Burns. 2014;40(4):702–7.
45. Purdue GF, Hunt JL. Electrocardiographic monitoring after electrical injury: necessity or luxury. J Trauma. 1986;26(2):166–7.
46. Waldmann V, Narayanan K, Combes N, et al. Electrical cardia injuries: current concepts and management. Eur Heart J. 2018;39:1459–65.
47. Bailey B, Gaudreault P, Thivierge RL. Experience with guidelines for cardiac monitoring after electrical injury in children. Am J Emerg Med. 2000;18(6):671–5.
48. Wallace BH, Cone JB, Vanderpool RD, et al. Retrospective evaluation of admission criteria for paediatric electrical injuries. Burns. 1995;21(8):590–3.
49. Zubair M, Besner GE. Pediatric electrical burns: management strategies. Burns. 1997;23(5):413–20.
50. Nolan JP, Soar J, Cariou A, et al. European Resuscitation Council and European Society of Intensive Care Medicine guidelines for post-resuscitation care 2015: section 5 of the

European Resuscitation Council guidelines for resuscitation 2015. Resuscitation. 2015;95:202–22.

51. Boyd AN, Hartman BC, Sood R, Walroth TA. A voltage-based analysis of fluid delivery and outcomes in burn patients with electrical injuries over a 6-year period. Burns. 2019;45:869–75.

52. Bhavsar P, Rathod KJ, Rathod D, Chamania CS. Utility of serum creatinine, creatine kinase and urinary myoglobin in detecting acute renal failure due to rhabdomyolysis in trauma and electrical burns patients. Indian J Surg. 2013;75(1):17–21.

53. Melli G, Chaudhry V, Cornblath DR. Rhabdomyolysis: an evaluation of 475 hospitalized patients. Medicine (Baltimore). 2005;84(6):377–85.

54. Coban YK. Rhabdomyolysis, compartment syndrome and thermal injury. World J Crit Care Med. 2014;3(1):1–7.

55. Elliott KG, Johnstone AJ. Diagnosing acute compartment syndrome. J Bone Jt Surg Br. 2003;85(5):625–32.

56. Burton AC. On the physical equilibrium of small blood vessels. Am J Phys. 1951;164(2):319–29.

57. d'Amato TA, Kaplan IB, Britt LD. High-voltage electrical injury: a role for mandatory exploration of deep muscle compartments. J Natl Med Assoc. 1994;86(7):535–7.

58. Hussmann J, Kucan JO, Russell RC, Bradley T, Zamboni WA. Electrical injuries—morbidity, outcome and treatment rationale. Burns. 1995;21(7):530–5.

59. Lee RC. Injury by electrical forces: pathophysiology, manifestations, and therapy. Curr Probl Surg. 1997;34(9):677–764.

60. Barillo DJ, Arabitg R, Cancio LC, Goodwin CW. Distant pedicle flaps for soft tissue coverage of severely burned hands: an old idea revisited. Burns. 2001;27(6):613–9.

61. Boozalis GT, Purdue GF, Hunt JL, McCulley JP. Ocular changes from electrical burn injuries. A literature review and report of cases. J Burn Care Rehabil. 1991;12(5):458–62.

62. Van Johnson E, Kline LB, Skalka HW. Electrical cataracts: a case report and review of the literature. Ophthalmic Surg. 1987;18(4):283–5.

63. Saffle JR, Crandall A, Warden GD. Cataracts: a long-term complication of electrical injury. J Trauma. 1985;25(1):17–21.

64. Mutlu FM, Duman H, Cil Y. Early-onset unilateral electric cataract: a rare clinical entity. J Burn Care Rehabil. 2004;25(4):363–5.

65. Petty PG, Parkin G. Electrical injury to the central nervous system. Neurosurgery. 1986;19(2):282–4.

66. Singerman J, Gomez M, Fish JS. Long-term sequelae of low-voltage electrical injury. J Burn Care Res. 2008;29(5):773–7.
67. Theman K, Singerman J, Gomez M, Fish JS. Return to work after low voltage electrical injury. J Burn Care Res. 2008;29(6):959–64.
68. Ko SH, Chun W, Kim HC. Delayed spinal cord injury following electrical burns: a 7-year experience. Burns. 2004;30(7):691–5.
69. Shih J, Shahrokhi S, Jeschke M. Review of adult electrical burn injury outcomes worldwide: an analysis of low-voltage versus high-voltage electrical injury. J Burn Care Res. 2017;38(1):e293–w298.
70. Kelley KM, Tkachenko TA, Pliskin NH, Fink JW, Lee RC. Life after electrical injury. Risk factors for psychiatric sequelae. Ann N Y Acad Sci. 1999;888:356–63.
71. Helm PA, Walker SC. New bone formation at amputation sites in electrically burn-injured patients. Arch Phys Med Rehabil. 1987;68(5 Pt 1):284–6.

Chapter 13
Chemical Burns

Henry B. Huson and Herb A. Phelan

Background

There are a wide variety of compounds that have the potential to cause cutaneous and ocular burns, as well as systemic side effects requiring the need for medical care. These compounds can be found in the occupational environment or the home, with an estimated 25,000 chemicals identified as potential sources of burns [1]. According to the American Association of Poison Control Centers, in 2019 alone, 7.1% of all exposures were due to household cleaning substances with an additional 6.2% of cases being related to cosmetics or personal care products, which is consistent with prior years [1, 2]. For pediatric exposures, 11.4% of exposures are related to cosmetic/personal care products, and 10.5% related to household cleaning substances with 43% of cases being children under the age of 5 [1]. While the rate of exposure within the

H. B. Huson
Department of Surgery, LSUHSC-New Orleans,
New Orleans, LA, USA
e-mail: hhuson@lsuhsc.edu

H. A. Phelan (✉)
University Medical Center-New Orleans Burn Unit,
New Orleans, LA, USA
e-mail: hphel1@lsuhsc.edu

© The Author(s), under exclusive license to Springer Nature Switzerland AG 2023   285
J. O. Lee (ed.), *Essential Burn Care for Non-Burn Specialists*,
https://doi.org/10.1007/978-3-031-28898-2_13

pediatric population is concerning, a more pressing matter is that the rate of serious complications such as major injury or death has increased by almost 5% each year since 2000 [1–3]. While these domestic exposures have a variety of causes, ranging from mislabeling and improper storage to intentional harm of others or suicide attempts, this growing threat is present with most products readily available to the general population.

According to data gathered by the American Burn Association, chemical burns account for 3% of hospital admissions but are related to approximately 30% of burn deaths [4]. Chemical burns carry a high morbidity, with 55% requiring surgical intervention, and most commonly involve the cosmetic areas of the body such as the face, neck, and hands [4]. Chemical burns present a dilemma to physicians given the difficulty in assessing the depth of burn as well as the timing of surgical excision. While the variety of chemical agents and their treatments is too vast to be covered in total, we will provide general principles for the treatment of chemical injuries, the most common agents, and an overview of the complications that may arise from exposure.

Pathophysiology

Burn injuries, whether as a result of a thermal or chemical insult, have a common pathophysiologic pathway: they result in the denaturation of proteins. A protein's three-dimensional structure is responsible for its biological activity and is dependent on forces such as hydrogen bonding or Van der Waal's forces. While thermal energy breaks these bonds causing the protein to unfold, chemical influences such as changes in pH or the dissolution of surrounding lipids may stabilize a protein resulting in a change in its biologic activity. These mechanisms continue as long as the offending agent is present, which is particularly important in chemical injuries where exposures are typically longer than those seen with thermal injuries. In addition, chemical agents may act systemically if their components, with their potential toxicity, end up in the circulation.

Several factors determine the severity of a chemical burn injury. The concentration and quantity of the offending agent determine the scope of injury, as do the manner and the duration of contact. The depth to which the chemical is capable of penetrating tissues has an obvious impact as does the agent's phase, as many chemicals behave differently as solids, liquids, or gases. Finally, the chemical's mechanism of action has a significant influence on tissue damage. Generally speaking, chemical agents in biological systems can be broken down into six mechanisms of action:

1. *Reduction*: Reducing agents denature proteins via the binding of free electrons within the tissue proteins. This chemical reaction may also produce a thermal effect causing a mixed picture. The most common agents encountered include hydrochloric acid, nitric acid, ferrous iron, alkyl mercuric compounds, and sulfite compounds.
2. *Corrosion*: Corrosive agents denature proteins via contact. They produce a soft eschar, typically progressing to shallow ulceration. The most common agents encountered include phenols, cresols, white phosphorus, sodium metals, lyes, sulfuric acid, dichromate salts, and hydrochloric acid.
3. *Oxidation*: Oxidizing agents denature proteins via the insertion of an oxygen, sulfur, or halogen atom to a viable body protein. The by-products produced are toxic and can continue to cause a reaction on the surrounding tissues. The most common agents encountered include sodium hypochloride, chromic acid, peroxide, and potassium permanganate.
4. *Vesication*: Vesicant agents act via the induction of tissue ischemia with anoxic necrosis at the site of contact. This results in a cytokine release with resultant cutaneous blister formation. The most common agents encountered include cantharides, mustard gas (nitrogen and sulfur), Lewisite, and dimethyl sulfoxide (DMSO).
5. *Desiccation*: Desiccant agents act via the dehydration of tissues resulting in an exothermic reaction causing the

release of heat within the tissues, exacerbating the tissue damage. The most common agents encountered include sulfuric acid, calcium sulfate, silica gel, and muriatic acid.

6. *Protoplasmic poisons*: These agents act via the formation of esters with proteins or via the binding/inhibiting of calcium or other organic ions that are necessary for tissue function and viability. The most common agents encountered include ester formers such as "alkaloidal" acids, acetic acid, and formic acid as well as the metabolic competitors/inhibitors such as hydrofluoric acid, oxalic acid, and hydrazoic acid.

The chemical agents can be classified by the chemical reaction they produce. The chemical agent's most important characteristic is that of its influence on pH, while its concentration will also affect its reactivity. Chemical burns can be described as either acidic or alkaline and while individual acids and alkali differ, the resultant injuries are similar enough to be broken down into groups as a whole.

Acids act as proton donors, releasing hydrogen ions and reducing the pH. Acids with a pH below 2 are regarded as strong acids and produce coagulation necrosis and precipitation of protein on skin contact. A better reflection of the strength of the acid than pH alone is the needed amount of alkali to restore a neutral pH.

Bases, on the other hand, are proton acceptors, removing hydrogen ions from the protonated amine groups and carboxylic groups, with the potential of injuring tissue at a pH above 11.5. Typically, alkali cause more injury than their acidic counterparts through liquefaction necrosis, allowing the alkali deeper penetration into the tissues. The hydroxyl ions within the tissues increase the solubility, allowing alkali proteinates to be formed after alkali dissolves the tissue proteins.

Organic solutions act via the dissolution of the lipid membrane within the cell walls, thus causing disruption of the cellular protein architecture.

Finally, *inorganic solutions* damage tissue by directly binding to the exterior of the cell wall, acting as a transporter for the previously mentioned agents, as well as forming salts with the proteins themselves. These reactions can also be associated with an exothermic reaction, resulting in additional tissue injury.

General Management

When treating the chemical burn patient, the principles of the primary and secondary assessments of trauma care are applicable. Beyond that generality, however, chemical burns also mandate removing the offending agent from the skin surface as quickly as possible, and tailoring subsequent care to the individual agent.

The clinician should elicit a thorough history in order to identify the offending agent and expedite appropriate treatment to minimize tissue damage. A valuable resource in this endeavor is the Material Safety Data Sheets (MSDS) required by law to be available for all chemicals present in the occupational setting. The MSDS sheets provide information on agent hazardous effects as well as systemic toxicities. Additional assistance can be acquired through the regional poison control centers for household chemicals or unidentified agents.

The importance of the duration of a chemical's contact and its direct correlation to the severity of injury cannot be overstated. As long as the inciting agent is present on the skin surface, tissue damage/destruction will be ongoing. The immediate removal of the offending agent is vital. This requires removal of any potentially contaminated clothing, copious irrigation at the scene of injury, and repeat irrigation upon arrival to the hospital. Irrigation of chemical burns should be carried out with large volumes of fluid and should occur in an environment that allows runoff of the irrigant. Tubs and tanks should be avoided as these can contain the chemical and spread the injurious material to previously unaffected tissues. Irrigation should be carried out with the safety of the healthcare provider in mind. For chemical burns, immediate copious irrigation has been shown to reduce the extent and depth of the injury and shorten hospital stay [5]. While there is currently no measure to grade the efficacy of the irrigation, the monitoring of the effluent's pH can provide a quantitative measure for adequacy. Irrigation ranging from 30 min to 2 h may be necessary to attain a normal pH. While copious irrigation is a mainstay in the treatment of virtually all chemical burns, there are some exceptions such as phenol, dry lime, and muriatic acid as these chemicals create a significant exothermic reaction when combined with water.

A point of contention within chemical burn care is the use of neutralizing agents. Theoretically, a neutralizing solution should eliminate the active chemical compound from the wound bed and prevent any further injury. As such, when the identity of an injurious agent is known as one that has a specific antidote, some benefit to the use of neutralization has been demonstrated [6]. However, the control over the quantity of the neutralizing agent is problematic as use may provoke an exothermic reaction, thus exacerbating the thermal injury in addition to creating a potential delay in the initiation of hydrotherapy. One must also take into account the fact that neutralizing agents may themselves cause toxicities. Due to these complicating factors, the use of neutralizing agents is discouraged as no single agent has been shown to be more efficacious than plain water irrigation [7].

Conventional burn formulas for resuscitation are used when appropriate, and urine output should be monitored to assess end organ perfusion and thus resuscitation. Due to the effects on systemic pH, blood gas and electrolyte analysis should be obtained,. In addition, the room should be maintained between 28 and 31 °C as the large volume lavage typically required for chemical burns puts the patient at risk for hypothermia. This risk is exacerbated by the use of unwarmed fluids and thus the irrigation water should be as near to body temperature as possible.

Principles in wound care for chemical burns are usually the same as those of thermal injuries. Following irrigation and debridement of blisters, chemical burns can be treated via coverage with antibiotic agents, creams, and/or dressings. The clinical assessment of the depth and extent of a chemical burn is difficult due to the unusual tanning and local anesthetic properties of some agents, resulting in some deep burns appearing to be more superficial. Due to this, chemical burns also tend to heal slower than their thermal counterparts.

Special Agents for Consideration

Acetic Acid

Acetic acid is a mild chelating agent that is usually found diluted to concentrations less than 40% (such as in products like table vinegar or hair products). At this concentration, it is usually harmless, however, if used inappropriately it may cause partial thickness burns. Some other names for acetic acid are ethanoic acid, ethylic acid, and methane carboxylic acid.

Carbolic Acid

Carbolic acid (otherwise known as phenol) is derived from coal tar. When concentrated, it acts as a caustic agent, causing partial or full thickness burns based off duration of skin contact. Ingestion of carbolic acid is also dangerous, as ingested amounts as small as 1 g can be lethal due to systemic effects such as ventricular arrhythmias and pulmonary edema. Prompt irrigation is required. In addition, polyethylene glycol as well as intravenous sodium bicarbonate has been shown to have some benefit [8, 9] but should not delay irrigation.

Chromic Acid

Chromic acid is responsible for corrosive ulcerations upon skin contact. Blood levels peak within 5 h of exposure and can be symptomatic with only 1% total body surface area (TBSA) burns, while burns greater than 10% TBSA are typically fatal due to systemic effects. As with other chemical burns, copious irrigation is the initial treatment of choice, yet a more specific antidote consists of rinsing with a dilute solution of sodium hyposulfite followed by additional rinsing in a buffered phosphate solution. Early excision of a chromic acid burn has also been shown to potentially help avoid the systemic effects [10, 11]. In order to treat the systemic effects, dimercaprol may be used for 7 days (4 mg/kg IM Q4H for 2 days, followed by 2–4 mg/kg/day). Early dialysis (defined as initiation within 24 h of the exposure) for the removal of any circulating chromium may be of benefit. In addition, exchange transfusion may be necessary.

Formic Acid

Formic acid is an agent used extensively in the glue and tanning industries. After skin contact, eschar formation occurs but systemic circulation is still possible resulting in metabolic acidosis, intravascular hemolysis, renal failure, pulmonary complications, and necrotizing pancreatitis. All formic acid injuries should mandate hospitalization due to the possibility of these systemic complications.

Epichlorohydrin Acid

Epichlorohydrin acid is rare, colorless, and known for its garlic-like odor. It is an agent typically found in glue, plastic, glycerol, and resin production as well as paper and water purification processes and the creation of explosives. As with other chemical burns, initial management involves copious irrigation.

Hydrochloric Acid/Muriatic Acid/Sulfuric Acid

Hydrochloric acid can be found diluted within many household cleaners. It causes local coagulation necrosis and ulceration leading to connective tissue consolidation and intramural vessel thrombosis, fibrosis, and hemolysis. Management consists of quick and continuous irrigation. The fumes from hydrochloric acid, if inhaled, can lead to upper airway edema and pulmonary inflammation.

Muriatic acid is an industrial-grade version of concentrated hydrochloric acid. Upon skin contact, it denatures proteins to form chloride salts. Similar to its less-concentrated counterpart, copious irrigation is the treatment of choice but with the addition of consideration for early excision.

Sulfuric acid is one of the more common agents responsible for chemical burns, typically seen in the occupational environment but also found in the domestic setting as it is found within household drain cleaners. Sulfuric acid and its precursor, sulfur trioxide, are strong acids, causing dehydration damage in addition to creating a thermal effect within the tissues. This leads to a coagulation necrosis and necrotic eschars with microvascular thrombus formation. Immediate irrigation with excision of any deep burns are the mainstays of treatment.

Hydrofluoric Acid

Hydrofluoric acid is typically found within the petroleum industry, as well as in materials for glass etching, germicides, dyes, tanning, and fireproofing materials. This agent is particularly lethal as it causes severe burns with tremendous systemic toxicity. Hydrogen ions produce superficial burns, while the fluoride ion penetrates the tissues resulting in the chelation of calcium and magnesium. This in turn causes cell death and liquefaction necrosis of the soft tissues. In addition, the free fluoride ions inhibit the Na–K ATPase allowing the loss of cellular potassium. This is thought to be the cause of the extreme pain associated with hydrofluoric acid injuries.

Hydrofluoric acid burns are classified based on the concentration of the exposure. At concentrations less than 20%, injuries may take up to 24 h to fully manifest. At 20–50% concentration, the injury becomes apparent within several hours. At over 50% concentration, immediate tissue destruction and pain occur.

The clinical presentation of a hydrofluoric acid burn depends on the route of exposure, concentration, duration of exposure, and the resistance of the tissue affected. Fingers are the most commonly injured structures. Death, however, is typically secondary to the systemic toxicity, with symptoms such as acidemia, hypocalcemia, hypomagnesemia, and hyperkalemia resulting in cardiac dysrhythmias. Due to the difficulty in the restoration of normal cardiac rhythm, hemodialysis may be necessary to eliminate fluoride ions and restore electrolyte imbalances.

Initial treatment consists of copious irrigation for a minimum of 30 min. With higher concentration exposures, calcium gluconate can be used. Topically, 3.5 g of 2.5% calcium gluconate mixed with a water-soluble lubricant can be applied to the wound 4–6 times daily over the course of 3–4 days. Alternatively, 0.5 mL/cm^2 of 10% calcium gluconate can be injected subcutaneously or intradermally in the area of the injury. Finally, 10 mL of 10% calcium gluconate and 40 mL of D5W can be infused intra-arterially but should occur within 6 h of the exposure to minimize the tissue necrosis and pain. Treatment should continue until the patient is symptom free.

Nitric Acid

Nitric acid is typically found in fertilizer, the iron and steel industries, and engraving products. It acts via oxidation, combining with proteins to form organonitrates, which are metabolic poisons. Upon skin contact, a yellow/brown stain will develop followed by eschar. Burn depth is difficult to assess due to the slow progression of the injury. Irrigation and topical treatments are the initial management.

Oxalic Acid

Oxalic acid is typically found within bleaching products and rust removers. It acts via combination with calcium which limits its bioavailability and thus limits muscle contraction. In addition to irrigation, treatment consists of intravenous calcium as well as the inclusion of cardiac monitoring and the frequent measurement of renal function and serum electrolytes.

Phosphoric Acid/Phosphorus

Phosphorus is an incendiary agent typically found within fireworks and fertilizers as well as in hand grenades and artillery shells. White phosphorus ignites upon contact with air and continues to burn until the oxygen source is removed, therefore copious irrigation and the removal of any macroscopic particles is the mainstay of treatment. Soaked dressings should be used during any transportation. In addition, ultraviolet light can be used to help identify embedded particles. Additionally, a 0.5% copper sulfate topical solution can be applied which will turn the particulates black, thus aiding in their identification and removal. Systemic effects include hypocalcemia, and hyperphosphatemia as well as cardiac arrythmias.

Alkalis

Alkalis, typically found in household cleaners in the form of lime, sodium hydroxide and potassium hydroxide, are commonly ingested as a means of suicide. Typically burns may appear superficial, but tissue destruction occurs long after exposure and thus may become full thickness over 2–3 days. Alkalis bind lipids and proteins, allowing passage of hydroxyl ions into the tissue, allowing deep penetration of the chemical and systemic absorption. Alkali injuries to the eyes are of specific concern as quick corneal penetration leads to scarring, opacification of the cornea, and perforation. Initial management requires prompt removal of any contaminated clothing, the removal of any dry residue and prompt large volume irrigation until the alkali is completely removed from the wound. As water cannot eliminate the alkali from the deeper layers of the wounds, excision of deep burns with immediate coverage should be considered.

Cement

Cement is one of the most commonly used chemical agents in the world. Calcium oxide accounts for 65% of the weight of cement, which when exposed to water becomes calcium hydroxide. Injury is the result of this hydroxyl ion and acts as both an alkali and a desiccant. Injury might not be noticed until several hours after exposure, and most commonly involves the lower extremities. Treatment consists of removal of cement-covered clothing and shoes. The practitioner must keep in mind that cement burns can be quite dangerous when ocular exposure occurs from a lack of proper safety eyewear. Similarly, the respiratory tract may become injured as a result of aerosolized calcium oxide dust.

Metals

Metals are typically involved with occupational injuries when molten metals are in use, most commonly involving sodium, lithium, potassium, magnesium, aluminum, and calcium. For chemical burns related to metals, water is contraindicated as it can lead to an explosive exothermic reaction. As such, sand and Class D fire extinguishers are treatments of choice. Mineral oil has also been shown to be effective [12].

Hydrocarbons

Hydrocarbons are typically found within plants, animal fats, and fuel oils. With prolonged contact, they act as corrosives causing the dissolution of the lipid cell membrane and thus cell death. The chemical burn associated is typically superficial. Early use of soap and water is most effective. Respiratory depression is a common systemic toxicity.

Hypochlorite Solutions

Hypochlorite solutions typically are found within household cleaners as well as bleaches. Systemic toxicity can lead to confusion, airway edema, vomiting, cyanosis, cardiovascular collapse, and coma. As little as 30 mL of a 15% solution can be fatal. Similar to other compounds, initial treatment is copious irrigation.

Alkyl Mercuric Compounds

Alkyl mercuric compounds react upon contact with skin, creating blisters in which free mercury can be found within the blister fluid. Over time, mercury can be absorbed leading to systemic toxicity. Initial treatment involves debridement of the blisters followed by repeat irrigation to remove the blister fluid.

Tar

Tar is a mineral product created from petroleum and coal. Also known as crude oil or asphalt, upon cooling it will produce a liquefaction injury that may require debridement. Hence immediate removal should be undertaken. Antibiotic ointments in addition to some household products such as mayonnaise, butter, or mineral oil have been shown to assist in the agent's removal [12, 13].

Vesicant Chemical Warfare Agents (Mustard, Lewisite, Nitrogen)

Historically used during trench warfare in World War I, these agents affect all of the epithelial layers. Exposure to mustard gas leads to burning of the eyes and throat as well as a feeling of suffocation. Depending on the dosage, symptoms may not arise until 24 h after exposure. Erythema of the skin occurs followed by blister formation and pruritus. The blisters then rupture, leaving shallow ulcerations. Owing to its disruption of cell replication, cutaneous lesions may take several months to heal. Lewisite is more powerful than mustard gas, and symptoms tend to appear sooner.

Clothing must be removed immediately followed by large volume irrigation. Benzodiazepines, antihistamines, and phenothiazines may be used to aid with pruritus. Blisters must be debrided/deroofed with topical antimicrobial and sterile dressing application. Dimercaprol has been used as an antidote in Lewisite poisoning, while sodium thiosulfate and N-acetylcysteine can help with mustard gas if administered early [14]. Keep in mind that most patients exposed to these agents have multiple sites of injury and these agents may also cause agranulocytosis or aplastic anemia. As such, bone marrow transplantation may be required.

Conclusion

While chemical burns account for only a small proportion of total burn injuries, their lethal implications mandate a special attention. While the prevention of such injuries is of the utmost importance, the gold standard of treatment remains copious irrigation with removal of the offending agents. Wound care for chemical burns can be carried out in a similar manner to that of thermal injuries, keeping in mind that chemical burns tend to be deeper than initially appear. Patients should be treated by specialized practitioners with referral to a Burn Center as soon as possible.

References

1. Gummin DD, Mowry JB, Beuhler MC, Spyker DA, Brooks DE, Dibert KW, Rivers LJ, Pham NPT, Ryan ML. 2019 Annual report of the American Association of Poison Control Centers' National Poison Data System (NPDS): 37th annual report. Clin Toxicol (Phila). 2020;58(12):1360–541. https://doi.org/10.1080/15 563650.2020.1834219.
2. Gummin DD, Mowry JB, Spyker DA, Brooks DE, Beuhler MC, Rivers LJ, Hashem HA, Ryan ML. 2018 Annual report of the American Association of Poison Control Centers' National Poison Data System (NPDS): 36th annual report [Erratum in: Clin Toxicol (Phila). 2019 Dec;57(12):e1.]. Clin Toxicol (Phila). 2019;57(12):1220–413. https://doi.org/10.1080/15563650.2019.16 77022.
3. Gummin DD, Mowry JB, Spyker DA, Brooks DE, Osterthaler KM, Banner W. 2017 Annual report of the American Association of Poison Control Centers' National Poison Data System (NPDS): 35th annual report. Clin Toxicol (Phila). 2018;56(12):1213–415. https://doi.org/10.1080/15563650.2018.1533727.
4. Robson MC, Smith DJ Jr, Jurkiewicz IN, et al. Plastic surgery: principles and practice. St Louis: CV Mosby; 1990. p. 1355–410.
5. Leonard LG, Scheulen JJ, Munster AM. Chemical burns: effect of prompt first aid. J Trauma. 1982;22:420–3.
6. Cope Z. General treatment of burns. Medical history of the second world war: surgery. London: HMSO; 1953. p. 288–312.
7. Pike J, Patterson A Jr, Arons MS. Chemistry of cement burns: pathogenesis and treatment. J Burn Care Rehabil. 1988;9(3):258–60.
8. Vesicants (Blister Agents). Part III-Chemical. Amended final draft (NATO Unclassified). NATO handbook on the medical effects of NBC defensive operations AMedP-6(B). 1996. p. 3–1.
9. Parpmeister B, Feister AJ, Robinson SI, et al. The sulfur mustard injury: description of lesions and resulting incapacitation. In: Medical defense against mustard gas. Boca Raton: CRC Press; 1990. p. 13–42.
10. Cason JS. Report on three extensive industrial chemical burns. Br Med J. 1959;1(5125):827–9.
11. Matey P, Allison KP, Sheehan TM, et al. Chromic acid burns: early aggressive excision is the best method to prevent systemic toxicity. J Burn Care Rehabil. 2000;21(3):241–5.

12. Harchelroad FP, Rottinghaus DM. Chemical burns. In: Emergency medicine: a comprehensive study guide. 6th ed. Amsterdam: Elsevier; 2004. p. 1226–30.
13. Consoli RJM. Emergency medicine. In: Rakel RE, editor. Textbook of family medicine. 7th ed. Amsterdam: Elsevier; 2007. p. 807–34.
14. Devereaux A, Amundson DE, Parrish JS, et al. Vesicants and nerve agents in chemical warfare. Decontamination and treatment strategies for a changed world. Postgrad Med. 2002;112(4):90–6.

Chapter 14
ICU Care of Burn Patients

Molly Hunter and David T. Harrington

Introduction

As burn care has improved, patients with severe burn injury have had improved survival [1]. However, severe burn injury requires care in specialized intensive care unit (ICU) due to the profound impact of burn injury on the body. Patients with burns >20% total body surface area (TBSA) require admission to a burn ICU because they are at risk for complications such as resuscitation failure, infection, sepsis, and multi-organ failure due to their injury [2]. Some patients with smaller burns also require ICU care because of significant medical comorbidities or either very young or advanced age. This chapter will address some of the special concerns in caring for severe burns in the ICU. Many topics discussed in this chapter are reviewed in more extensive detail in other chapters.

M. Hunter · D. T. Harrington (✉)
Department of Surgery, Warren Alpert Medical School of Brown University, Providence, RI, USA
e-mail: david.harrington@brownphysicians.org

© The Author(s), under exclusive license to Springer Nature Switzerland AG 2023
J. O. Lee (ed.), *Essential Burn Care for Non-Burn Specialists*,
https://doi.org/10.1007/978-3-031-28898-2_14

Cardiovascular System

Severe burns create a mixed picture of shock in the first days after the injury. Due to release of inflammatory mediators, cardiac contractility is decreased, and cardiac output will be impaired. In addition, patients are simultaneously losing free fluid from wounds through evaporation as well as losing intravascular volume through capillary leak into tissue causing edema. In short, severely burned patients can have a mix of distributive, hypovolemic, and cardiogenic shock in the first 24–48 h after their injury [3]. In this setting, burn resuscitation is a lifesaving intervention for the severely burned patient.

Burn Resuscitation

The most important components of burn resuscitation are quick initiation of crystalloid resuscitation and a closed loop protocol that allows intensive care providers to titrate the resuscitation to each patient. A formula like the modified Brooke Formula (2 mL/kg/%TBSA burned) estimates the amount of fluid required in the first 24 h with half to be given in the first 8 h. Providers can use this formula to calculate an initial fluid rate, but the hourly titration of the intravenous rate is based on the patient's response including urine output. Recommended urine output is 0.5 mL/kg/h in adults and 1.0 mL/kg/h in children. Many centers have adopted a closed loop, computer supported protocol to assist providers with resuscitation [4]. The importance of having a protocol, written or computer-assisted, that can adjust to the fluid demands of each patient cannot be overstated. Burn patients with inhalation injury, significant electrical injury, or intoxication with alcohol or drugs will require more resuscitation [5].

Invasive Monitoring

In order to facilitate burn resuscitation, patients should have a Foley catheter placed to monitor urine output and an arterial line to monitor mean arterial pressure (MAP). Arterial lines are often needed as blood pressure cuffs can be inaccurate due to tissue edema. In addition, tissue edema can cause issues with placement and maintenance of peripheral intravenous catheters, and some severely burned patients will require placement of a central venous catheter. These should be placed through unburned skin if possible to reduce risk of infection, but can go through burned skin if necessary [2]. Catheters placed through burned skin need to be changed more frequently than catheters placed through unburned skin.

In the first 24–48 h, most severely burned patients will not have normal hemodynamics. Due to the decreased cardiac output, a MAP between 50 and 60 mmHg can be tolerated if urine output and mental status are adequate. Due to the systemic inflammatory response to injury, severely burned patients will have a baseline tachycardia. Goal heart rate should be less than about 130 beats/minute [4].

Fluid Creep

While it is important to quickly escalate fluid resuscitation to combat shock in severely burned patients, it is equally important to consider de-escalation of fluid infusions to avoid complications from over-resuscitation as the patient's burn shock physiologic changes abate over the 18–24 h post-burn period. Due to the high fluid requirements needed, patients with large TBSA burns are at risk of compartment syndrome, pulmonary edema, and even cerebral edema in the setting of burn resuscitation. This phenomenon of excess fluid resuscitation that was seen in many burn centers from 1990 to 2010 was called "Fluid Creep" [5]. In order to prevent this, many burn centers utilize "colloid rescue" in the first 24 h to reduce volume of fluid. In addition to colloid use, protocols for burn resuscitation should have a feedback system that has providers turning down fluid rates as patients reach goal parameters [4]. Other factors that have been associated with fluid creep are the potential overuse of mechanical ventilation in the first 48 h after burn and overzealous use of narcotics. Both interventions should be thoughtfully used in the acute burn setting.

Pulmonary

The effect of severe burns on the pulmonary system can be from direct effect due to inhalation injury, from systemic injury from the systemic inflammatory response to injury or impairment of oxidative metabolism from cyanide and carbon monoxide poisoning. Here, we will cover some topics specific to burn patients in the intensive care unit.

Airway Injury

Inhalation injury can cause significant concern for upper airway edema. Thermal injury will be absorbed in the upper airway, except in the case of steam which can reach further down the respiratory tract. Traditionally, patients with evidence of facial burns or soot around mouth and nares were considered at risk for inhalation injury. However, these signs have been shown to have a poor correlation with need for intubation. While the best assessment of upper airway injury is a nasolaryngoscopy for direct visualization [6], often providers must rely on patient history and clinical exam to determine the likelihood of upper airway injury and need for intubation.

Airspace Injury

Oxygenation can be compromised in severe burns due to direct injury from inhaled soot, mists, and fumes or indirect injury from systemic factors. Inhalation of chemicals or irritants in smoke can damage lungs leading to hypoxia and need for intubation. Inhalation injury is associated with an increased need for resuscitation as well as an increased risk of mortality. Diagnosis relies on clinical judgment and should be supported by evidence of inhalation injury on bronchoscopy. Treatment for lower airway inhalation injury is supportive. Patients will have significant sloughing of mucosa and formation of fibrin casts requiring aggressive pulmonary toilet. For those requiring intubation, lung protective ventilation is recommended, and bronchodilators may have some benefit [7].

In addition to direct injury, severely burned patients are at risk for acute respiratory distress syndrome (ARDS) from the significant systemic inflammatory response to their injury. This can occur in up to 30% of burn patients requiring intensive care [2]. This presents as increasing hypoxia occurring days after the injury with bilateral opacities on chest radiograph as defined by the Berlin Criteria. Treatment is supportive with lung protective mechanical ventilation aiming for target tidal volumes of 6 mL/kg of predicted body weight and plateau pressures of <30 cmH_2O. For patients with severe ARDS, other strategies such as paralysis and proning can improve oxygenation. If all else fails, providers can consider extracorporeal membrane oxygenation (ECMO) [8]. Therapy for ARDS is also to look for and treat any potential underlying drivers of this inflammatory insult. Identifying and treating sepsis and expeditious removal of any residual eschar should also be performed [5].

Ventilation

Ventilation is an important consideration in the severely burned patient. Patients will be compensating for a metabolic acidosis from tissue hypoperfusion in the setting of shock. Patients with large burns or circumferential burns to the torso may require escharotomies to allow for improved ventilation [2].

Toxins

Fire environments produce cyanide and carbon monoxide. Both these toxins poison the ability of the cell to use oxygen in oxidative metabolism. Direct measurement of the percentage of hemoglobin bound with carbon monoxide is readily available by blood gas measurement or co-oximeter but measurement of cyanide levels often takes 24–36 h in many centers. Development of a metabolic acidosis or unexpected decrease in mental status should prompt a workup and treatment for these potentially life-threatening toxins.

Infection and Sepsis

Skin is an important part of our defense against infection. Severe burn injury not only causes direct destruction of a barrier to infection but also a global depression of the immune system leading to an increased risk of infection [9]. Infections account for 51% of deaths in burn patients with pneumonia, cellulitis, urinary tract infection, and burn wound infection as the top sources [10]. However, in the setting of a systemic inflammatory response to injury, diagnosis can be difficult in the severely burned patient. For each type of infection, it is important to consider early source control and early empiric antibiotics with narrowing according to culture data as soon as possible. Below are some considerations for common infections in severely burned patients.

Prevention

The most important part of infection control in critically ill burn patients is prevention. First, treatment of burn wounds with early excision and skin grafting reduces the systemic inflammatory effects as well as restoring a barrier against infection. While wounds are open, topical antimicrobials can combat bacterial growth [10].

Burn patients with greater than 20% TBSA burns should have a private room with an elevated ambient temperature to prevent hypothermia. In addition to strict hand hygiene, providers and visitors should wear gowns, gloves, hats, and masks to reduce the risk of contamination. These measures have been shown to reduce the risk of nosocomial infection in the burn patient [11]. These precautions should be maintained until less than 20% TBSA burns are open.

To prevent catheter associated infections, it is important to assess the need for these catheters daily and remove central lines and Foley catheters as soon as they are no longer needed. Central lines through intact skin can be changed as per routine institutional protocols, but catheters through burn skin may need to be replaced every 3–5 days [12].

Sepsis

Detecting sepsis in the severely burned patient requires providers to pay close attention to the patient's overall condition to see changes in hemodynamics, metabolism, and laboratory values. Providers cannot rely on absolute values alone to differentiate sepsis from the background of a systemic inflammatory response to injury which most all burn patients manifest. In 2007, the American Burn Association Consensus Conference found that the definition of sepsis used for non-burned patients did not describe sepsis in burn patients adequately. This consensus conference defined sepsis as "a change in the burn patient that triggers the concern for infection" [13]. Sepsis requires three or more of the following criteria:

- Temperature >39 °C or <36.5 °C
- Progressive tachycardia >110 beats/minute
- Progressive tachypnea >25 breaths per minute or minute ventilation >12 L/min
- Thrombocytopenia <100,000/mcL

- Hyperglycemia in the absence of pre-existing diabetes mellitus
- Inability to continue enteral feeding >24 h

  AND

- Culture positive infection *OR* pathologic tissue source identification *OR* clinical response to antimicrobials

Pneumonia

The diagnosis of pneumonia can be obscured with a presence of ARDS and/or inhalation injury. Scoring systems such as the Clinical Pulmonary Infection Score (CPIS) can guide providers on screening ventilated patients for ventilator-associated pneumonia (VAP) [14]. For ventilated patients where pneumonia is suspected, providers can obtain culture data with bronchoalveolar-lavage (BAL) to help confirm the diagnosis and narrow antibiotic coverage.

Burn Wound Infections

Diagnosing a burn wound infection takes careful clinical judgment. Wounds will become colonized with bacteria within 24 h of burn injury; therefore, the presence of bacteria does not equate with an infection. In order to diagnose a wound infection, a quantitative wound culture should be taken and show >10^5 bacteria/gram of tissue in the setting of infection or sepsis. Clinical suspicion can also be used. Cellulitis, early tinctorial change of the burn eschar, and premature separation of the burn eschar should raise a clinical suspicion for burn wound infection or sepsis. Treatment includes intravenous antibiotics and urgent debridement of infected tissue [13]. In some cases, due to use of broad spectrum antibiotics and the immunocompromised state of major burns, patients can develop invasive fungal infections. Yeast infections can be treated with topical and systemic antifungals as well as debridement. However, fungal infections carry a high mortality and need to be treated with radical debridement and possible amputation for source control [10].

Metabolism

The body's metabolic response to a large burn is activated by pro-inflammatory cytokines and creates a profound hypermetabolic and catabolic state which approaches double the basal rate [9]. As a result, patients have an increased caloric need that can approach as high as 110–150% of non-burned patients [6]. This leads to breakdown of proteins and weight loss. Significant weight loss can lead to immune dysfunction and delayed wound healing [15].

Nutrition

The importance of adequate nutrition in burn patients cannot be overstated. The best measurement of a burn patient's caloric need is through indirect calorimetry. However, if this is not available, caloric needs can be estimated using equations such as the Harris Benedict equation to estimate basal energy expenditure and adjust for demands of burn injury by using a multiplier of 1.5 [15]. Enteral feeding should be initiated as early as is feasible and routinely within the first 24 h. In large burn injury, diets and tube feedings should be high in protein and carbohydrates and low in fat [16]. Burn patients are at risk for swallowing dysfunction. Inhalation injury, long-term intubation, placement of a tracheostomy tube, long-term use of nasogastric tubes, and extensive burns to the neck are risk factors for swallowing dysfunction. Patients with any of these risk factors should have a comprehensive bedside swallowing evaluation. Aspiration detected on bedside evaluation should lead to a nothing by mouth status. If no aspiration is detected on bedside evaluation, then the patient should have a definitive test to rule-out aspiration such as a modified barium swallow (MBS) or fiberoptic endoscopic evaluation of swallowing (FEES). These definitive evaluations of swallowing are necessary because bedside evaluation alone has a false negative rate and subsequent silent aspiration of up to 25–30%.

Hyperglycemia

Due to the profound stress response in large burn injuries, many patients develop insulin resistance resulting in hyperglycemia. This can lead to poor wound healing and loss of skin grafts. This insulin resistance can persist for months after a large burn injury. Blood glucose should be followed closely in all patients with large burns, even those without a history of diabetes. Subcutaneous insulin can be used to control blood glucose, and in severe cases continuous intravenous insulin can be used in the acute setting [16].

Renal

Patients with severe burn injuries are at risk for acute kidney injury at different phases of their course. About 30% of severely burned patients will develop acute kidney injury, and this is associated with an increased mortality [6]. Early kidney injury is related to burn shock or in some cases compartment syndrome or direct injury to muscles leading to rhabdomyolysis. In both cases, a robust burn resuscitation is the best response to early kidney injury. Acute kidney injury that develops after the initial resuscitation is most often related to sepsis. Source control and treatment of infection are necessary to prevent ongoing injury.

Renal Replacement Therapy

Rarely, burn patients will progress to renal failure and require renal replacement therapy. However, progression to renal failure is a poor prognostic indicator and is associated with up to 80% mortality in the burn population. Intermittent hemodialysis can be used for patients with adequate blood pressure. However, more often burn patients in the ICU require continuous renal replacement therapy (CRRT) due to hemodynamic instability [17].

Palliative Care

Palliative care is an important concept in the treatment of severely burned patients. Burn patients have significant pain and stress both from the injury and from the treatment in the intensive care unit. It is important to have good communication with patients and their families about the prognosis and course of their treatment as well as understand the goals of each patient [17]. The use of palliative care teams have been used in some burn centers with positive effects.

Prognosis

While there are several models for determining mortality in burn patients, three factors are crucial in determining prognosis: patient age, TBSA burned, and the presence of inhalation injury [18]. One of the most widely used is the Revised Baux Score [Age + Percent Burn + 17 × (Inhalation Injury, with 1 = yes, 0 = no)] which takes into account these factors [19]. In addition to mortality, burn providers should discuss the expectations of rehabilitation.

Goals of Care

Discussions about what to expect and overall prognosis should begin when a patient is admitted to the ICU. Often, patients are unable to participate in the discussions due to intubation or burn shock. Providers should identify and involve the appropriate surrogate decision-makers [20]. In determining when to withhold or withdraw life sustaining treatment, health care providers should participate in shared decision-making taking into account the patient's advance directives or living will if available. Factors related to burn mortality are the same that correlate with withdrawal of care [21].

References

1. Pruitt BA, Wolf SE. An historical perspective on advances in burn care over the past 100 years. Clin Plast Surg. 2009;36(4):527–45. https://doi.org/10.1016/j.cps.2009.05.007.
2. Guzman EP, Oropello JM. Critical care of burn patients. In: Oropello JM, Pastores SM, Kvetan V, editors. Critical care. New York: McGraw-Hill Education; 2022. http://accessmedicine.mhmedical.com/content.aspx?aid=1136417932.
3. Wurzer P, Culnan D, Cancio LC, et al. Pathophysiology of burn shock and burn edema. In: Total burn care. 5th ed. Amsterdam: Elsevier Inc.; 2018. p. 66–76.e3. https://doi.org/10.1016/B978-0-323-47661-4.00008-3.
4. Cancio LC, Bohanon FJ, Kramer GC. Burn resuscitation. In: Total burn care. 5th ed. Amsterdam: Elsevier; 2018. p. 77–86.e2. https://doi.org/10.1016/B978-0-323-47661-4.00009-5.
5. Latenser BA. Critical care of the burn patient. Crit Care Med. 2010;38(4):1225–6. https://doi.org/10.1097/ccm.0b013e3181d453fd.
6. Woodson LC, Sherwood ER, Kinsky MP, et al. Anesthesia for burned patients. In: Total burn care. 5th ed. Amsterdam: Elsevier Inc.; 2018. p. 131–157.e4. https://doi.org/10.1016/B978-0-323-47661-4.00013-7.
7. Walker PF, Buehner MF, Wood LA, et al. Diagnosis and management of inhalation injury: an updated review. Crit Care. 2015;19(1):1–12. https://doi.org/10.1186/s13054-015-1077-4.

8. Fan E, Brodie D, Slutsky AS. Acute respiratory distress syndrome advances in diagnosis and treatment. JAMA J Am Med Assoc. 2018;319(7):698–710. https://doi.org/10.1001/jama.2017.21907.

9. Demling RH. Burns and other thermal injuries. In: Doherty GM, editor. Current diagnosis and treatment: surgery. New York: McGraw-Hill Education; 2015. http://accessmedicine.mhmedical.com/content.aspx?aid=1105485667.

10. Cambiaso-Daniel J, Gallagher JJ, Norbury WB, et al. Treatment of infection in burn patients. In: Total burn care. 5th ed. Amsterdam: Elsevier Inc.; 2018. p. 93–113.e4. https://doi.org/10.1016/B978-0-323-47661-4.00011-3.

11. Raes K, Blot K, Vogelaers D, et al. Protective isolation precautions for the prevention of nosocomial colonisation and infection in burn patients: a systematic review and meta-analysis. Intensive Crit Care Nurs. 2017;42:22–9. https://doi.org/10.1016/j.iccn.2017.03.005.

12. Rafla K, Tredget EE. Infection control in the burn unit. Burns. 2011;37(1):5–15. https://doi.org/10.1016/j.burns.2009.06.198.

13. Greenhalgh DG, Saffle JR, Holmes JH, et al. American burn association consensus conference to define sepsis and infection in burns. J Burn Care Res. 2007;28(6):776–90. https://doi.org/10.1097/BCR.0b013e3181599bc9.

14. Shan J, Chen HL, Zhu JH. Diagnostic accuracy of clinical pulmonary infection score for ventilator-associated pneumonia: a meta-analysis. Respir Care. 2011;56(8):1087–94. https://doi.org/10.4187/respcare.01097.

15. Clark A, Imran J, Madni T, et al. Nutrition and metabolism in burn patients. Burn Trauma. 2017;5(1):1–12. https://doi.org/10.1186/s41038-017-0076-x.

16. Porter C, Tompkins RG, Finnerty CC, et al. The metabolic stress response to burn trauma: current understanding and therapies. Lancet. 2016;388(10052):1417–26. https://doi.org/10.1016/S0140-6736(16)31469-6.

17. Carson JS, Goverman J, Fagan SP. Acute renal failure in association with thermal injury. In: Total burn care. 5th ed. Amsterdam: Elsevier Inc.; 2018. p. 318–327.e2. https://doi.org/10.1016/B978-0-323-47661-4.00031-9.

18. Hussain A, Choukairi F, Dunn K. Predicting survival in thermal injury: a systematic review of methodology of composite prediction models. Burns. 2013;39(5):835–50. https://doi.org/10.1016/j.burns.2012.12.010.

19. Williams DJ, Walker JD. A nomogram for calculation of the revised Baux score. Burns. 2015;41(1):85–90. https://doi.org/10.1016/j.burns.2014.05.001.
20. Pham TN, Otto A, Young SR, et al. Early withdrawal of life support in severe burn injury. J Burn Care Res. 2012;33(1):130–5. https://doi.org/10.1097/BCR.0b013e31823e598d.
21. Bartley CN, Atwell K, Cairns B, et al. Predictors of withdrawal of life support after burn injury. Burns. 2019;45(2):322–7. https://doi.org/10.1016/j.burns.2018.10.015.

Chapter 15
Pain Management in Burn Patients

Jordan B. Starr, Paul I. Bhalla, and Sam R. Sharar

Introduction

Pain management is a critical component of burn care. Pain control acutely after a burn injury mitigates the physiologic stress response. In the long term, reduced pain intensity and interference are associated with improved mobility, psychosocial outcomes, quality of life, and chronic pain severity [1–3]. Despite the importance of pain control after burns, pain in this population is difficult to treat and vulnerable to under-treatment [4–7].

This is partly due to the multiple sources of pain from burns. After a burn injury, patients have background pain from the trauma. This can be exacerbated with breakthrough pain from physical therapy or even smaller tasks, such as turning in bed. In addition to these constant threats, burn patients are subjected to procedure related pain from dressing changes and post-operative pain from more significant debridements and grafting.

Pain mechanisms in burn patients are also diverse, complicating which therapies are best to choose for any given patient. Because full-thickness burns destroy afferent nerves, there is primary pain from the initial injury and secondary

J. B. Starr (✉) · P. I. Bhalla · S. R. Sharar
Department of Anesthesiology and Pain Medicine, University of Washington, Seattle, WA, USA
e-mail: starrj@uw.edu; pbhalla@uw.edu; sharar@uw.edu

pain from healing and reinnervation of previously destroyed tissues. These different stages lead to nociceptive pain from tissue damage and inflammation as well as neuropathic pain from damage to neurologic structures [8].

Further complicating pain management in burn patients is that pre-injury psychiatric disorders and substance use disorders are risk factors for burn injuries [9–11]. Patients are also at risk for developing mood disorders, anxiety, post-traumatic stress disorder (PTSD), and addiction after their burns, all of which can affect pain and engagement with care [11, 12].

Pain Assessment

The first step in the management of pain is regular, adequate assessment of pain intensity and its interference with function. Multiple tools measuring pain intensity exist, with the simplest being the 10-point numeric rating scale (NRS) and visual analog scale (VAS) in patients who can communicate. Though simple to use, interpretation of patient-reported scores can be difficult in patients with comorbid psychiatric or substance abuse disorders. For this reason, pain score trends combined with behavioral cues are often more clinically informative than absolute cut-offs (e.g., NRS greater than 4/10 indicating moderate pain) for altering treatment strategies. In non-communicating adults, the critical-care pain observation tool (CPOT) is a validated measure to assess pain that relies on observable physiological and behavioral indicators [13]. Scores greater than two suggest the presence of pain [14].

In children, there are many age and developmental-level appropriate pain scales. One of the most well studied is the FLACC (Face, Legs, Activity, Cry, Consolability) scale for nonverbal children up to age seven [15]. Scores greater than three are indicative of at least moderate pain [15]. In children 3 years and older who can communicate, but who cannot reliably report on the NRS or VAS, the Wong-Baker FACES pain rating scale is another validated metric. On the Wong-Baker FACES scale, a score of six or "hurts even more" is consistent with a VAS greater than four [16]. After determining a patient is in pain, the primary interventions involve pharmacological (Table 15.1) and

TABLE 15.1 Summary of medications for pain after burns

Class	Prototypical agents	Typical dosing	Primary mechanism	Side effects	Contraindications
Acetaminophen	Acetaminophen	1000 mg PO q6h PRN	Central COX inhibition	Hepatotoxicity	Acute or chronic liver injury
NSAIDs	Ibuprofen	600 mg PO q6h PRN	COX inhibition	Bleeding, GI ulcers, renal injury	Renal dysfunction, CNS hemorrhage
Gabapentinoids	Gabapentin	300–600 mg PO TID	Calcium channel blockade	Sedation	Dosed renally
Alpha-2 agonists	Tizanidine	4 mg PO TID	Alpha-2 agonism	Hypotension, sedation, withdrawal	Hypotension, bradycardia
TCAs/SNRIs	Duloxetine	60 mg daily	SNRI	Nausea, sedation (TCAs)	Other serotonergic meds, arrythmias
Muscle relaxants	Methocarbamol	1000 mg PO q6h	CNS depressant	Sedation	None

(continued)

TABLE 15.1 (continued)

Class	Prototypical agents	Typical dosing	Primary mechanism	Side effects	Contraindications
Opioids	Oxycodone	5 mg PO q4h PRN	mu-opioid agonism	Constipation, pruritus, nausea, sedation, tolerance, addiction	Respiratory depression
NMDA antagonists	Ketamine	1–3 mcg/kg/min IV	NMDA antagonism	Nightmares, hallucinations	Schizophrenia, hepatic injury
Local anesthetics	Lidocaine	1 mg/kg/h IV	Sodium channel blockade	Nausea, CNS and cardiac toxicity	Local anesthetic allergy, hypotension, arrhythmia
Anxiolytics	Midazolam	2 mg IV PRN	GABA agonism	Respiratory depression, delirium, addiction	Respiratory compromise, delirium
Anesthetics	Nitrous oxide	50% inhaled gas	Unknown	Nausea, dysphoria	Hypoxia, cytopenia

CNS central nervous system, *COX* cyclooxygenase, *GABA* gamma aminobutyric acid, *GI* gastrointestinal, *NMDA* N-methyl-D-aspartate, *NSAID* nonsteroidal anti-inflammatory drug, *SNRI* serotonin-norepinephrine reuptake inhibitor, *TCA* tricyclic antidepressant non-pharmacological treatment to reduce its intensity, along with strategies to restore the function and well-being of burn injured patients.

Medications

Acetaminophen

Acetaminophen is a mainstay of multimodal analgesia. It acts centrally via COX enzyme inhibition, cannabinoid agonism, and inhibition of nitric oxide pathways [17]. It can be given orally (PO), rectally (PR), or intravenously (IV), with differences in time to efficacy but not potency. In adults, the maximum daily dose is 4 g, with reductions in the elderly and patients with hepatic disease.

Nonsteroidal Anti-inflammatory Drugs

Nonsteroidal anti-inflammatory drugs (NSAIDs) are useful analgesics with opioid sparing effects. They inhibit COX-1 and COX-2, except for celecoxib, which is a selective COX-2 inhibitor. Ibuprofen is the prototypical NSAID with a maximum dose of 600 mg every 6 h or 800 mg every 8 h. Ketorolac is useful as an IV agent that can be given for up to 5 days. All NSAIDs can cause renal injury. COX-1 inhibition more strongly inhibits platelet aggregation and gastric mucosal protection. COX-2 inhibition has a stronger association with thrombosis [17].

Gabapentinoids

Gabapentin and pregabalin are also adjuncts with evidence for efficacy in burn pain [18]. They both act via blockade of nerve calcium channels. Gabapentin is typically the first-line agent, with a therapeutic dose around 600 mg every 8 h in healthy adults. Because gabapentin has high variability in gastric absorption, it is recommended to start at a lower dose and increase every few days either to effect or sedation. Pregabalin is usually reserved for patients with inadequate pain relief or excessive sedation from gabapentin, with a therapeutic dose around 150 mg every 12 h.

Alpha-2 Receptor Agonists

Clonidine, tizanidine, and dexmedetomidine are alpha-2 receptor agonists, which reduce norepinephrine release and sympathetic outflow [18]. These medications have an opioid sparing effect, reduce delirium, and have even been associated with a survival benefit in sepsis [19, 20]. Clonidine and tizanidine can be given orally, while dexmedetomidine is an infusion useful for sedation during mechanical ventilation or procedures. If clonidine or tizanidine is used as scheduled medications, they should be tapered off to prevent withdrawal symptoms. Tizanidine 2–4 mg every 8 h is useful as a first-line agent given its reduced side-effect profile compared to clonidine.

Tricyclic Antidepressants and Serotonin-Norepinephrine Reuptake Inhibitors

These classes of medications have excellent evidence in chronic, neuropathic pain conditions [21, 22]. Their evidence in acute pain and burns specifically is weaker [22, 23]. Nevertheless, they can be considered in patients with poorly controlled pain, predominantly neuropathic pain from burns or another injury, or concomitant depression. Both medication classes increase serotonin and norepinephrine in the synaptic cleft, while tricyclic antidepressants (TCAs) are also antagonists on cholinergic, muscarinic, and histaminergic receptors [21, 22]. Given its improved side-effect profile, duloxetine is often started at 30 mg daily. This can be increased weekly to a goal dose of 60 mg daily for pain or 120 mg daily for pain and depression. The primary adverse effect is nausea during the initial week of treatment. If a TCA is selected, desipramine tends to have the fewest anticholinergic side effects.

Muscle Relaxants

Muscle relaxants are a diverse group of medications used in chronic and acute pain conditions, though evidence in burn pain is lacking. Benzodiazepines, tizanidine, and cyclobenzaprine, essentially a TCA, are discussed elsewhere. Carisoprodol and metaxalone are usually avoided due to their addictive properties and sedation. Though it is a general CNS depressant, methocarbamol is included in this class, as well as baclofen, which is a centrally acting GABA-B receptor agonist. Methocarbamol is typically first line as its only common side effect is mild sedation. Doses range from 500 to 1500 mg every 6 h as tolerated. Baclofen is usually reserved for patients with upper motor neuron lesions causing spasticity, and it can cause potentially lethal withdrawals if abruptly discontinued.

Opioids

Opioids play a critical role in burn care. They act primarily via mu-opioid receptor agonism, with contributions via kappa-opioid and delta-opioid receptor agonism [18]. The most commonly employed oral opioids include morphine, oxycodone, hydrocodone, and hydromorphone prescribed as needed for background pain. Morphine or hydromorphone IV is often added for breakthrough pain. For patients with unknown opioid requirements or who have rapid changes in their opioid needs, such as after surgery, utilizing patient-controlled analgesia (PCA) can improve patient satisfaction and care.

In patients who are able to communicate or use a PCA, continuous opioid infusions increase the risk of respiratory depression. Nevertheless, they have a role in young children and intubated patients, typically in the form of a fentanyl infusion.

Methadone also plays a unique role in burn care. In addition to long-acting mu-receptor agonism, it causes N-methyl-D-aspartate (NMDA) antagonism and serotonin and norepinephrine reuptake inhibition [18]. It can be prescribed up to four times daily for pain, with starting doses of 5–10 mg. It is especially useful for non-opioid naïve patients. It is important to monitor the QTc in patients on methadone, with a QTc over 500 ms necessitating a dose reduction. Buprenorphine, a partial mu-agonist, can also play a role in burn patients with opioid use disorders.

Regardless of the opioid chosen, side effects include pruritus, nausea, vomiting, constipation, respiratory depression, opioid induced hyperalgesia, along with tolerance and addiction. It is therefore important to provide multimodal analgesia and reduce opioid dosing as soon as tolerated.

Ketamine

Ketamine, either in high doses for procedures or in low-dose infusions for background pain, is a useful adjunct for burn pain management. It is an NMDA receptor antagonist that functions synergistically with opioids. Analgesic infusions range from 1 to 3 mcg/kg/min with negligible adverse effects. Dosing for procedures is associated with unpleasant hallucinations although this can be mitigated with coadministration of benzodiazepines [18].

Lidocaine

Topical and IV lidocaine are adjunct options that can be offered to burn patients. For small burns, topical lidocaine can be effective, though systemic toxicity becomes a concern for larger burns [24]. IV lidocaine can be used for background or procedural pain, albeit with limited evidence [25]. Dosing at 1 mg/kg/h for up to 48 h has been used safely at our institution in patients without hepatic compromise. The primary adverse effect is nausea.

Anxiolytics

Anxiolytics for burns includes benzodiazepines and hydroxyzine. Benzodiazepines are the standard for anxiolysis and amnesia for painful procedures, but they are associated with respiratory depression, delirium, tolerance, and addiction. Hydroxyzine is an antihistamine, FDA approved for anxiety. With a reduced side-effect profile compared to benzodiazepines, it can be used for background anxiety symptoms, typically at 25–50 mg every 6 h as needed.

Anesthetics

For particularly painful procedures and operations, monitored anesthesia care (MAC) or general anesthesia will be necessary. However, inhaled nitrous oxide has been used by non-anesthesia personnel. It is typically inhaled via a mask held by the patient in a 50:50 mixture with oxygen. It can be used for procedures, but it is associated with nausea, dysphoria, spontaneous abortion, and bone marrow suppression [24].

Regional Anesthesia

Regional anesthesia involves placing local anesthetic near specific nerves in order to anesthetize a large area of the body. The nerves that are targeted can be central, near to the spinal cord, or peripheral. Regional anesthesia can be used as the sole anesthetic for surgery, as a supplement to general anesthesia for surgery, or for analgesia of the targeted area of the body. Its use for perioperative pain is well-established and has been shown to reliably improve early quality of pain relief, reduce the need for opioid medication, and improve patient satisfaction [26].

Regional anesthesia can involve a single injection of local anesthetic ("single shot block") or the placement of a catheter that allows for continuous infusion of local anesthetic over several days. Other variables to consider when discussing regional anesthesia include the type of local anesthetic used, the volume and concentration of the drug, and the addition of other drugs into the injectate (Table 15.2).

Burn injury pain should be amenable to regional anesthesia as it is mediated by peripheral nociceptors at the injury site as well as by injuries to the nerves themselves (peripheral neuropathic pain) and by the peripheral inflammatory response to the injury. Furthermore, local anesthetics have some intrinsic anti-inflammatory properties and can modulate steps of the inflammatory cascade [27, 28]. Pain from surgical debridement of a burn injury and from graft donor sites should therefore respond well to regional anesthesia. However, the available evidence for the effectiveness of regional anesthesia specifically in burn injured patients is limited to a small number of randomized controlled trials.

TABLE 15.2 Factors influencing regional anesthesia

Variable		Notes on effect
Local anesthetic drug		Change in duration of numbness
Dose of local anesthetic	Concentration	Density of block
	Volume	Spread of local anesthetic
Additives	Dexamethasone	Increase duration of block
	Dexmedetomidine	Increase duration of block
	Epinephrine	Marker for intravascular injection, increase duration of short-acting local anesthetics

Despite limited high quality trials, regional analgesia seems to be a useful potential adjunct to systemic analgesia, with very few adverse effects [29]. The reason it remains underused as an analgesic modality in the burn injured population is probably due to the added complexity of care relating to regional anesthesia. Nerve blocks are usually performed by a specially trained anesthesiologist, meaning availability of expertise may be inconsistent. If peripheral nerve catheters are used, appropriate nursing care must be available to identify and manage potential problems, and systems must be in place to manage complications. Nonetheless, although further randomized control trials are warranted, regional analgesia is currently recommended by consensus expert opinion where possible [30].

Neuraxial Anesthesia

Centrally acting, or neuraxial, local anesthetic techniques include spinal (intrathecal) anesthesia, epidural anesthesia, and paravertebral anesthesia. Spinal and epidural techniques involve injections into appropriate areas of the back using blind landmark techniques. Paravertebral blocks are traditionally performed blind, but, more recently, ultrasound guided techniques have been described and used depending on practitioner skill and comfort [31]. Neuraxial blocks require specific patient positioning and may be technically challenging to place. As sympathetic and motor nerves are also affected, patients can often experience hypotension, urinary retention, and lower extremity weakness. Rare but serious adverse events include epidural abscess and spinal cord ischemia secondary to hematoma.

Peripheral Nerve Blocks

Peripheral nerve blocks are most commonly performed using ultrasound to visualize specific structures of interest and guide the needle to a precise location. The upper extremity can be blocked by a number of approaches to the brachial plexus, and common blocks of the lower extremity target the femoral nerve, lateral femoral cutaneous nerve, and the sciatic nerve. Peripheral blocks that target fascial planes rather than nerves have also been described, and their use has grown as ultrasound imaging technology has allowed these planes to be more easily identified. Transverse abdominus plane (TAP) blocks and quadratus lumborum (QL) blocks target the abdomen and anterior lower thorax; serratus anterior plane blocks (SAPB) target the anterolateral thoracic wall; erector spinae plane blocks (ESPB) target the posterolateral hemithorax. One advantage of fascial plane blocks is that the needle is not placed near a nerve or blood vessel, reducing the risk of neural injury or toxicity from intravascular injection of local anesthetic.

Upper extremity blocks and plane blocks of the trunk have been successfully reported in burn injured patients [32, 33]. The use of lateral femoral cutaneous nerve block and fascia iliaca plane blocks for donor site pain have also been shown to be reliable for reducing pain scores and opioid use by both single shot and nerve catheter techniques, in children and adults, when compared to local anesthetic infiltration [34–36].

Non-pharmacological Modalities

Pharmacological therapy for pain is often limited by actual or potential adverse effects, and even with maximal pharmacological pain therapy, patients with severe burns may experience high or intolerable pain levels. Analgesic medications and regional anesthesia target the sensory nociceptive component of pain, but the overall pain experience also consists of an experiential component (the individual experience of pain), a cognitive component (an individual's thoughts about pain), and a behavioral component (how an individual acts in response to pain), all of which are influenced by an individual's perception, expectations, and past experiences [37, 38].

A number of non-pharmacological interventions are available that have been shown to help with pain management in the burn population. While there is significant heterogeneity in methodology and outcome measures, there are also no adverse effects associated with them other than cost. Broadly, non-pharmacological analgesia falls into two categories. *Distraction techniques* work on the principle that non-noxious stimuli can suppress pain and redirect attention. *Cognitive techniques* work by mitigating anxiety and addressing the affective component of pain and downregulating sympathetic tone. In reality, many non-pharmacological techniques work in more than one of these categories.

These techniques are safe and effective as adjuncts in the analgesic management of burn patients. Despite this, these interventions are likely underused because of the expertise, time, and overall expense [39]. Current American Burn Association guidelines recommend every patient should be offered non-pharmacological analgesia, at least as an adjunct to their pain management regimen, and that cognitive behavioral therapy (CBT), hypnosis, and virtual reality have the strongest evidence base [40].

Distraction Techniques

Music is easily available, portable, and customizable to patients' preferences. It inhibits pain by gate-control block of sensory fibers, while also stimulating endorphin secretion. It has been shown to improve pain, anxiety, and relaxation in background pain and pain during dressing changes [41–43]. More interactive forms of music therapy such as music-based imagery (MBI) and music alternate engagement (MAE) also show significant reduction in pain, but not opioid use, during dressing changes [44, 45].

Virtual reality (VR) uses an immersive visual and auditory experience usually delivered through a headset to distract a patient's attention from painful stimuli. VR use during dressing changes and other procedures appears to have a significant effect on pain scores, but not opioid consumption [46]. Functional MRI suggests that although distraction is the predominant mechanism of action, VR also may modulate the pain experience [47]. Interactive video gaming can be considered a subset of VR in terms of mechanism and efficacy [39, 48].

A number of other distraction techniques have been examined for burn pain, including massage therapy, aromatherapy, and acupuncture [49–51]. All of them generally show a moderate positive effect on pain scores but with small sample sizes and significant heterogeneity.

Cognitive Techniques

Hypnosis causes an altered state of consciousness to a more suggestible state, facilitating changes in pain perception, along with increasing relaxation. Reduction in pain quality and anxiety has been shown in adults and children although not a reduction in pain intensity [39, 52, 53].

CBT aims to modify patients' thought processes relating to their pain experience [54]. Both hypnosis and CBT require highly trained personnel to be a viable modality for burn pain management.

Initial Treatment Approach

Although there are many options for pain management, it is useful to have a standardized approach for all patients and adjust as necessary. We recommend ensuring all of a patients home psychoactive and chronic pain medications are restarted. Assuming there are no contraindications, add basic adjuncts such as acetaminophen and an NSAID. In patients with moderate pain, start an oral opioid for background pain and an IV opioid for breakthrough pain. In those with severe pain, starting an IV opioid delivered via PCA can be more effective initially. For procedures, ensure short-acting, quick-onset opioids or benzodiazepines are available. Non-pharmacologic techniques—particularly distraction techniques such as music and VR that are simple, inexpensive, and widely available—should be included in the multimodal analgesia plan for all burn patients, regardless of the size or severity of their burn. Once these interventions are enacted, continually assess pain control and safety. If treatment goals are not being met, then consider pain management specialist consultation.

Other useful consultants include addiction medicine in patients with substance use disorders, child life for pediatric patients, palliative care for those at the end of life, and psychiatry for patients with coexisting mental health disorders. If available, engaging specialists in non-pharmacological modalities can be helpful, including acupuncture, massage therapy, rehabilitation psychology, and spiritual care.

References

1. Nelson S, Uhl K, Wright LA, Logan D. Pain is associated with increased physical and psychosocial impairment in youth with a history of burn injuries. J Pain. 2020;21(3–4):355–63. S1526-5900(19)30774-6.
2. Saxe G, Stoddard F, Courtney D, et al. Relationship between acute morphine and the course of PTSD in children with burns. J Am Acad Child Adolesc Psychiatry. 2001;40(8):915–21. S0890-8567(09)60339-7.
3. Gauffin E, Öster C, Sjöberg F, Gerdin B, Ekselius L. Health-related quality of life (EQ-5D) early after injury predicts long-term pain after burn. Burns. 2016;42(8):1781–8. http://www.sciencedirect.com/science/article/pii/S030541791630167X. https://doi.org/10.1016/j.burns.2016.05.016.
4. Schechter NL, Allen DA, Hanson K. Status of pediatric pain control: a comparison of hospital analgesic usage in children and adults. Pediatrics. 1986;77(1):11–5.
5. Choinière M, Melzack R, Girard N, Rondeau J, Paquin MJ. Comparisons between patients' and nurses' assessment of pain and medication efficacy in severe burn injuries. Pain. 1990;40(2):143–52. 0304-3959(90)90065-L.

6. Carrougher GJ, Ptacek JT, Sharar SR, et al. Comparison of patient satisfaction and self-reports of pain in adult burn-injured patients. J Burn Care Rehabil. 2003;24(1):1–8. https://doi.org/10.1097/00004630-200301000-00003.

7. Melzack R. The tragedy of needless pain. Sci Am. 1990;262(2):27–33. https://doi.org/10.1038/scientificamerican0290-27.

8. Schneider JC, Harris NL, El Shami A, et al. A descriptive review of neuropathic-like pain after burn injury. J Burn Care Res. 2006;27(4):524–8. 01253092-200607000-00017.

9. Brezel BS, Kassenbrock JM, Stein JM. Burns in substance abusers and in neurologically and mentally impaired patients. J Burn Care Rehabil. 1988;9(2):169–71. https://doi.org/10.1097/00004630-198803000-00009.

10. Logsetty S, Shamlou A, Gawaziuk JP, et al. Mental health outcomes of burn: a longitudinal population-based study of adults hospitalized for burns. Burns. 2016;42(4):738–44. S0305-4179(16)30011-0.

11. Duke JM, Randall SM, Boyd JH, Wood FM, Fear MW, Rea S. A population-based retrospective cohort study to assess the mental health of patients after a non-intentional burn compared with uninjured people. Burns. 2018;44(6):1417–26. S0305-4179(18)30369-3.

12. Carrougher GJ, Ptacek JT, Honari S, et al. Self-reports of anxiety in burn-injured hospitalized adults during routine wound care. J Burn Care Res. 2006;27(5):676–81. 01253092-200609000-00018.

13. Buttes P, Keal G, Cronin SN, Stocks L, Stout C. Validation of the critical-care pain observation tool in adult critically ill patients. Dimens Crit Care Nurs. 2014;33(2):78–81. https://doi.org/10.1097/DCC.0000000000000021.

14. Gélinas C, Fillion L, Puntillo KA, Viens C, Fortier M. Validation of the critical-care pain observation tool in adult patients. Am J Crit Care. 2006;15(4):420–7. 15/4/420.

15. Merkel SI, Voepel-Lewis T, Shayevitz JR, Malviya S. The FLACC: a behavioral scale for scoring postoperative pain in young children. Pediatr Nurs. 1997;23(3):293–7.

16. Garra G, Singer AJ, Taira BR, et al. Validation of the Wong-Baker FACES pain rating scale in pediatric emergency department patients. Acad Emerg Med. 2010;17(1):50–4. https://doi.org/10.1111/j.1553-2712.2009.00620.x.

17. Hanna MN, Ouanes JP, Tomas VG. Postoperative pain and other acute pain syndromes. In: Benzon H, Rathmell J, Wu C, Turk D, Argoff C, Hurley R, eds. Practical management of pain. St. Louis: Mosby; 2013:271–297.

18. Brookman JC, Kumar K, Wu C. Burn pain. In: Benzon H, Rathmell J, Wu C, Turk D, Argoff C, Hurley R, editors. Practical management of pain. St. Louis: Mosby; 2013. p. 1003–1008.

19. Pandharipande PP, Sanders RD, Girard TD, et al. Effect of dexmedetomidine versus lorazepam on outcome in patients with sepsis: an a priori-designed analysis of the MENDS randomized controlled trial. Crit Care. 2010;14(2):R38. https://doi.org/10.1186/cc8916.

20. Blaudszun G, Lysakowski C, Elia N, Tramèr MR. Effect of perioperative systemic α2 agonists on postoperative morphine consumption and pain intensity: systematic review and meta-analysis of randomized controlled trials. Anesthesiology. 2012;116(6):1312–22. https://doi.org/10.1097/ALN.0b013e31825681cb.

21. Moraczewski J, Aedma KK. Tricyclic antidepressants. In: StatPearls [Internet]. Treasure Island: StatPearls Publishing; 2020. https://www.ncbi.nlm.nih.gov/books/NBK557791/.

22. de Oliveira Filho GR, Kammer RS, Dos Santos HC. Duloxetine for the treatment acute postoperative pain in adult patients: a systematic review with meta-analysis. J Clin Anesth. 2020;63:109785. S0952-8180(19)31858-6.

23. Friedman BW, Dym AA, Davitt M, et al. Naproxen with cyclobenzaprine, oxycodone/acetaminophen, or placebo for treating acute low back pain: a randomized clinical trial. JAMA. 2015;314(15):1572–80. https://doi.org/10.1001/jama.2015.13043.

24. Sharar SR, Patterson DR. Burn pain. In: Ballantyne JC, Fishman SM, Rathmell JP, editors. Bonica's management of pain. Baltimore: Lippincott Williams & Wilkins; 2018. p. 754–766.

25. Wasiak J, Spinks A, Costello V, et al. Adjuvant use of intravenous lidocaine for procedural burn pain relief: a randomized double-blind, placebo-controlled, cross-over trial. Burns. 2011;37(6):951–7. https://doi.org/10.1016/j.burns.2011.03.004.

26. Bugada D, Ghisi D, Mariano ER. Continuous regional anesthesia: a review of perioperative outcome benefits. Minerva Anestesiol. 2017;83(10):1089–100. https://doi.org/10.23736/S0375-9393.17.12077-8.

27. Lirk P, Picardi S, Hollmann MW. Local anaesthetics: 10 essentials. Eur J Anaesthesiol. 2014;31(11):575–85. https://doi.org/10.1097/EJA.0000000000000137.

28. Picardi S, Cartellieri S, Groves D, et al. Local anesthetic-induced inhibition of human neutrophil priming: the influence of structure, lipophilicity, and charge. Reg Anesth Pain Med. 2013;38(1):9–15. https://doi.org/10.1097/AAP.0b013e31827a3cbe.

29. Anderson TA, Fuzaylov G. Perioperative anesthesia management of the burn patient. Surg Clin North Am. 2014;94(4):851–61. S0039-6109(14)00071-1.

30. Town CJ, Johnson J, Van Zundert A, Strand H. Exploring the role of regional anesthesia in the treatment of the burn-injured patient: a narrative review of current literature. Clin J Pain. 2019;35(4):368–74. https://doi.org/10.1097/AJP.0000000000000680.

31. Krediet AC, Moayeri N, van Geffen GJ, et al. Different approaches to ultrasound-guided thoracic paravertebral block: an illustrated review. Anesthesiology. 2015;123(2):459–74. https://doi.org/10.1097/ALN.0000000000000747.

32. Ueshima H, Otake H. Continuous erector spinae plane block for pain management of an extensive burn. Am J Emerg Med. 2018;36(11):2130.e1–2. S0735-6757(18)30571-0.

33. Cordts T, Horter J, Vogelpohl J, Kremer T, Kneser U, Hernekamp JF. Enzymatic debridement for the treatment of severely burned upper extremities—early single center experiences. BMC Dermatol. 2016;16(1):8–2. https://doi.org/10.1186/s12895-016-0045-2.

34. Shteynberg A, Riina LH, Glickman LT, Meringolo JN, Simpson RL. Ultrasound guided lateral femoral cutaneous nerve (LFCN) block: safe and simple anesthesia for harvesting skin grafts. Burns. 2013;39(1):146–9. S0305-4179(12)00059-9.

35. Shank ES, Martyn JA, Donelan MB, Perrone A, Firth PG, Driscoll DN. Ultrasound-guided regional anesthesia for pediatric burn reconstructive surgery: a prospective study. J Burn Care Res. 2016;37(3):213. https://doi.org/10.1097/BCR.0000000000000174.

36. Cuignet O, Pirson J, Boughrouph J, Duville D. The efficacy of continuous fascia iliaca compartment block for pain management in burn patients undergoing skin grafting procedures. Anesth Analg. 2004;98(4):1077–81, table of contents. https://doi.org/10.1213/01.ane.0000105863.04140.ae.

37. Cassell EJ. Diagnosing suffering: a perspective. Ann Intern Med. 1999;131(7):531–4. 199910050-00009.

38. Fordyce WE. Behavioural science and chronic pain. Postgrad Med J. 1984;60(710):865–8. https://doi.org/10.1136/pgmj.60.710.865.
39. Kim DE, Pruskowski KA, Ainsworth CR, Linsenbardt HR, Rizzo JA, Cancio LC. A review of adjunctive therapies for burn injury pain during the opioid crisis. J Burn Care Res. 2019;40(6):983–95. https://doi.org/10.1093/jbcr/irz111.
40. Romanowski KS, Carson J, Pape K, et al. American burn association guidelines on the management of acute pain in the adult burn patient: a review of the literature, a compilation of expert opinion, and next steps. J Burn Care Res. 2020;41(6):1129–51. raa119.
41. Najafi Ghezeljeh T, Mohades Ardebili F, Rafii F, Haghani H. The effects of music intervention on background pain and anxiety in burn patients: randomized controlled clinical trial. J Burn Care Res. 2016;37(4):226–34. https://doi.org/10.1097/BCR.0000000000000266.
42. Hsu KC, Chen LF, Hsiep PH. Effect of music intervention on burn patients' pain and anxiety during dressing changes. Burns. 2016;42(8):1789–96. S0305-4179(16)30131-0.
43. Zhang XH, Gao XX, Wu WW, Yu JA. Impact of orally administered tramadol combined with self-selected music on adult outpatients with burns undergoing dressing change: a randomized controlled trial. Burns. 2020;46(4):850–9. S0305-4179(19)30513-3.
44. Tan X, Yowler CJ, Super DM, Fratianne RB. The efficacy of music therapy protocols for decreasing pain, anxiety, and muscle tension levels during burn dressing changes: a prospective randomized crossover trial. J Burn Care Res. 2010;31(4):590–7. https://doi.org/10.1097/BCR.0b013e3181e4d71b.
45. Li J, Zhou L, Wang Y. The effects of music intervention on burn patients during treatment procedures: a systematic review and meta-analysis of randomized controlled trials. BMC Complement Altern Med. 2017;17(1):158–4. https://doi.org/10.1186/s12906-017-1669-4.
46. Scapin S, Echevarría-Guanilo ME, Boeira Fuculo Junior PR, Gonçalves N, Rocha PK, Coimbra R. Virtual reality in the treatment of burn patients: a systematic review. Burns. 2018;44(6):1403–16. S0305-4179(17)30602-2.
47. Bermo MS, Patterson D, Sharar SR, Hoffman H, Lewis DH. Virtual reality to relieve pain in burn patients undergoing imaging and treatment. Top Magn Reson Imaging. 2020;29(4):203–8. https://doi.org/10.1097/RMR.0000000000000248.

48. Voon K, Silberstein I, Eranki A, Phillips M, Wood FM, Edgar DW. Xbox kinect™ based rehabilitation as a feasible adjunct for minor upper limb burns rehabilitation: a pilot RCT. Burns. 2016;42(8):1797–804. S0305-4179(16)30178-4.

49. Najafi Ghezeljeh T, Mohades Ardebili F, Rafii F. The effects of massage and music on pain, anxiety and relaxation in burn patients: randomized controlled clinical trial. Burns. 2017;43(5):1034–43. S0305-4179(17)30023-2.

50. Choi J, Lee JA, Alimoradi Z, Lee MS. Aromatherapy for the relief of symptoms in burn patients: a systematic review of randomized controlled trials. Burns. 2018;44(6):1395–402. S0305-4179(17)30563-6.

51. Cuignet O, Pirlot A, Ortiz S, Rose T. The effects of electroacupuncture on analgesia and peripheral sensory thresholds in patients with burn scar pain. Burns. 2015;41(6):1298–305. S0305-4179(15)00062-5.

52. Jafarizadeh H, Lotfi M, Ajoudani F, Kiani A, Alinejad V. Hypnosis for reduction of background pain and pain anxiety in men with burns: a blinded, randomised, placebo-controlled study. Burns. 2018;44(1):108–17. S0305-4179(17)30348-0.

53. Chester SJ, Tyack Z, De Young A, et al. Efficacy of hypnosis on pain, wound-healing, anxiety, and stress in children with acute burn injuries: a randomized controlled trial. Pain. 2018;159(9):1790–801. https://doi.org/10.1097/j.pain.0000000000001276.

54. Wiechman Askay S, Patterson DR, Sharar SR, Mason S, Faber B. Pain management in patients with burn injuries. Int Rev Psychiatry. 2009;21(6):522–30. https://doi.org/10.3109/09540260903343844.

Chapter 16
Outpatient Burn Care

Barclay T. Stewart and Nicole S. Gibran

Introduction

The vast majority of the 11 million people globally who sustain burn injuries that require medical attention each year have small burns that can be safely and effectively managed in the outpatient setting (see Chap. 1) [1]. However, careful care planning and organization are required to achieve excellent outcomes. Outpatient burn care involves emergency units, primary and wound care clinics, mental health clinics, physiotherapy programs, and interdisciplinary burn centers. Each of these environments plays a vital role in the care of individuals who sustained smaller burn injuries and follow-up care of patients living with larger burn injuries after hospital discharge.

B. T. Stewart (✉)
Division of Trauma, Burn and Critical Care Surgery, UW Medicine Regional Burn Center, University of Washington, Harborview Medical Center, Seattle, WA, USA
e-mail: barclays@uw.edu

N. S. Gibran
Washington Research Foundation, Seattle, WA, USA

University of Washington, Seattle, WA, USA
e-mail: nicoleg@uw.edu

335
J. O. Lee (ed.), *Essential Burn Care for Non-Burn Specialists*, https://doi.org/10.1007/978-3-031-28898-2_16

Burn clinics within regional burn centers are interdisciplinary and provide comprehensive wound management, burn therapy, psychological treatment, functional activities, social support, and vocational rehabilitation. Given that most people in the world live far from an interdisciplinary burn center where these resources are available, coordinating community-based care is a core function of a regional burn center. Telemedicine now plays an important role as a triage, education, and care delivery platform [2–4].

Burn injuries, even small ones, can be devastating and lead to scarring, pain, itch, disfigurement, dysfunction, and distress. People living with even small burn injuries experience anxiety, depression, pain interference, acute stress symptoms, and difficulty with re-integration that can manifest in many ways and be subtle even to experienced burn care providers. Therefore, systematic screening of patients to detect concerning signs, symptoms, and impairments using patient-reported outcome (PRO) measures can identify those patients who need specialized care. Similarly, PRO measures can be used to track patient recovery over time, evaluate the effectiveness of care, and identify service delivery gaps.

Value of Interdisciplinary Outpatient Burn Care

Integrated, interdisciplinary outpatient care within a burn center can ensure quality care, reduce hospital lengths of stay, bolster inpatient care capacity, and reduce overall costs of care [1, 5, 6]. By concentrating burn-injured patients to a high-volume center, patients and healthcare systems benefit coupling patient volume and care quality through concentrating infrastructure, expertise, and resources [7, 8]. However, regional burn centers should also plan and organize outpatient burn care with collaborating outpatient therapy and mental health care providers within their catchment areas to facilitate encounters that are easier for patients and their support system in certain circumstances.

The multiple and complex sequelae of burn injuries can often be anticipated by experienced, interdisciplinary burn care teams. These sequelae include physical and psychosocial complications, poor community integration, and inability to return to work or school. When risk factors are recognized early, these sequelae can often be prevented or reduced with a combination of interdisciplinary management and follow-up coordination. However, reports from survivors have demonstrated that the clinical manifestations of these sequelae vary from patient to patient, can be subtle, and are often challenging to manage as an outpatient without dedicated burn care providers, nurses, therapists, psychologists, and vocational rehabilitation counselors [9].

Patients benefit from concentrated services. The burden of multiple outpatient care visits can be significantly reduced when all necessary interdisciplinary services (i.e., burn surgeons, nurses, therapists, mental health professionals, vocational rehabilitation specialists, physiatrists, social workers) are provided in a single encounter. Patients often prefer expert burn care delivered during interdisciplinary encounters and often by providers with whom they are familiar. Therefore, the added time and monetary costs associated with travel to regional centers often are sometimes valued greater than less organized or experienced burn care closer to home. Given the growing capacity for telemedicine, reducing travel-related burdens on patients and ensuring access to interdisciplinary burn care services no longer need to be competing interests.

Telemedicine (e.g., phone consultation, videoconference, use of photos to inform remote care) is technically feasible, and cost-effective for all burn care-related disciplines in the outpatient setting, including psychology and burn therapy (see Chap. 18) [10]. Telemedicine can play an important triage tool to identify patients who might benefit from in-person burn expert consultation and those who would be better served by care within their communities, avoiding unnecessary transfers [2, 11, 12]. Additionally, telemedicine review of patients and wounds at a burn center can be used to guide care by non-burn providers and serve to increase community-based burn care capacity over time [2, 10, 12]. Among the bright spots of the COVID-19 pandemic include increased use and acceptance of telemedicine. Telemedicine, when planned and organized within a burn center, is not associated with lower patient satisfaction or decreased wound and scar assessment fidelity compared with in-person care [3, 13]. Detailed guidelines produced by American Telemedicine Association for teleburn care can be found at american-telemed.org [14].

Although the costs of developing and maintaining integrated, interdisciplinary regional outpatient burn care are high, they are markedly lower than the costs associated with longer hospital stays, delays in diagnosis of outpatient complications (e.g., wound infections, range of motion impairment), and unplanned hospital readmissions [1]. Therefore, maintenance of regional, interdisciplinary burn centers, and increasing community-based care partnerships in a hub and spoke model can mitigate costs and improve local capacity for outpatient burn care [15].

Identifying Patients Who Are Appropriate for Outpatient Burn Care

Selecting patients with an acute burn injury who can achieve an excellent outcome without hospitalization is the first and most critical step in outpatient burn care. Four sets of factors determine whether or not a patient is appropriate for outpatient management:

1. Injury factors—size, depth, and location of injury, pain
2. Patient factors—age, comorbidities, functional status
3. Social factors—social support, concern for abuse or neglect, access to clean wound care environment and transportation
4. Local burn care capacity and interdisciplinary burn center outreach

Generally speaking, patients must have injuries that do not require inpatient care (e.g., no need for fluid resuscitation, complex wound care, or advanced pain management; no advanced comorbidities), the resources to manage their injuries and daily needs at home (e.g., clean wound care environment, social support), and ability to access burn care services when needed [16].

Commonly considered patient and injury characteristics that should prompt consultation with a burn center and possible inpatient management are listed in Table 16.1. Although these criteria were developed for well-resourced health systems, they can be used to inform decisions and protocols regarding appropriateness of outpatient care in any setting.

TABLE 16.1 Criteria for burn center referral adapted from American Burn Association Burn Center referral criteria

---

Example criteria for referral to an interdisciplinary burn center

Partial thickness burns ≥20% Total Body Surface Area (TBSA) in patients aged 10–50 years old

Partial thickness burns ≥10% TBSA in children aged 10 or adults aged 50 years old

Full-thickness burns ≥5% TBSA in patients of any age

Patients with partial or full-thickness burns of the hands, feet, face, eyes, ears, perineum, and/or major joints

Patients with high-voltage electrical injuries, including lightning injuries

Patients with significant burns from caustic chemicals

Patients with burns complicated by multiple trauma

Patients with burns who sustained inhalation injury

Patients with comorbidities that could complicate management, recovery, or mortality risk (e.g., substance use)

Burn injury in patients who will require special social, emotional and/or long-term rehabilitative support

Suspected child abuse

Regardless of setting and resource availability, it may be necessary to hospitalize a patient briefly until a more in-depth assessment of their injury, functional status, social support system, and access to transportation can be completed to facilitate successful outpatient care.

Thorough assessment of psychosocial comorbidities and social support is a key component of the decision-making process that may lead to proceeding with outpatient care. Patients must have a safe environment to live in, e.g., home, transitional housing, medical respite at a shelter. There can be no suspicion of abuse, neglect, or psychological conditions that may jeopardize the patient's safety or possibility to achieve a good outcome. Family and/or friends must be available to support the patient, particularly those who need assistance with mobility, wound care, and/or transportation.

Special Injury Considerations

Patients with combined burns and other trauma require a thorough evaluation at a trauma center. The combination of these injuries results in high risk of complications and mortality, even for smaller burn injuries. As an example, a retrospective analysis of the National Trauma Data Bank determined that the non-burn trauma exerts a negligible increase in the risk of a poor outcome; however, increase in the burn size, even for small burns, results in a stepwise increase in the rate of poor outcomes for patients with these combined injuries [17].

About one-third of burn patients sustain one or more types of inhalation injury (i.e., upper airway heat injury, tracheobronchial steam or chemical injury, parenchymal smoke irritant injury, and systemic toxicity—carbon monoxide, cyanide, as examples). Patients with a history of injury within an enclosed space or associated with exposure to heat, smoke, or chemicals and supporting clinical signs and symptoms should be managed at a burn center.

Although electrical and chemical injuries generally warrant consultation with a burn center, patients with smaller injuries can usually be managed as outpatients (see Chap. 13). Low-voltage household current (110–220 volts) electrical injuries typically cause only minor tissue damage. Patients who do not experience syncope and who have normal screening electrocardiogram (ECG) may be treated as outpatients without concern for subsequent cardiac events. However, anticipatory guidance is sometimes needed. As example, a toddler who chews on a live wire and sustains an injury to the oral commissure is at risk of delayed labial artery bleeding, particularly as the scab lifts off. Parents or caregivers should be educated about this risk and how to manage it by pinching the corner of the mouth and presenting to an emergency department.

Small chemical injuries can also be treated in the outpatient setting depending on the type of chemical, ability to perform decontamination, and location of the injury (see Chap. 14). Certain chemicals, such as powder alkalis and hydrofluoric acid, require serial decontamination and treatment that is often best suited for the inpatient setting. For those who can achieve adequate decontamination by brushing off dry powders and thorough irrigation of injuries until a normal skin pH is achieved, an outpatient plan can be created. Given that wound depth progression is common with chemical injuries, patients must be closely followed for infection, contracture, and need for surgical care.

Inpatient to Outpatient Transitions

Patients who require inpatient management for their injury and are nearing hospital discharge should be prioritized for follow-up at a burn center, particularly those with large burns or other significant injuries. The transition between inpatient and outpatient care is a vulnerable time for patients and their families, often characterized by competing feelings of joy to be leaving the hospital and new or exacerbated acute stress symptoms, fear, isolation, and anxiety [18]. Additionally, the functional gains achieved during inpatient care must be consolidated in the days and weeks after hospital discharge. Therefore, these patients are often best supported by close, interdisciplinary follow-up with providers within a known system.

Functions of an Outpatient Burn Clinic

When possible, care of patients with burn injuries in the outpatient setting should be interdisciplinary with careful attention paid to patients' physical, psychological, and social well-being. Specifically, nursing and wound care, scar management, functional activities, psychosocial therapy, and vocational rehabilitation services should be available for patients when needed either in-person or via telemedicine. Even small burns can have significant biopsychosocial impacts.

Burn Surgery Services

Burn surgeons play important roles in outpatient burn care, including clinical care, acute wound management, scar reconstruction, and long-term follow-up. Burn surgeons often guide the overall care of burn injured patients. During an outpatient encounter, the surgeon will assess the patient, wound and their broader psychosocial context for opportunities to reduce the risk of hypertrophic scar and contracture formation with surgical care. Over the long term, surgeons work with patients and the interdisciplinary team to mitigate the impacts that scars, contractures, and other sequelae of burn injury have on patients through a reconstruction plan. The array of specialist skills to manage acute burn injuries and burns as a chronic condition is extensive [19]. Surgeons must be aware of their limitations and seek consultation and co-management with other specialist colleagues when needed.

Wound Care and Nursing Services

Wound care and education comprise a significant proportion of burn clinic resources and nursing responsibilities. Successful wound management facilitates timely healing, minimizes the risk of infection, reduces pain, and prevents the need for inpatient care (see Chap. 6). Burn clinics should offer a variety of dressing options to achieve these goals depending on the patient and wound characteristics. As an example, some patients prefer daily dressing changes so that they can shower frequently, and others prefer longer term dressing options that minimize pain and anxiety of wound care. Importantly, wounds must be assessed during the first days and weeks from injury to evaluate and predict wound closure. Patients whose wounds are not anticipated to heal within 2–3 weeks should be evaluated for surgical wound closure to mitigate the risk of hypertrophic scar formation. Wound assessments should be timed such that decisions about benefits and risks of early excision and grafting can be made with the patient and their family. Concerns about wound infection, including patient-reported change in wound appearance or increased pain with wound care, should trigger expert wound assessment.

The American Burn Association (ABA) published *Burn Nursing: Scope and Standards of Practice* reflects a focused effort to establish specific guidelines for the specialty of burn nursing in both the inpatient and outpatient settings. Consensus-based burn nursing competencies should be applied to build nursing and wound care capacity in burn centers and to support regional education outreach programs [20].

Burn Therapy Services

Burn therapy is central to successful mobility, resumption of activities of daily living, and range of motion and strength (see Chap. 22). Burn therapists assess range of motion and risk of contracture, prescribe stretching and exercise programs, create custom splints and casts, recommend assistive devices and home and work adaptations, and coordinate care for new amputees. Like nurses, therapists provide critical educational services to patients and their families. In 2011, the Rehabilitation Committee of the ABA published clinical competencies for burn rehabilitation therapists [21]. These guidelines provide recommended standards of performance for therapists caring for burn patients. Given that many patients require community-based outpatient therapy to counteract contracture and improve range of motion and independence, expansion of burn therapy competency training to non-specialists and development of teletherapy programs are potentially valuable opportunities for burn center outreach and education to improve patient functional outcomes.

Psychology and Social Services

Burn injuries have a high prevalence of pain, pruritus, acute and post-traumatic stress symptoms, anxiety, depression, opioid misuse and abuse, changes in sexuality and intimacy and challenges with body image [22–28]. These symptoms constitute physical and mental function and often negatively impact social connectedness, community integration, and post-traumatic growth. Further, individual symptoms can be difficult to identify and can amplify one another, which complicates their management. National consensus has concluded that outpatient screening for pain interference, depression, and post-traumatic stress are critical for optimal care of burn patients [29, 30]. Furthermore, access to psychology and social services is critical in the outpatient burn setting to directly address burn-related mental health issues. Burn clinic psychologists commonly employ motivational interviewing, cognitive behavioral therapy (CBT), and relaxation exercises. [31, 32] In particular, CBT is a psychological intervention that improves people's ability to manage pain, acute stress symptoms, anxiety, and depression [33]. CBT generally focuses on challenging and changing unhelpful cognitive distortions, such as catastrophizing. It also targets maladaptive behaviors, improves emotional regulation, and aides in the development of personal coping strategies. The most common treatment dose of CBT involves 6–10, 60-min outpatient sessions. However, 4 sessions have been shown to have significant and similar benefits but with markedly less burden on patients in the outpatient setting [34]. CBT delivered through telemedicine has also been demonstrated to be safe and effective [35].

Non-surgical Scar Management Services

In addition to the care and planning provided by a burn surgeon, clinics should provide scar management services or referral opportunities for consultation and counseling about scar and treatment options, clinic-based treatments (e.g., intralesional therapies such as steroid injection, microneedling), fitting for custom pressure garments, scar massage, and coordination for surgical management. Management of scar in the outpatient setting is beyond the scope of this chapter (see Chap. 21).

Vocational Rehabilitation Services

Return to work has been identified as a core functional outcome for burn care and rehabilitation. Burn injury causes significant interruption of work, with an average time away from work of 17 weeks and only 66% of patients working at 6 months post-injury [36]. A significant number of patients may never return to work, with reported rates of only 60 to 80% of previously employed patients working at 1 year [37]. Vocational rehabilitation is essential for graduating patients back to the work environment. A key member of the outpatient burn care team is a vocational counselor who coordinates return to work with both patients and employers, including the need for duty modifications. Published evidence-based guidelines [37] for comprehensive return to work programs following burns include having a vocational counselor who [38]:.

1. Advocates for workers' rights and focuses on *ability*, not *disability*
2. Liaises between patient, employer burn center, workers' compensation, and labor and industry
3. Completes and updates the Activity Prescription Form
4. Encourages active patient participation in the return-to-work process
5. Provides a toolkit of activities for recovering patients to facilitate return to work
6. Distributes the Burn Model System *Employment After Burn Injury* factsheet.

Child Life and Scholastic Support Services

For children, return to school is an important goal for outpatient burn care and, on average, occurs 8–10 days following injury [39]. Despite a fast return, children may experience difficulty with managing pain at school, integration due to appearance, physical limitations, and the reactions of their peers [40]. Efforts should be made to help children keep up with schoolwork. School visits or videoconferences from the clinic may help reintroduce children who have changes in appearance or assistive devices to their teachers and peers. A comprehensive return to school program with a child-life specialist to educate peers and teachers and encourage acceptance represents best practice for burn centers that care for children [41]. These services are well-suited for telemedicine, particularly in virtual school settings.

General Principles of Outpatient Burn Care

The outpatient burn care plan for acute injuries should incorporate the following principles:

1. Screen for concerning signs, symptoms, and impairments
2. Perform patient and wound assessment
3. Cleanse the wound and develop a dressing plan
4. Manage pain, anxiety and acute stress symptoms
5. Assess range of motion and create a stretching and exercise plan
6. Educate patients and their support system
7. Define return conditions and schedule
8. Consider long-term follow-up to assess the patient and their scars

Screen for Concerning Signs, Symptoms, and Impairments

Identifying patients who need specific or additional services is a core function of outpatient burn care. People living with burn injuries experience a range of physical, psychological, and social morbidity. Further, morbidities can manifest in subtle ways that can go undetected if not systematically assessed with objective and valid measures [42–44]. Burn clinic staff can use brief measures to assess for overall physical and mental health and function and specific conditions common among people living with burn injuries, such as poor range of motion, significant pain interference, pruritus, anxiety, depression, isolation, and acute and post-traumatic stress disorder (ASD/PTSD). As an example, the International Society for Burn Injuries (ISBI) and other national burn associations (e.g., ABA, Australian, and New Zealand Burns Association [ANZBA]) recommend screening for ASD/PTSD, anxiety, depression, and alcohol abuse [1, 30, 45]. Examples of measures currently used by burn clinics include Patient-Reported Outcomes Measurement Information

System® (PROMIS) Global-10, Patient Health Questionnaire-2 (PHQ-2), CAGE Alcohol Questionnaire, and PTSD Checklist 5-Civilian (PCL-C).

ASD/PTSD are particularly common following burn injury. The presence of ASD early after injury predicts the development of PTSD, indicating that early diagnosis and treatment is beneficial [27, 46]. The prevalence of PTSD ranges from 2 to 40% by 6 months post-injury, 9 to 45% in the year post-injury, and 7 to 25% more than 2 years post-injury [46]. This prevalence is more than twice that of the general population. Symptoms including intrusive thoughts, nightmares, flashbacks, and hypervigilance are common among people living with both conditions. Standardizing screening and the use of validated tools can identify patients in need of treatment early. The PCL-C has been used for this purpose, although other tools are available [47, 48]. The Primary Care PTSD screen is a short, four-item test designed for use in the primary care setting [49]. Patients who screen positive should either receive psychological treatment or be referred to a mental health provider for evaluation and treatment. Systematic use of PRO measures as screening tools allows for efficient application of the intensive resources required to manage severe physical and psychosocial comorbidities to the patients who need them most.

Perform Patient and Wound Assessment

In addition to performing a standard history and physical examination, the outpatient provider should examine the wound and consider its size, distribution, depth, and stage of healing. Interpreting burn wounds, particularly early after injury, can be challenging since the wound depth may progress or become more apparent 72–96 h after injury. Photos and videoconferencing can be used to support consultation with an experienced burn care provider and/or track changes in the wound appearance and healing over time, particularly when incorporated into the medical record [3]. Burn wound assessment is covered in detail elsewhere in Chap. 6.

Cleanse the Wound and Develop a Dressing Plan

Wounds should be washed with soap and water, and loose blisters and non-viable skin remnants should be debrided. Opinions about the optimal management of and dressing plan for burn wounds vary. Numerous randomized controlled trials and observational studies have demonstrated that no single technique is superior [50]. It is important to consider wound characteristics, patient / family ability to manage the wound and execute the dressing plan, and the general dressing principles. A cross-sectional survey of 121 burn providers from 39 countries provided insight into the ideal burn dressing qualities [51]. Respondents recommended that the ideal dressing would establish an optimum micro-environment for wound healing, maintain the wound temperature and moisture level, allow epithelial migration, exclude environmental bacteria, minimize pain, not require daily changes, and be affordable. Although there is no ideal dressing to date, many of these qualities are satisfied by the use of non-stick gauze and antibiotic ointment, silver-impregnated dressings, and biological dressings [52]. All wounds should be supported with gentle compression to minimize swelling and pain from vascular engorgement and reduce the risk of infection [53].

Manage Pain, Anxiety, and Acute Stress Symptoms

Patients should undergo a systematic assessment to understand their pain, anxiety, and acute stress symptoms (see Chap. 16). Most patients will require pain medication for wound care. Acetaminophen and/or non steroidal anti-inflammatory drugs (NSAIDs) are often sufficient, but low doses of opioids may be needed in some cases. Pain medications with or without a low dose of anxiolytic medication can be provided for patients to take ~30 min prior to their outpatient visit to facilitate more comfortable and less traumatic wound care in the outpatient setting, particularly for their first dressing removal or when conservative debridement is anticipated.

Multimodal analgesia should be prescribed for patients who have background and breakthrough pain despite use of the medications above or who are living with significant pain interference. Multimodal analgesia consists of targeted pharmacological therapies with varying mechanisms combined with non-pharmacological techniques [54]. In addition to acetaminophen, NSAIDs, and opioids, patients with more complex pain needs may also be prescribed gabapentinoids, α–adrenergic agonists, tricyclic antidepressants (TCA), and serotonin-norepinephrine reuptake inhibitors (SNRI) (e.g., duloxetine) [29]. The goal of multimodal analgesia is to reduce pain intensity and interference while minimizing side effects from any one class of medication. Although theoretically useful and commonly employed, observational studies of burn pain management have demonstrated that multimodal analgesia that includes gabapentin ± duloxetine did not consistently reduce pain intensity [55].

Opioid misuse, abuse, and diversion can occur after burn injury. However, the vast majority of patients do not use opioids 30 days after injury [56]. Therefore, efforts to identify those at high risk of opioid misuse and abuse and provision of supportive strategy for opioid tapering in the outpatient setting are required [57]. Given the frequency of preinjury substance use disorder, collaboration with addiction and pain medicine specialists is often needed to achieve excellent outcomes for these vulnerable patients [29, 58].

Most patients will not have anxiety or acute stress symptoms that require pharmacological therapy. Instead, non-pharmacological techniques can be taught to patients and used when needed (e.g., relaxation, distraction, cognitive restructuring, time- or quota-based activity pacing, sleep hygiene) [27, 31, 32, 59–61]. Patients with significant anxiety, depression, and acute stress symptoms should be referred for cognitive behavioral therapy at a burn center or with a mental health provider close to their home [31, 62].

Pruritus can occur after a burn injury during the wound healing and scar remodeling phases [55, 63–65]. Postburn pruritus may begin early after a burn injury and can persist

afterward. Itch affects more than 40% of long-term burn survivors [64]. Despite this high prevalence, the pathophysiology
of pruritus following burn injury is poorly understood.
Although itch of cutaneous origin shares a common neural
pathway with pain, the afferent nerve fibers conducting itch
are a distinct subset: they respond to histamine, acetylcholine,
and other pruritogens, but are generally insensitive to
mechanical stimuli [66]. An elegant hypothesis proposes four
classes of itch: cutaneous (proprioceptive), neuropathic, neurogenic, and psychogenic [66]. Treatment of postburn itch,
like pain, should be approached in a systematic way that
acknowledges the aforementioned classes of itch using multimodal protocols [67]. Although numerous treatments are
prescribed for postburn pruritus (e.g., moisturizer, topical
lidocaine, anti-histamines, gabapentinoids, ondansetron, μ
opioid antagonists, κ opioid agonists, TCA, SSNRI, steroid
injection, laser therapy), there is no consensus on the best
protocol or biomarkers for use of specific agents. Some trial
and error and time are typically required to achieve satisfactory relief.

Assess Range of Motion and Create a Stretching and Exercise Plan

Providers and/or therapists should assess the range of motion
of joints affected by a burn and develop a stretching and exercise plan that mitigates contractures. Regardless of whether a
wound heals on its own or is skin grafted, a scar is formed: all
scars contract. Although wound contraction is a normal
response to injury, a major goal of therapy is to prevent contracture formation, the complication of excessive contraction,
usually across joints or areas with lax skin. Contracture limits
range of motion by forming scar bands that span joints.
Stretching and exercise increase or maintain range of motion
by applying force across scar and, through repetition, increase
the resting length of the tissue. Exercises should begin during
the acute phase of injury and continue throughout the period

of scar remodeling, which may last up to 24 months. The principles of stretching and exercise plans include the following:

1. Observe tissue reaction without dressings or garments
2. Monitor blanching of the wound to avoid prolonged vascular compromise
3. Slow, sustained stress is more tolerable and effective for lengthening tissue than quick, short stretches
4. Elongate skin, scar, and muscle with combined joint movements
5. Use functional exercises that mimic daily and work-related activities
6. Position limbs and joints to maintain increased range of motion after exercise

Splinting and casting can be used to prevent or modify scar contracture formation (See Chap. 21) [68]. Indications for splinting include the prevention of deformity, lengthening of tissue, preservation of length, and protection of skin grafts. Splints allow the application of low force over long periods of time, which maintains range of motion and function during periods of immobility, such as sleep. Splints may be static, static progressive, or dynamic; the latter is employed if exercise and static splinting fail to gain adequate range of motion.

The indications for splinting change with the phase of outpatient burn care. In the acute phase, splinting focuses on edema control, maintaining position, and relief of pressure points to facilitate uniform healing. In the intermediate phase, protection of grafts and maintaining adequate range of motion become more important. In the long term, emphasis is on the mitigation of scar contracture. It should be explicitly stated that splints and casts are not substitutes for range of motion exercises.

Serial casting also allows application of low force over time to stretch tissue [69]. Casts may be useful for patients with low adherence to a rehabilitation plan, as they are more difficult to remove than splints. However, casting eliminates the ability to perform regular range of motion exercises and causes muscle atrophy of the casted extremity. Additionally, casts require reapplication at regular intervals to apply equal and adequate forces over time.

Educate Patients and Their Support System

There are few injuries and conditions that require as much participation from patients and families to achieve a good outcome than burn injuries. It is vital to educate patients and their support systems and incorporate them into the care process as collaborators. Clinic visits should include ample time for education to maintain their understanding of and participation in the recovery processes. Education can be augmented by factsheets (https://msktc.org/burn/factsheets), videos, and augmented reality tools. The Model Systems Knowledge Translation Center (MSKTC) has factsheets for burn-injured patients and their providers on topics such as wound care, pain, psychological distress, exercise, itchy skin, employment after injury, scar management, sleep problems, sexuality and intimacy, social interaction, sun protection, and body image. Additionally, survivorship communities, like the Phoenix Society for Burn Survivors (https://www.phoenix-society.org), provide people living with burn injury and their providers with resources to improve care and understanding and connects survivors to others who have experienced similar injuries.

Define Return Conditions and Schedule

In the acute phase, specific signs and symptoms that mandate early reassessment should be discussed. Such issues include increasing pain or anxiety associated with dressing changes, signs of infection, functional decline, inability to sleep, and safety concerns. Frequency of clinic visits varies based upon the needs of the patient. Generally, patients with an acute injury should be evaluated 1–2 times per week. Patients who live close to a clinic could be seen daily for wound care if needed, and those who liver further away could be managed with a combination of in-person and telemedicine visits during the healing process.

Consider Need for Long-Term Follow-Up to Assess the Patient and Their Scar

Patients with wounds that do not heal within 14 days have increased scarring risk; the majority of wounds that remain open for longer than 21 days develop some degree of hypertrophic scarring [26]. A hypertrophic scar is a raised, erythematous, pruritic, and inelastic mass of tissue that results from a large amount of extracellular matrix of altered composition and organization compared to normal dermis. Hypertrophic scarring is common, with a prevalence that ranges between 32 and 72% depending on factors such as presence of specific genes, TBSA burn, location of injury, and time to healing [70–72]. Scar formation can result in contracture, pain, itch, loss of thermal regulation, stigmatization, and psychological distress [26]. Some patients develop hypertrophic scar without risk factors. Therefore, follow-up visits should be planned for patients to return to the clinic or send photographs of their wounds within 1–3 months after wound closure and until the scar has matured, which may be a year or more after injury. During these encounters, providers can assess the scar, discuss its impact on the patient's function and quality of life, and develop a scar management plan (see Chap. 21).

Outreach to Support Community-Based Burn Care

There will be circumstances when patients are unable or unwilling to travel the long distances necessary to access interdisciplinary burn centers for in-person care. Additionally, some patients, injuries, and problems need initial consultation and close surveillance by an interdisciplinary burn team but not the intensity of an in-person encounter. Therefore, burn centers should establish outreach programs to support community-based providers, particularly in regions and contexts where travel can be long or burdensome. These programs have taken the form of satellite clinics managed and staffed by a regional burn center or indirectly by identifying, training, and supporting community-based care providers. Ways in which burn centers have optimized outpatient care include the creation of specific care and consultation pathways, implementation of locoregional quality improvement programs, continuing education opportunities, and dissemination of best-practice guidelines.

Pathways

With a mature trauma system with established referral practices, burn care pathways can streamline consultation and transfer requests, reduce under- and over-triage rates, extend burn care expertise within a geographic region, increase the efficiency of burn center services, and improve patient satisfaction. As an example, the UW Medicine Regional Burn Center developed four pathways (Table 16.2) to make referring practitioners comfortable with emergency care of burn wounds and facilitate burn expert assessment of burn wounds. Practitioners at emergency departments and clinics within the region call UW Medicine Transfer Center and provide information regarding the patient, injury, local capacity, and specific request. Nurses at the Transfer Center then determine which of four pathways the patient should follow and enact the respective protocol. In addition to collating information, the Transfer Center coordinates photos of the injury to inform recommendations by a burn surgeon at the UW Medicine Regional Burn Center. When appropriate, the Transfer Center notifies the Burn Clinic via an electronic platform and the Burn Clinic calls the patient the next busi-

TABLE 16.2 Example of regional consultation and transfer pathways adapted from UW Medicine Regional Burn Center

Pathway	Consulting practitioner request	Indications	Protocol highlights
Black	Urgent consult with a burn surgeon	Airway concerns, >5% TBSA and full-thickness injuries, electrical and chemical injuries, concomitant burn and other injuries, and/or a social concern (e.g., abuse or neglect)	Transfer Center connects the referring practitioner to the on-call burn surgeon. Depending on the case, the patient is then either transferred for inpatient care at the Burn Center or a Burn Clinic follow-up plan is made.
Red	Transfer due to inadequate capacity for inpatient or outpatient care	Patient and/or burn injury that exceeds local capacity	Transfer Center connects the referring practitioner to the on-call burn surgeon. Patient transfer to the Burn Center is arranged.
Blue	Brief consultation to facilitate local care without transfer to the Burn Center	Patient and injury that can be managed locally with the consultation with and support of an experienced burn care provider	Burn Clinic coordination is provided based on the patient and injury.
Green	Outpatient follow-up at the Burn Center	Small burn injuries and patients who otherwise meet outpatient criteria	Transfer Center and Burn Clinic create a follow-up plan.

ness day with appointment details. This system manages about 150 consultations per month, 75% of which are treated locally with guidance by the Burn Center. This triage tool has significantly reduced under- and over-triage of patients to the Burn Center.

Quality Improvement

Local and burn center quality improvement (QI) programs should systematically collect burn care metrics (e.g., under- and over-triage, adherence to best-practice guidelines, wound infection rate, unplanned hospital admission rates, patient satisfaction) and review them individually and within the context of a wider burn care system. Such QI programs serve to identify opportunities to improve triage performance and the quality of care provided to inpatients and outpatients. Detailed guidance for local and regional burn care quality improvement programming in low- and middle-income coun-

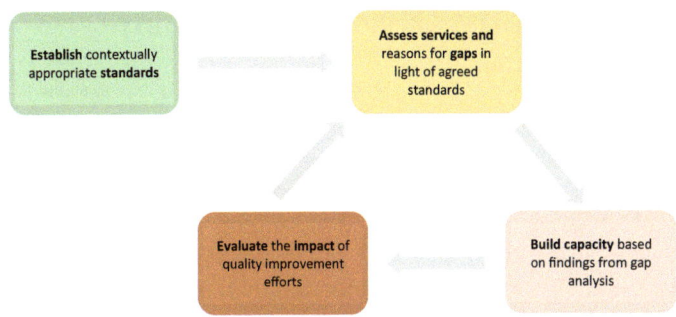

Fig. 16.1 Framework for local and regional burn care quality improvement programs adapted from Interburns (International Network for Training, Education and Research in Burns) [73]

tries has been published by Interburns (International Network for Training, Education and Research in Burns) [73]. The Interburns framework describes the steps to define clinical standards, evaluate service delivery and perform a gap analysis, build targeted capacity, and assess the impact of the efforts (Fig. 16.1). Ethiopia, Ghana, Malawi, India, Bangladesh, Cote D'Ivoire, Pakistan, Palestine, and Nepal have taken part in all or parts of this process to improve care for burn patients [73, 74].

Training

Burn center outreach should include training programs for community practitioners that strengthen their ability to triage burn-injured patients, provide outpatient care, and recognize the need for consultation and referral. Training programs might take the form of continuing medical education courses, workshops to target specific capacity deficiencies, and/or webinars. The use of social media platforms can extend burn prevention, first aid and care messaging and support outreach initiatives. Over time, the cumulative effect of these activities will increase burn care knowledge and capacity in communities more proximate to patient homes.

Use of Outcome Measures for Quality Improvement

Assessing the performance of clinical services using PRO measures is a core function of burn care. People living with small or large burn injuries may sustain temporary or irreparable loss of function due to the injury, burn care system dysfunction, failure of social support, and/or patient characteristics. When burn care and rehabilitation efforts fail to return patients to a preinjury functional state, it is imperative that patients retain a good quality of life. Quality of life data can determine the effectiveness of the care being provided and inform long-term expectations of patients and their support systems.

A United States program (Burn Model System, BMS) was established in 1993 by the predecessor of the National Institute of Disability, Independent Living and Rehabilitation Research (NIDILRR). The BMS National Database now includes >7200 participants from six major interdisciplinary burn centers with follow-up ranging from 6 months to 20 years. Reports from the BMS have contributed valuable information about participants' experiences during recovery from a burn injury, risk factors for poor outcomes, and opportunities to engineer burn care systems to be more responsive to patients' needs. Additionally, BMS and the NIDILRR Model Systems Knowledge Translation Center have produced resources and educational materials for patients and providers that are essential to outpatient burn care and improving outcomes for burn survivors [75].

The challenge for burn care systems becomes incorporating the systematic use of PRO measures into clinical care and using those data to inform individual patient care needs, opportunities for quality improvement, and the impacts of specific burn care system interventions. These challenges are even greater where care is distributed across multiple environments and when it is delivered across multiple platforms. However, these changes in the delivery of outpatient burn care are all the more reasons to ensure patients receive the services they need and achieve optimal outcomes.

Conclusion

The goal of outpatient burn care is to manage acute injuries and return patients to their preinjury level of function. To maximize this potential, an interdisciplinary team approach with specific, measurable functional goals is needed. This approach can be achieved at a regional burn center or at non-specialty clinics with incorporation of burn expert outreach, consultation, and telemedicine. Regular assessment of patient progress, wound healing, scar formation, and creation of personalized treatment plans is essential. Given the lack of strong evidence-based guidelines for outpatient burn management, care should be performed in consultation with experienced providers from interdisciplinary burn centers [1,45]. Regardless of the burn care system structure, use of PROs should define therapeutic requirements, referral to advanced specialty care, and evaluate burn care performance.

References

1. Committee IPG, Advisory S, Steering S. ISBI practice guidelines for burn care, part 2. Burns. 2018;44(7):1617–706.
2. Martinez R, et al. The value of WhatsApp communication in paediatric burn care. Burns. 2018;44(4):947–55.
3. Cai LZ, et al. Accuracy of remote burn scar evaluation via live video-conferencing technology. Burns. 2017. https://doi.org/10.1016/j.burns.2016.11.006.
4. Atiyeh B, Dibo SA, Janom HH. Telemedicine and burns: an overview. Ann Burns Fire Disasters. 2014;27(2):87–93.

5. Wiechman SA, et al. An expanded delivery model for outpatient burn rehabilitation. J Burn Care Res. 2015;36(1):14–22.

6. Kastenmeier A, et al. The evolution of resource utilization in regional burn centers. J Burn Care Res. 2010;31(1):130–6.

7. Caputo LM, et al. The relationship between patient volume and mortality in American trauma centres: a systematic review of the evidence. Injury. 2014;45(3):478–86.

8. Palmieri TL, et al. Burn center volume makes a difference for burned children. Pediatr Crit Care Med. 2015;16(4):319–24.

9. Wiechman S, Holavanahalli R. Burn survivor focus group. J Burn Care Res. 2017;38(3):e593–5.

10. Boccara D, et al. Ongoing development and evaluation of a method of telemedicine: burn care management with a smartphone. J Burn Care Res. 2018;39(4):580–4.

11. Curtis EE, et al. Early patient deaths after transfer to a regional burn center. Burns. 2019;46(1):97–103.

12. Wiktor AJ, et al. Multiregional utilization of a Mobile device app for triage and transfer of burn patients. J Burn Care Res. 2018;39(6):858–62.

13. Yenikomshian HA, et al. Evaluation of burn rounds using telemedicine: perspectives from patients, families, and burn center staff. Telemed J E Health. 2019;25(1):25–30.

14. Theurer L, et al. American Telemedicine Association guidelines for Teleburn. Telemed J E Health. 2017;23(5):365–75.

15. Mandal A. Quality and cost-effectiveness—effects in burn care. Burns. 2007;33(4):414–7.

16. Warner PM, Coffee TL, Yowler CJ. Outpatient burn management. Surg Clin North Am. 2014;94(4):879–92.

17. Grigorian A, et al. Rising mortality in patients with combined burn and trauma. Burns. 2018;44(8):1989–96.

18. Gotlib Conn L, et al. Trauma patient discharge and care transition experiences: identifying opportunities for quality improvement in trauma centres. Injury. 2018;49(1):97–103.

19. Al-Mousawi AM, et al. Burn teams and burn centers: the importance of a comprehensive team approach to burn care. Clin Plast Surg. 2009;36(4):547–54.

20. Carrougher GJ, et al. Burn nurse competencies: developing consensus using E-Delphi methodology. J Burn Care Res. 2018;39(5):751–9.

21. Parry I, Esselman PC, A. Rehabilitation Committee of the American Burn, clinical competencies for burn rehabilitation therapists. J Burn Care Res. 2011;32(4):458–67.

22. Amtmann D, et al. Pain across traumatic injury groups: A National Institute on Disability, Independent Living, and Rehabilitation Research model systems study. J Trauma Acute Care Surg. 2020;89(4):829–33.

23. Grant GG, et al. Exploring the burn model system national database: burn injuries, substance misuse, and the CAGE questionnaire. Burns. 2020;46(3):745–7.

24. Pham TN, et al. The impact of discharge contracture on return to work after burn injury: a burn model system investigation. Burns. 2020;46(3):539–45.

25. Amtmann D, et al. Satisfaction with life over time in people with burn injury: a National Institute on Disability, Independent Living, and Rehabilitation Research burn model system study. Arch Phys Med Rehabil. 2020;101(1S):S63–70.

26. Goverman J, et al. The presence of scarring and associated morbidity in the burn model system national database. Ann Plast Surg. 2019;82(3 Suppl 2):S162–8.

27. Wiechman SA, et al. Reasons for distress among burn survivors at 6, 12, and 24 months postdischarge: a burn injury model system investigation. Arch Phys Med Rehabil. 2018;99(7):1311–7.

28. McAleavey AA, et al. Physical, functional, and psychosocial recovery from burn injury are related and their relationship changes over time: a burn model system study. Burns. 2018;44(4):793–9.

29. Romanowski KS, et al. American Burn Association guidelines on the management of acute pain in the adult burn patient: a review of the literature, a compilation of expert opinion, and next steps. J Burn Care Res. 2020;41(6):1129–51.

30. Gibran NS, et al. Summary of the 2012 ABA burn quality consensus conference. J Burn Care Res. 2013;34(4):361–85.

31. Cukor J, et al. The treatment of posttraumatic stress disorder and related psychosocial consequences of burn injury: a pilot study. J Burn Care Res. 2015;36(1):184–92.

32. Seehausen A, et al. Efficacy of a burn-specific cognitive-behavioral group training. Burns. 2015;41(2):308–16.

33. Hajihasani A, et al. The influence of cognitive behavioral therapy on pain, quality of life, and depression in patients receiving physical therapy for chronic low back pain: a systematic review. PM R. 2019;11(2):167–76.

34. Jensen MP, et al. Psychosocial factors and adjustment to chronic pain in persons with physical disabilities: a systematic review. Arch Phys Med Rehabil. 2011;92(1):146–60.

35. Dent L, et al. Using telehealth to implement cognitive-behavioral therapy. Psychiatr Serv. 2018;69(4):370–3.
36. Brych SB, et al. Time off work and return to work rates after burns: systematic review of the literature and a large two-center series. J Burn Care Rehabil. 2001;22(6):401–5.
37. Mason ST, et al. Return to work after burn injury: a systematic review. J Burn Care Res. 2012;33(1):101–9.
38. Carrougher GJ, et al. An intervention bundle to facilitate return to work for burn-injured workers: report from a burn model system investigation. J Burn Care Res. 2017;38(1):e70–8.
39. Esselman PC. Community integration outcome after burn injury. Phys Med Rehabil Clin N Am. 2011;22(2):351–6, vii.
40. Christiansen M, et al. Time to school re-entry after burn injury is quite short. J Burn Care Res. 2007;28(3):478–81; discussion 482–3.
41. Blakeney P, et al. Efficacy of school reentry programs. J Burn Care Rehabil. 1995;16(4):469–72; discussion 466–8.
42. Amtmann D, et al. National Institute on Disability, Independent Living, and Rehabilitation Research burn model system: review of program and database. Arch Phys Med Rehabil. 2020;101(1S):S5–S15.
43. Wiechman S, Hoyt MA, Patterson DR. Using a biopsychosocial model to understand long-term outcomes in persons with burn injuries. Arch Phys Med Rehabil. 2020;101(1S):S55–62.
44. Amtmann D, et al. Psychometric properties of the satisfaction with life scale in people with traumatic brain, spinal cord, or burn injury: a National Institute on Disability, Independent Living, and Rehabilitation Research model system study. Assessment. 2017;26(4):695–705.
45. ISBI Practice Guidelines Committee; Steering Subcommittee; Advisory Subcommittee. ISBI practice guidelines for burn care. Burns. 2016;42(5):953–1021.
46. Giannoni-Pastor A, et al. Prevalence and predictors of posttraumatic stress symptomatology among burn survivors: a systematic review and meta-analysis. J Burn Care Res. 2016;37(1):e79–89.
47. Falder S, et al. Core outcomes for adult burn survivors: a clinical overview. Burns. 2009;35(5):618–41.
48. Wiechman SA. Psychosocial recovery, pain, and itch after burn injuries. Phys Med Rehabil Clin N Am. 2011;22(2):327–45, vii.
49. Prins A, et al. The primary care PTSD screen for DSM-5 (PC-PTSD-5): development and evaluation within a veteran primary care sample. J Gen Intern Med. 2016;31(10):1206–11.

50. Wasiak J, et al. Dressings for superficial and partial thickness burns. Cochrane Database Syst Rev. 2013;(3):CD002106.

51. Selig HF, et al. The properties of an "ideal" burn wound dressing—what do we need in daily clinical practice? Results of a worldwide online survey among burn care specialists. Burns. 2012;38(7):960–6.

52. Douglas HE, Wood F. Burns dressings. Aust Fam Physician. 2017;46(3):94–7.

53. Webb E, et al. Compression therapy to prevent recurrent cellulitis of the leg. N Engl J Med. 2020;383(7):630–9.

54. McGreevy K, Bottros MM, Raja SN. Preventing chronic pain following acute pain: risk factors, preventive strategies, and their efficacy. Eur J Pain Suppl. 2011;5(2):365–72.

55. Kneib CJ, et al. The effects of early neuropathic pain control with gabapentin on long-term chronic pain and itch in burn patients. J Burn Care Res. 2019;40(4):457–63.

56. Yenikomshian HA, et al. Outpatient opioid use of burn patients: a retrospective review. Burns. 2019;45(8):1737–42.

57. Kim DE, et al. A review of adjunctive therapies for burn injury pain during the opioid crisis. J Burn Care Res. 2019;40(6):983–95.

58. Leazer ST, et al. Analgesic use in contemporary burn practice: applications to burn mass casualty incident planning. Burns. 2020;46(1):90–6.

59. Patterson DR, et al. Virtual reality hypnosis for pain associated with recovery from physical trauma. Int J Clin Exp Hypn. 2010;58(3):288–300.

60. Fauerbach JA, et al. Psychological distress after major burn injury. Psychosom Med. 2007;69(5):473–82.

61. Bryant RA, et al. Treatment of acute stress disorder: a randomized controlled trial. Arch Gen Psychiatry. 2008;65(6):659–67. https://doi.org/10.1001/archpsyc.65.6.659.

62. Knoerl R, Lavoie Smith EM, Weisberg J. Chronic pain and cognitive behavioral therapy: an integrative review. West J Nurs Res. 2016;38(5):596–628.

63. Schneider JC, et al. Pruritus in pediatric burn survivors: defining the clinical course. J Burn Care Res. 2015;36(1):151–8.

64. Carrougher GJ, et al. Pruritus in adult burn survivors: postburn prevalence and risk factors associated with increased intensity. J Burn Care Res. 2013;34(1):94–101.

65. Otene CI, Onumaegbu OO. Post-burn pruritus: need for standardization of care in Nigeria. Ann Burns Fire Disasters. 2013;26(2):63–7.

66. Twycross R, et al. Itch: scratching more than the surface. QJM. 2003;96(1):7–26.
67. Richardson C, Upton D, Rippon M. Treatment for wound pruritus following burns. J Wound Care. 2014;23(5):227–8, 230, 232-3.
68. Jang KU, et al. Multi-axis shoulder abduction splint in acute burn rehabilitation: a randomized controlled pilot trial. Clin Rehabil. 2015;29(5):439–46.
69. Bennett GB, et al. Serial casting: a method for treating burn contractures. J Burn Care Rehabil. 1989;10(6):543–5.
70. Agabalyan NA, et al. Comparison between high-frequency ultrasonography and histological assessment reveals weak correlation for measurements of scar tissue thickness. Burns. 2017;43(3):531–8. https://doi.org/10.1016/j.burns.2016.09.008. Epub 2017 Jan 18.
71. Lawrence JW, et al. Epidemiology and impact of scarring after burn injury: a systematic review of the literature. J Burn Care Res. 2012;33(1):136–46.
72. Sood RF, et al. Genome-wide association study of postburn scarring identifies a novel protective variant. Ann Surg. 2015;262(4):563–9.
73. Potokar T, et al. A comprehensive, integrated approach to quality improvement and capacity building in burn care and prevention in low and middle-income countries: an overview. Burns. 2020;46(8):1756–67.
74. Potokar T, et al. Training of medical and paramedical personnel in burn care and prevention. Indian J Plast Surg. 2010;43(Suppl):S121–5.
75. Carrougher GJ, et al. 'Living Well' after burn injury: using case reports to illustrate significant contributions from the burn model system research program. J Burn Care Res. 2020;42(3):398–407.

Chapter 17
Telemedicine

Lauren B. Nosanov and Amalia Cochran

Effective prevention efforts have resulted globally in a lower incidence of burn injury. An unforeseen consequence of this success in the United States is an overall decrease in centers providing regionalized burn care, with only 70 American Burn Association (ABA) verified centers in the United States as of 2020 [1–3]. Remaining centers have developed progressively larger catchment areas, often necessitating air transport when interfacility transfers are needed [4–7]. Disparities in access to specialized burn care persist nationally, particularly in rural regions [3, 8]. Global access is sparse and is a major challenge as 90% of burns occur in developing or underdeveloped countries, with the majority of those burned being children [1]. Telemedicine has become one of the major modes used to bridge these gaps at a local, locoregional, regional, national, and international level [9, 10].

The Institute of Medicine defines telemedicine as "the use of electronic information and communications technologies to provide and support health care when distance separates

L. B. Nosanov
Department of Surgery, University of Wisconsin,
Madison, WI, USA

A. Cochran (✉)
Department of Surgery, University of Florida, Gainesville, FL, USA
e-mail: amalia.cochran@surgery.ufl.edu

participants" [11]. Earlier forms of telemedicine technologies were asynchronous, consisting of storing and forwarding images and communications. While this approach remains popular, synchronous interactive platforms have become more widely used. Associated technologies are numerous and include a variety of modalities including web-based platforms, proprietary communication systems, encrypted text, and video messaging services such as WhatsApp, Facebook Portal, FaceTime, and Skype, non-encrypted texting from personal phones, and publicly and privately available burn-specific applications for mobile devices such as Burn App and Teleburn App [12–17]. Standard digital cameras and smartphones provide adequate image resolution for accurate diagnosis and clinical decision-making [18].

The medical community has long appreciated the value of telemedicine, citing diminished unnecessary travel, increased cost savings, availability of specialty services, improved rates of post-operative follow-up, expediency of "real time" communication, and teleconferencing and education across large distances and even across national borders [12, 19]. The benefits of telemedicine have been established in studies of multiple surgical subspecialties, with application to both adult and pediatric patient populations [20, 21]. Telemedicine is a crucial tool for triage and management in the setting of natural disasters and can be used during triage, resuscitation, and evacuation from military settings in remote front-line austere environments [1].

Within burn care, telemedicine has been used for over 20 years. Current technology allows for provider-to-provider consultation as well as direct patient-provider communication. A 2012 survey of ABA burn center directors showed that 84% were using at least one form of telemedicine as a part of their practice [22]. Patient portals enable outpatient consultation, post-operative or post-discharge monitoring, guidance and troubleshooting of home wound care, long-term scar monitoring, rehabilitative care, and ongoing psychosocial support that draws on the multidisciplinary resources provided by burn centers [12, 20, 23, 24].

Widespread adoption of telemedicine for burn care has been slow, due in part to a dearth of high-level evidence supporting efficacy, patient satisfaction, cost effectiveness, and safety. Initially, Massman et al. published a small case series out of Regions Hospital Burn Center, finding that telemedicine follow-up improved access to rural and underserved areas and diminished travel time and costs [25]. A subsequent publication from the same group evaluated a larger cohort of patients with similar findings [26]. The body of supporting literature has since grown, as demonstrated in a 2012 systematic review by Wallace et al. [18]. The authors identified 24 studies, eight of which assessed technical feasibility and clinical validation, seven of which looked at clinical decision-making in acute burn care, and nine that focused on outpatient care. Although some have expressed concern as to burn provider capacity to accurately evaluate burn injuries by photographic images alone, data show that addition of a visual component to consultation improves estimation of burn total body surface area (TBSA) [1, 18, 20, 23, 27].

With the diminishing prevalence of burn injuries, non-specialist providers are experiencing less exposure to burns both in training and in practice. Misestimation of burn size and severity can lead to both under-triage and over-triage, which can be ameliorated by utilization of telemedicine [4, 13, 28, 29]. Lack of familiarity most often leads to overestimation of burn size and underestimation of burn depth [3]. A recent systematic review on burn size estimation by Pham et al. found that TBSA burn miscalculations between 5 and 339% were reported within the 26 articles evaluated [28]. It has been demonstrated elsewhere that overestimation of burn TBSA occurs in up to 70% of patients transferred to burn centers [5, 30]. One retrospective analysis of all burn patients transferred by air to a regional burn center found that referring physicians' analyses of burn size differed from burn center measures by 9% TBSA, comprising 75% of the total burn size [7]. There are numerous, significant consequences of burn size misestimation including unnecessary healthcare costs, misappropriation of limited resources, and delay in providing appropriate patient care. Further, burn TBSA overestimation is linked with over-resuscitation, which in turn results in increased morbidity and mortality from complications such as abdominal compartment syndrome [18, 28, 29].

Lack of familiarity with inhalation injury is similarly a major source of avoidable morbidity as well as cost. Although there is a risk of underappreciation of airway edema and potential for airway loss, the tendency is toward overestimation of this risk. Romanowski et al. showed that more than one-third of intubations in patients transferred to burn centers could be considered unnecessary, in that many patients were extubated within 24 h of arrival to the burn center [31]. Similarly, Wibbenmeyer et al. found that while only 5% of patients were intubated in a pre-hospital or pre-transfer setting, nearly two-thirds were extubated within 24 h of transfer [30]. Kashefi et al. reported a 14.5% rate of intubation among over-triaged patients which they attributed to potential over-diagnosis of inhalation injury or airway compromise [6].

Recent updated burn center referral criteria aid in identifying patients with injuries who benefit from telehealth consultation for triage (Table 17.1) [32]. These include full-thickness burns greater than 5% TBSA, adults older than 55, children with burns greater than 10% TBSA, chemical burns, inhalation injury, high-voltage and lightening electrical injuries, and those with injury due to frostbite. Patients with epidermal skin sloughing disorders such as Stevens-Johnson syndrome (SJS), toxic epidermal necrolysis (TEN), and necrotizing soft tissue infection (NSTI) are also recommended for transfer given that they benefit from nursing expertise and multidisciplinary support more readily available at a burn center. Beyond this, patients who benefit from burn center consultation include full-thickness burns of any size, children with burns smaller than 10% TBSA, and low-voltage electrical injuries. Referring providers caring for patients not in need of transfer can acquire guidance as to initial management including wound dressing choice and can establish a plan for follow-up with either local providers, burn center outpatient clinics, or burn center telemedicine [20, 33].

TABLE 17.1 Recommendations for burn center transfer and consultation [with permission from Oxford University Press]

	Patient transfer potentially indicated[a, b]	Telemedicine consultation recommended[c]	Outpatient burn center referral recommended[b, c]
Thermal burns	• Full thickness >5% TBSA	• Recommended for all potentially deep burns of any size	• Full-thickness burns <5% TBSA
	• Partial thickness >10% TBSA		• Partial-thickness burns <10% TBSA
	• Any deep partial- or full-thickness burns involving the face, hands, genitalia, feet, perineum, or over any joints		
Inhalation injury	• All patients with true inhalation injury	• Recommended for flash burns to the face without inhalation injury	• Not specifically indicated
	• Patients smoking on oxygen with other comorbidities such as COPD may benefit from burn center admission		

(continued)

TABLE 17.1 (continued)

	Patient transfer potentially indicated[a,b]	Telemedicine consultation recommended[c]	Outpatient burn center referral recommended[b,c]
	• Facial flash burns do not need burn center admission unless they have thermal burns meeting above criteria		
Pediatrics (≤16 years)	• Same %TBSA thresholds as adults	• Recommended for all potentially deep burns of any size	• Same thresholds as adults
	• Children with <10%TBSA full or partial thickness burns may benefit from burn center admission due to dressing change, rehabilitation, or parent/caregiver needs		• Outpatient consultation at a burn center should occur within 7 days of injury
Older adults (≥55 years)	• Same %TBSA thresholds as other adults	• Recommended for all potentially deep burns of any size	• Same thresholds as other adults
	• Older adult (>55 years) burn patients may particularly benefit from the multi-disciplinary team resources available at a burn center		

Chemical injuries	• All chemical injuries should be cared for in a burn center	• Recommended if available	• Not specifically indicated
Electrical injuries	• All high voltage electrical injuries	• Recommended if available	• Low voltage electrical injuries should receive, at minimum, one follow-up visit to a burn center to screen for delayed symptom onset and vision problems
	• Lightning injury		
Cold injury	• Grades II–IV frostbite	• Recommended if available	• Not specifically indicated
	• All cold injured patients may benefit from the multidisciplinary team resources available in a burn center		

(continued)

TABLE 17.1 (continued)

	Patient transfer potentially indicated[a, b]	Telemedicine consultation recommended[c]	Outpatient burn center referral recommended[b, c]
Non-burn skin disorders	• Stevens–Johnson syndrome (SJS) or Toxic Epidermal Necrolysis (TENS) with epidermal slough • Necrotizing Soft-Tissue Injury (NSTI) – These patients benefit from the wound care, rehabilitation, and healing expertise of the multidisciplinary burn team.	• Recommended if available	• Not specifically indicated

[a] This document represents the consensus of burn care stakeholders' experience and opinion on which patients likely benefit from burn center care. It is NOT intended to replace throughtful provider-to-provider conversation based on the individual needs of each patient and is not prescriptive. Many factors, including geography and patient preferences, must be considered when making triage decisions

[b] Burn centers contain specialist providers of all kinds, including specialty trained nurses, rehabilitation therapists, dieticians, physicians, and psychosocial support staff. The availability of these resource should be a factor in all patient triage decisions, based on the patient's needs

[c] Telemedicine is an effective tool to improve the triage and care of burn patients. It should be used to support the triage and transfer decision-making process between providers whenever possible and is particularly helpful in reducing over-triage of small deep burns and in promoting accurate %TBSA estimation

Much of the current literature on utilization of telemedicine for management of burn injuries focuses on reduction of unnecessary transfers through improved triage [6, 17, 20, 21]. Transfers are costly and utilize scare resources, particularly those that are long distance and require air transport. It is not uncommon that inappropriately triaged patients undergo unnecessary travel to a burn center to be discharged immediately or after a brief hospital stay. While over-triage is reported in both adult and pediatric patients, the rate is significantly higher among children than adults [6]. Specifically, Reiband et al. found that the over-triage rate was highest among children less than 2 years old suffering scald burns [34]. McWilliams et al. performed an eight-year retrospective study of rural pediatric patients evaluated by telemedicine showing that improved triage of 4068 patients whose burn wounds that were reviewed resulted in only 364 acute transfers [20].

In a retrospective review of patients with small burns, Boccara et al. found telemedicine consultation was highly effective for identification of the presence of injuries with a surgical need that therefore warranted transfer [35]. In this study only 34.7% of patients required transfer, of which 3.4% were deemed unnecessary in that patients did not ultimately undergo surgery. A telemedicine quality improvement effort at a regional burn center serving a catchment including eight states found that the addition of image review to initial phone consultations changed transfer decisions for 24.5% of the study population [5]. Of these, 60.5% were down-triaged while 39.5% were up-triaged.

A recent study by Carmichael et al. evaluated the effect of a mobile phone app on triage and transfer of patients to a burn center from regional referring institutions [33]. Comparisons were made to patients referred during the same time frame via a call center without use of the burn mobile phone app. Patients were considered "down-triaged" after telemedicine evaluation if they were determined to be appropriate for outpatient management or transport by personal vehicle as opposed to ground ambulance or helicopter.

Overall, one-third of patients evaluated with the burn mobile phone app were able to be down-triaged, with a resultant average cost savings of $634 per patient. In comparison, no patients managed without telemedicine were able to be down-triaged. Based on their experience, the authors concluded that telemedicine most greatly impacted the triage of patients with burns greater than 1% TBSA and less than 10% TBSA.

A similar investigation by Saffle et al. compared triage and transfer of patients managed prior to implementation of a telemedicine referral program and after [4]. All patients determined to require transfer prior to the telemedicine program implementation were transported to the regional burn center by air. In comparison, approximately half of the patients evaluated initially by telemedicine consultation were able to avoid the need for air transport. While a small proportion were transferred via private vehicles, several were determined not to require transfer at all and were able to receive all care locally. The authors additionally concluded that telemedicine consultation enhanced the allocation of critical care resources and expedited transfer of severely injured patients. Rapid and accurate identification of these critical patients was also felt to help justify the risks and cost of air transport.

With the diminished need for travel and a decrease in travel-related costs without a perceived compromise in delivered care, multiple studies have found high levels of patient satisfaction [21, 23, 36]. One study demonstrated that based on medicare reimbursement rates, an average of $910 could be saved for those transferred by private vehicle or local management and $83 could be saved in driving costs for those who could be managed by their local primary care physician [33]. Hickey et al. performed a retrospective review of patients participating in interactive home telehealth visits for follow-up burn care and identified a travel distance save of 188 miles per patient, equivalent to 201 min of travel time, resulting in an average savings of $108.50 [23].

A satisfaction survey administered by Liu et al. noted that respondents were pleased with both diminished time and money spent to achieve follow-up with their burn providers [24]. They also found that providers' ability to share their screen through their telemedicine interface was positively received by patients. Allowing patients to view images of their own wounds and grafts facilitated conversation and increased patients' sense of active participation in their own care. Similar benefits can also be observed through study of the rehabilitative phase of care [20, 24]. Liu et al. found that utilization of a telemedicine rehabilitation program saved 146 ambulance transports (for a cost of $101,110), 6.8 outpatient burn clinic days, and 2–3 days of patient travel. Beyond these measurable outcomes, the authors felt that incorporating telemedicine improved burn center providers' relationships with care team members at the local rehabilitation hospital.

With introduction and maintenance of telemedicine programs, there are a number of administrative considerations. All telemedicine must follow both ethical and legal best practices [15]. The American Telemedicine Association recently published a policy guide for the use of telemedicine in the practice of burns [37]. Emphasis is placed on compliance with relevant local, state, federal, and international laws and regulations, including prescription practices. Providers must follow policies and standard operating procedures of governing institutions or otherwise establish appropriate policies and procedures if functioning within a private or solo practice. Documentation standards require careful review, particularly given their application to billing purposes.

Systems must be secure and prioritize privacy and confidentiality of patient data in accordance with the Health Insurance Portability and Accountability Act (HIPAA) [22]. Providers need to be appropriately credentialed and trained and clinical oversight must be provided where applicable. Programs designed for referral and consultation should have adequate staffing to allow for availability at any time of the day or night. Platforms should be designed to keep up with technological advancement. System function and performance must have ongoing monitoring and evaluation. Further, burn center management should facilitate processes of quality assurance, audit, and research for a telemedicine program to thrive.

Reimbursement for telemedicine services provided has remained an ongoing challenge. While the 1997 Balanced Budget Act required Medicare reimbursement of telemedicine visits, this did not translate into direct remuneration of providers. Required reimbursement by Medicare, Medicaid, and the State Children's Health Insurance program was expanded by the 2000 Benefits Improvement and Protection Act, though applicability was limited. Current regulation is primarily on a state-by-state basis. A roadblock for institutions looking to establish and maintain a telemedicine program is the need to determine a plan for solvency. Notably, Russell et al. found that in transitioning support for a telemedicine program beyond a grant reimbursement was similar for in-person and telemedicine patients [38]. Familiarity with coding specific to telemedicine is also crucial [1].

A number of barriers to successful adoption and usage of a telemedicine in burns exist. The main obstacles to implementation of a burn telemedicine program cited by Monte Soldado et al. were the need to maintain a reliable and complex technical infrastructure, establishment of a training program for involved providers, and ongoing coordination and logistics [39]. The most common barriers to successful establishment and maintenance of a telemedicine program cited by burn center directors were licensure, credentialing, and malpractice considerations [22]. These issues become increasingly problematic if a center's catchment area extends beyond state borders, raising the potential need for practitioners to obtain and maintain licensure in multiple states.

There is significant provider and healthcare system reluctance to adopt new technology [4]. In a 2014 review of telemedicine in burn care, Atiyeh et al. note that the culture of medicine has created a trend for healthcare providers to be suspicious and fearful of new technology [1]. While this road-block has resolved gradually over time, the most significant catalyst for adoption and propagation of telemedicine programs has been the emergence of the 2019 novel coronavirus (COVID-19). The pandemic has indelibly changed practice patterns surrounding use of telemedicine in burn care [40]. Burn centers have had to rework multidisciplinary management plans with wide adoption of telemedicine particularly in the outpatient setting due to limitations on direct personal contact [41]. One algorithm released several months into the pandemic included teleconsultation for guidance and follow-up of minor burn injury and also advocated for post-discharge recovery guidance; the same authors also emphasized the importance of using teleconsultation for triage and clinical decision-making prior to patient transfer during the pandemic [42].

However, not all clinical situations are appropriate for telemedicine. Patients requiring evaluation of concurrent non-burn injuries must be assessed in person with availability of required personnel and imaging technology. Scar assessment and management are highly challenging without the ability to consider palpation findings. Long-term scar management also typically requires measurement and fitting of custom compression garments, facemasks, and splints which necessitate face-to-face evaluation [1]. Evaluation for surgery for both acute burns and reconstruction can be initiated via telemedicine but ultimately requires in-person presentation for comprehensive planning.

Use of telemedicine, while imperfect, can contribute meaningfully to the care of burn patients. While COVID-19 has resulted in the more rapid and widespread adoption of telemedicine in burn care, these changes will hopefully prove to be durable care processes once the pandemic recedes. Telemedicine provides a powerful medium for certain aspects of burn care, particularly initial triage and management, and is an important adjunct for provision of high-value burn care.

References

1. Atiyeh B, Dibo SA, Janom HH. Telemedicine and burns: an overview. Ann Burns Fire Disasters. 2014;27:87–93.
2. American Burn Association. Burn center regional map [Internet]. 2020 [cited 2020 Dec 13]. http://ameriburn.org/public-resources/burn-center-regional-map/.
3. Saffle JR. Telemedicine for acute burn treatment: the time has come. J Telemed Telecare [Internet]. 2006;12:1–3. http://journals.sagepub.com/doi/10.1258/135763306775321353.
4. Saffle JR, Edelman L, Theurer L, Morris SE, Cochran A. Telemedicine evaluation of acute burns is accurate and cost-effective. J Trauma Inj Infect Crit Care [Internet]. 2009;67:358–365. http://journals.lww.com/00005373-200908000-00019.
5. Garber RN, Garcia E, Goodwin CW, Deeter LA. Pictures do influence the decision to transfer: outcomes of a telemedicine program serving an eight-state rural population. J Burn Care Res [Internet]. 2020;41:690–694. https://academic.oup.com/jbcr/article/41/3/690/5733697.
6. Liu YM, Mathews K, Vardanian A, Bozkurt T, Schneider JC, Hefner J, et al. Urban telemedicine. J Burn Care Res [Internet]. 2017;38:e235–e239. https://academic.oup.com/jbcr/article/37/5/e453-e460/4563498.
7. Saffle JR, Edelman L, Morris SE. Regional air transport of burn patients: a case for telemedicine? J Trauma Inj Infect Crit Care [Internet]. 2004;57:57–64. http://journals.lww.com/00005373-200407000-00013.
8. Carmichael H, Wiktor AJ, McIntyre RC, Lambert Wagner A, Velopulos CG. Regional disparities in access to verified burn center care in the United States. J Trauma Acute Care Surg [Internet]. 2019;87:111–116. http://journals.lww.com/01586154-201907000-00017.
9. Syed-Abdul S, Scholl J, Chen CC, Santos MDPS, Jian W-S, Liou D-M, et al. Telemedicine utilization to support the management of the burns treatment involving patient pathways in both developed and developing countries. J Burn Care Res [Internet]. 2012;33:e207–e212. https://academic.oup.com/jbcr/article/33/4/e207-e212/4588273.

10. Fuzaylov G, Knittel J, Driscoll DN. Use of telemedicine to improve burn care in Ukraine. J Burn Care Res [Internet]. 2013;34:e232–6. https://academic.oup.com/jbcr/article/34/4/e232-e236/4565967.

11. Institute of Medicine (US) Committee on Evaluating Clinical Applications of Telemedicine. Telemedicine: a guide to assessing telecommunications in health care [Internet]. Field MJ, editor. Washington, DC: National Academies Press (US); 1996. https://www.ncbi.nlm.nih.gov/books/NBK45448/?report=reader.

12. Garcia DI, Howard HR, Cina RA, Patel S, Ruggiero K, Treiber FA, et al. Expert outpatient burn care in the home through mobile health technology. J Burn Care Res [Internet]. 2018;39:680–684. https://academic.oup.com/jbcr/article/39/5/680/4942066.

13. Wiktor AJ, Madsen L, Carmichael H, Smith T, Zanyk S, Amani H, et al. Multiregional utilization of a mobile device app for triage and transfer of burn patients. J Burn Care Res [Internet]. 2018;39:858–862. https://academic.oup.com/jbcr/article/39/6/858/5070604.

14. Wurzer P, Parvizi D, Lumenta DB, Giretzlehner M, Branski LK, Finnerty CC, et al. Smartphone applications in burns. Burns [Internet]. Elsevier Ltd and International Society of Burns Injuries; 2015;41:977–989. https://doi.org/10.1016/j.burns.2014.11.010.

15. Martinez R, Rogers AD, Numanoglu A, Rode H. The value of WhatsApp communication in paediatric burn care. Burns [Internet]. Elsevier Ltd and International Society of Burns Injuries; 2018;44:947–955. https://doi.org/10.1016/j.burns.2017.11.005.

16. Wallis LA, Fleming J, Hasselberg M, Laflamme L, Lundin J. A smartphone app and cloud-based consultation system for burn injury emergency care. Efron PA, editor. PLoS One [Internet]. 2016;11:e0147253. https://doi.org/10.1371/journal.pone.0147253.

17. den Hollander D, Mars M. Smart phones make smart referrals. Burns [Internet]. Elsevier Ltd and International Society of Burns Injuries; 2017;43:190–194. https://doi.org/10.1016/j.burns.2016.07.015.

18. Wallace DL, Hussain A, Khan N, Wilson YT. A systematic review of the evidence for telemedicine in burn care: with a UK perspective. Burns [Internet]. Elsevier Ltd and International Society of Burns Injuries; 2012;38:465–80. https://doi.org/10.1016/j.burns.2011.09.024.

19. Turk E, Karagulle E, Aydogan C, Oguz H, Tarim A, Karakayali H, et al. Use of telemedicine and telephone consultation in decision-making and follow-up of burn patients: initial experience from two burn units, vol. 37. Burns [Internet]. Elsevier Ltd and International Society of Burns Injuries; 2011. p. 415–9. https://doi.org/10.1016/j.burns.2010.10.004.

20. McWilliams T, Hendricks J, Twigg D, Wood F, Giles M. Telehealth for paediatric burn patients in rural areas: a retrospective audit of activity and cost savings. Burns [Internet]. Elsevier Ltd and ISBI; 2016;42:1487–1493. https://doi.org/10.1016/j.burns.2016.03.001.

21. Asiri A, AlBishi S, AlMadani W, ElMetwally A, Househ M. The use of telemedicine in surgical care: a systematic review. Acta Inform Medica [Internet]. 2018;26:201. https://www.ejmanager.com/fulltextpdf.php?mno=302643394.

22. Holt B, Faraklas I, Theurer L, Cochran A, Saffle JR. Telemedicine use among burn centers in the United States. J Burn Care Res [Internet]. 2012;33:157–162. https://academic.oup.com/jbcr/article/33/1/157-162/4602127.

23. Hickey S, Gomez J, Meller B, Schneider JC, Cheney M, Nejad S, et al. Interactive home telehealth and burns: a pilot study. Burns [Internet]. Elsevier Ltd and International Society of Burns Injuries; 2017;43:1318–1321. https://doi.org/10.1016/j.burns.2016.11.013.

24. Liu YM, Mathews K, Vardanian A, Bozkurt T, Schneider JC, Hefner J, et al. Urban telemedicine. J Burn Care Res [Internet]. 2017;38:e235–e239. https://academic.oup.com/jbcr/article/38/1/e235-e239/4568933.

25. Massman NJ, Dodge JD, Fortman KK, Schwartz KJ, Solem LD. Burns follow-up: an innovative application of telemedicine. J Telemed Telecare [Internet]. 1999;5:52–54. http://journals.sagepub.com/doi/10.1258/1357633991932540.

26. Nguyen LT, Massman NJ, Franzen BJ, Ahrenholz DH, Sorensen NW, Mohr WJ, et al. Telemedicine follow-up of burns: lessons learned from the first thousand visits. J Burn Care Rehabil [Internet]. 2004;25:485–490. http://journals.lww.com/00004630-200411000-00009.

27. Jones OC, Wilson DI, Andrews S. The reliability of digital images when used to assess burn wounds. J Telemed Telecare [Internet]. 2003;9:22–24. http://journals.sagepub.com/doi/10.1258/135763303322196213.

28. Pham C, Collier Z, Gillenwater J. Changing the way we think about burn size estimation. J Burn Care Res [Internet]. 2019;40:1–11. https://academic.oup.com/jbcr/article/40/1/1/5104866.

29. Parvizi D, Giretzlehner M, Dirnberger J, Owen R, Haller HL, Schintler MV, et al. The use of telemedicine in burn care: development of a mobile system for TBSA documentation and remote assessment. Ann Burns Fire Disasters. 2014;27:94–100.

30. Wibbenmeyer L, Kluesner K, Wu H, Eid A, Heard J, Mann B, et al. Video-enhanced telemedicine improves the care of acutely injured burn patients in a rural state. J Burn Care Res [Internet]. 2016;37:e531–e538. https://academic.oup.com/jbcr/article/37/6/e531-e538/4563492.

31. Romanowski KS, Palmieri TL, Sen S, Greenhalgh DG. More than one third of intubations in patients transferred to burn centers are unnecessary: proposed guidelines for appropriate intubation of the burn patient. J Burn care Res [Internet]. 2013;37:e409–e414. http://www.ncbi.nlm.nih.gov/pubmed/26284640.

32. Bettencourt AP, Romanowski KS, Joe V, Jeng J, Carter JE, Cartotto R, et al. Updating the burn center referral criteria: results from the 2018 eDelphi consensus study. J Burn Care Res [Internet]. 2020;41:1052–1062. https://academic.oup.com/jbcr/article/41/5/1052/5775361.

33. Carmichael H, Dyamenahalli K, Duffy PS, Lambert Wagner A, Wiktor AJ. Triage and transfer to a regional burn center — impact of a Mobile phone app. J Burn Care Res [Internet]. 2020;41:971–975. https://academic.oup.com/jbcr/article/41/5/971/5863151.

34. Reiband HK, Lundin K, Alsbjørn B, Sørensen AM, Rasmussen LS. Optimization of burn referrals. Burns [Internet]. Elsevier Ltd and International Society of Burns Injuries; 2014;40:397–401. https://doi.org/10.1016/j.burns.2013.08.001.

35. Boccara D, Bekara F, Soussi S, Legrand M, Chaouat M, Mimoun M, et al. Ongoing development and evaluation of a method of telemedicine: burn care management with a smartphone. J Burn Care Res [Internet]. 2018;39:580–584. https://academic.oup.com/jbcr/article/39/4/580/4683477.

36. Redlick F, Roston B, Gomez M, Fish JS. An initial experience with telemedicine in follow-up burn care. J Burn Care Rehabil [Internet]. 2002;23:110–115. http://journals.lww.com/00004630-200203000-00007.

37. Theurer L, Bashshur R, Bernard J, Brewer T, Busch J, Caruso D, et al. American telemedicine association guidelines for Teleburn. Telemed e-Health [Internet]. 2017;23:365–375. https://www.liebertpub.com/doi/10.1089/tmj.2016.0279.

38. Russell KW, Saffle JR, Theurer L, Cochran AL. Transition from grant funding to a self-supporting burn telemedicine program in the western United States. Am J Surg [Internet]. Elsevier Inc; 2015;210:1037–1044. https://doi.org/10.1016/j.amjsurg.2015.08.003.

39. Monte Soldado A, López-Masrramon B, Aguilera-Sáez J, Serracanta Domenech J, Collado Delfa JM, Moreno Ramos C, et al. Implementation and evaluation of telemedicine in burn care: study of clinical safety and technical feasibility in a single burn center. Burns [Internet]. Elsevier Ltd and International Society of Burns Injuries; 2020;46:1668–1673. https://doi.org/10.1016/j.burns.2020.04.027.

40. Ilenghoven D, Hisham A, Ibrahim S, Mohd Yussof SJ. Restructuring burns management during the COVID-19 pandemic: a Malaysian experience. Burns [Internet]. 2020;46:1236–1239. https://linkinghub.elsevier.com/retrieve/pii/S0305417920303612.

41. Sharaf A, Muthayya P. Multidisciplinary management of the burn injured patient during a pandemic—the role of telemedicine. Burns [Internet]. Elsevier Ltd and International Society of Burns Injuries; 2021;47:252. https://doi.org/10.1016/j.burns.2020.04.028.

42. Saha S, Kumar A, Dash S, Singhal M. Managing burns during COVID-19 outbreak. J Burn Care Res [Internet]. 2020;41:1033–1036. https://academic.oup.com/jbcr/article/41/5/1033/5849079.

Chapter 18
Burn Disasters

Wendy Y. Rockne, Victor C. Joe, and James C. Jeng

Introduction: Disasters, Mass Casualty Incidents, and Burns

Disasters, which can generally be defined as sudden events that cause great damage or loss of life [1], are a part of the human experience to varying degrees. The intersection of hazards (natural, human-made, or a combination of both) with vulnerable populations resulting in severe damage or destruction will likely be witnessed, if not experienced, by most people during the course of their lifetimes [1].

Over the past two decades, disasters and specifically mass casualty incidents (MCIs) have been increasingly present in the public eye. Technologic advances such as the advent and now omnipresence of social media allow early and widespread dissemination of national and worldwide events, including photographs, eye-witness accounts, and even real-time video footage on a global scale as never before in human history.

Although these advances may have broadened our relationships and networks as a global community, disasters remain fundamentally local events that then expand to

W. Y. Rockne · V. C. Joe · J. C. Jeng (✉)
Department of Surgery, University of California Irvine,
Orange, CA, USA
e-mail: wrockne@hs.uci.edu; vcjoe@hs.uci.edu; jcjeng@hs.uci.edu

© The Author(s), under exclusive license to Springer Nature
Switzerland AG 2023
J. O. Lee (ed.), *Essential Burn Care for Non-Burn Specialists*,
https://doi.org/10.1007/978-3-031-28898-2_18

involve communities, regions, and nations [2, 3]. Because of this, robust MCI planning at the local level is crucial to minimize loss of life.

While the term MCI may be assumed to be synonymous with massive numbers of casualties, it is actually applied independently of casualty numbers. Rather it is used to denote an event that overwhelms the local healthcare system, i.e., where the number of casualties vastly exceeds the local resources and capabilities in a short period of time [4]. This is a threshold that can be quickly reached in the case of burn disasters; while burn mass casualty incidents (BMCIs) may not be common, they entail significant morbidity and mortality when they occur.

In light of this, practicing medical professionals should have a working knowledge of the available resources for burn disasters. This background knowledge enables appropriate response activation, early management, and adequate triage of injured patients in the event of a BMCI. The purpose of this chapter is not to offer detailed descriptions of how to care for burn patients in the acute setting, but rather to provide a brief synopsis of available resources for BMCIs.

Burn Disasters

The phrases "burn disaster" or "burn mass casualty incident" may bring to mind such events as structure fires, forest fires, or fires at the urban interface. However, it is worth bearing in mind that not all BMCIs result from catastrophic fires [5]. For example, the Oklahoma City bombing in 1995 is frequently precluded from BMCI analysis because no actual fire occurred after the explosion [6]. However, nine victims had thermal burns covering up to 70% of their body surface area, ranging from partial- to full-thickness burns [7], in essence meeting the criteria for a BMCI.

In addition to burns suffered during the initial disaster event, emergency responders commonly suffer burns during rescue operations. Rescue workers in both the Oklahoma

City bombing and 9/11 terrorist attacks sustained chemical and thermal burns while working on the rubble pile [8]. These additional injuries add to the strain on healthcare systems and can contribute to the evolution of a BMCI.

Many other types of disasters, including industrial accidents, earthquakes, and radiation-related disasters, can result in a BMCI despite not being directly associated with a catastrophic fire [9–13]. Typically, BMCIs can be stratified into four broad categories: mass gatherings with a sudden fire, natural disasters, industrial accidents, and purposeful hostilities [14, 15]. While it is important to remember that disaster planning needs to be developed first in terms of MCI, leaving more specialized planning tailored to specific disaster type as a secondary consideration [16], a general familiarity with major BMCIs that have occurred in the recent past is essential in understanding and developing a plan for future BMCI response.

Mass Gatherings

New Taipei Water Park Color Dust Fire: 2015

In June of 2015 a "Color Play Asia" party, inspired by the colored powder used in the Hindu Festival of Colors, was held at a water park in Taiwan. As nearly 4000 partygoers danced on a large stage and swimming pool emptied for the occasion, concert organizers deployed colored corn starch powder into the air over the crowd using air blowers and compressed gas canisters. The airborne corn starch caught fire resulting in a large deflagration. This was worsened when staff sprayed carbon-dioxide fire extinguishers toward participants, resulting in dispersal of the burning starch into multiple widespread dust clouds [17].

The fire reportedly lasted 40 s and burned approximately 500 people, killing 15 and leaving almost 200 in critical condition [18]. Patients were taken to over 50 hospitals across Taiwan, transported by nearly 300 emergency vehicles (including emergency medical services, military vehicles, personal vehicles, and taxis) and accompanied by a total of 1235 first responders [19]. The influx of hundreds of burn patients arriving at already busy hospitals created substantial difficulty for anyone to receive care consistent with the conventional standard of care (also known as the "crowd out effect") [20].

Despite these challenges, prompt and coordinated disaster response resulted in tremendous patient outcomes; after 3 months, the overall mortality rate was an unprecedented 2.4%, a stark comparison to the predicted 26.8% [19]. This incident demonstrated not only the incredible amount of resources needed to adequately respond to large-scale BMCIs but also the necessity for alternative transport means when standard EMS systems are overwhelmed. The impressive patient outcomes from this event further highlight the effectiveness of coordinated preparedness response, both on the national and international levels [18–20].

Station Night Club Fire: 2003

In February of 2003 at a nightclub in West Warwich, Rhode Island, pyrotechnics accompanying the evening's headlining band, Great White, ignited flammable acoustic foam in the ceiling and walls surrounding the stage. The fire reportedly reached flash point in under a minute, resulting in rapid fire growth and vision-obscuring toxic black smoke. This, when combined with illegally blocked egress points, resulted in the deaths of 100 people with an additional 230 injured [21, 22].

Natural Disasters

Black Saturday Bushfire: 2009

In February of 2009 in the State of Victoria, Australia, extreme heat, high winds, and the effects of years of drought combined to create one of the worst wildfire disasters world-wide, costing over four billion Australian dollars and claiming 173 lives. The majority of these fatalities were due to radiant heat and smoke inhalation. An additional 24 patients were sent to major burn centers in serious condition; three of these patients died [23, 24]. Notably, although an immense number of people were exposed to the bushfire and a fair percentage sustained major burns, it was later determined that only 10% of these received appropriate first aid for their injuries [25].

Industrial Accidents

Chernobyl Nuclear Power Plant Accident: 1986

In April of 1986 a nuclear accident occurred during a safety test on a nuclear reactor in the Chernobyl Nuclear Power Plant near the city of Pripyat in the Soviet Union. A combination of unstable conditions and reactor design flaws resulted in an uncontrolled nuclear chain reaction, causing two explosions which ruptured the nuclear reactor core and destroyed the reactor building. These were followed by an open-air reactor core fire that released airborne radioactive contamination for over a week, precipitating onto portions of the USSR and Western Europe before final containment.

In the disaster and immediate response, 134 people were hospitalized with acute radiation syndrome incurred from absorbing high doses of ionizing radiation. Of these, 28 died within days to months; all of the fatalities in this acute period were among station operators and firefighters, many who had sustained large total body surface area (TBSA) beta burns from the continued wearing of dust-soaked uniforms [11]. While it is impossible to know the overall fatalities due to this event, model predictions with the greatest confidence values of the eventual total death toll as a result of Chernobyl radiation exposure exceed 4000. Nuclear cleanup is ongoing and currently scheduled for completion in 2065 [12].

Purposeful Hostilities

9/11: 2001

On September 11, 2001, four commercial airliners traveling from the northeastern United States to California were hijacked midflight by al-Qaeda terrorists. Two of these planes were crashed into the World Trade Center towers in New York City, one was crashed into the west side of the Pentagon in Virginia, and one crashed into a field in Pennsylvania (diverted from its intended target in Washington, D.C.). This attack resulted in nearly 3000 fatalities with an additional 6000 injured and remains the deadliest terrorist attack in human history [25, 26]. Approximately one-third of those injured sustained severe burn injuries [27, 28]. These devastating attacks served as a "galvanizing calamity" of sorts, spurring interest in the development of national frameworks to respond to MCIs on a massive scale [16, 29].

The Atomic Bombings of Hiroshima and Nagasaki: 1945

Although infrequent, radiation-related disasters represent novel and challenging threats that can put health care systems at great risk [2]. The nuclear weapons detonated over the Japanese cities of Hiroshima and Nagasaki during World War II not only killed more than 100,000 people but also left an equal number of people with acute radiation illnesses [30]. As technology continues to advance, fissile weapons with similar yield can now be concealed in containers as small as a suitcase, raising the alarming potential for their use in terrorism [31]. Planning models demonstrate that with the detonation of such a device over a populated area, 30% of the surviving injured are expected to have burn wounds from a variety of mechanisms, including the initial blast, radiation injury, structure fires that occur as a result of the blast, and injuries incurred during the aftermath of such a disaster [32]. This could produce tens (and potentially hundreds) of thousands of patients with burn injuries which would rapidly overwhelm traditional resources for an extended period, even in countries with robust MCI/BMCI systems in place.

BMCI Response Requirements

Burn Injuries

Most BMCIs produce fewer patients than expected that will require inpatient burn center care [6]. Reviews of injury/fatality patterns from catastrophic fires resulting in multiple casualties over the past century show that most fatalities occur at the initial scene, en route to the hospital, or shortly after hospital arrival. Many of the injured are treated and released at the scene or after evaluation in the emergency department without involvement of a burn care team [6]. While it is tempting to interpret such data at face value, the impact of BMCIs on patients, communities, and health care systems extends far beyond fatalities.

While it is true that patients with significant burn injuries generally represent a small subset of injured patients in many MCIs, their higher injury severity and complexity result in a disproportionate impact on healthcare systems [2]. A disaster that results in "only" ten severely burned patients requiring hospitalization produces an immense drain on hospital resources that continues for months after the actual disaster has passed [6]. Unlike most traumatic injuries, burn trauma remains resource-intensive over an extended period of time, with ever-changing requirements that fluctuate throughout the course of each patient's treatment [33].

In order to create a relevant disaster plan, the point at which a local or regional healthcare system would be overwhelmed by a BMCI must be known. This necessitates developing a thorough understanding of resources required in both the acute phase of a BMCI (where operative requirements are greatest) and the more protracted phase (where rehabilitation needs increase) [33]. On average, a mean of 0.3 operations and 22.8 min of operating time is needed per percent TBSA burn, and length of inpatient stay roughly equates to 1.1 days per percent TBSA burn [33]. Additionally, although burn centers may not be directly involved with the cohort of "walking wounded" on the day of injury, the resulting need to locate and provide these patients with ongoing outpatient burn care creates a vast and ongoing logistical and personnel burden for burn centers [6, 34].

Capability

Two major determinants to success of disaster response are adequate assessment and planning for a healthcare system's capability and capacity. Capability refers to the types of clinician available to render appropriate care for the wounded and the specialized equipment for this care [2]. When discussing BMCI, this can specifically refer to burn specialty teams including experienced burn surgeons and nurses, staff familiar with the unique needs of burn patients, and experienced critical care personnel.

In contrast to trauma patients, seriously injured burn patients do not necessarily require expedient surgical intervention. As the major concern in large burn injuries is hypovolemic shock, the priorities of treatment for patients in the acute setting are stabilization, prevention of organ damage, and prevention of wound progression or infection [16].

Ideally, patients with serious burn injuries should be promptly sent to and managed at burn centers, where specialized burn care teams and resources are available [35]. However, during a disaster that involves significant numbers of burn patients, this may be difficult if not impossible to achieve, especially in the first hours and days following the inciting incident. The first receiver for most burn mass casualties will therefore likely be a hospital without a burn center, where it may be necessary for seriously burned patients to remain for days [33].

Previous incidents have demonstrated that burn patients from BMCIs tend to be distributed across several hospitals on the day of the disaster [6]. This offsets the initial burden on the burn center in the acute phase, but later adds to the workload as hospitals appropriately request transfer of burn patients to the burn center for specialized care. This may require secondary triage by burn centers, allowing redistribution of patients to other qualified burn centers and activation of multijurisdictional/multiagency response to augment burn center staff with experienced burn specialty teams [34].

Additionally, as burn trauma is a long disease process with complex treatment needs, a multidisciplinary approach is necessary for optimal care in both the short- and long term. Therefore, the development of a robust outpatient burn treatment capacity is vital to BMCI response [6].

Capacity and Burn Surge

The American Burn Association (ABA) defines burn surge as 50% more burn patients than normal capacity at any given time in a single burn center [16]. Capacity refers to the quantity of resources available for response, including staff, space, and supplies [2]. Key factors that determine capacity include both readily available, routinely used resources as well as key assets that can be flexed to accommodate MCI needs (e.g., outpatient facilities, conference rooms, temporary structures, and holding areas) [2]. One important measure of scalable capacity is the ability to increase hospital bed availability by expanding by 20% within 4 h to accommodate the highest acuity patients in an MCI [14].

When discussing capacity as it specifically relates to BMCIs, it includes such vital resources as ventilators, burn beds, and surgical suites [36]. In 2011, the American Hospital Association identified 5795 hospitals with 944,277 staffed beds, and 123 self-identified burn centers reported 1895 beds collectively, yielding a ratio of approximately one burn center for every 47 hospitals (or one "burn bed" out of every 498 hospital beds) [37]. While the number of burn centers has increased slightly in the interim (currently 133 [38]), the burn bed to hospital bed ratio remains largely unchanged [37].

Additionally, there is an increasing shortage of trained burn surgeons across the country. At present, there are only approximately 300 trained burn surgeons practicing at burn centers across the country [38], and burn care is no longer a part of the standard curriculum of surgical training in the United States. This, combined with the decline in frequency of major burns due to public safety and public health efforts/interventions, have made it increasingly difficult to preserve and pass on the collective expertise of existing burn experts for the future [38]. These factors are essential to be aware of during disaster planning, as the limited availability of resources necessary for optimal burn care can quickly become a critical bottleneck in the healthcare system response [38–40], requiring careful planning and strategy to circumvent.

Given the relative scarcity of resources and infrequency of BMCIs, it is both reasonable and prudent to consider and plan for these events as worst-case scenarios in modern health care systems [2]. While this strategy has been discussed intermittently in the American burn community for decades [41, 42], the various terrorist acts, military conflicts, and natural disasters that occurred with the commencement of the twenty-first century sparked a new focus on disaster research and improvement of disaster burn care systems [38]. In 2012, a National Burn Surge Strategy Meeting was convened by the Emergency Care Coordination Center (ECCC) of the Office of the Assistant Secretary for Preparedness and Response within the **U.S. Department of Health and Human Services (HHS)**. This meeting examined the foundations of a national framework to address the complex issues in facilitating a rapid, coordinated, and effective response to BMCIs, spurring further collaboration for and research into BMCI response [16]. Additionally, across the United States, both state and regional research and disaster preparedness efforts are advancing, adding to a growing repository of BMCI planning resources [41, 42].

National, Federal, and Military Resources for the BMCI

The American Burn Association

In burn disaster response, both geography and lines of political jurisdiction play a large part in ability to both plan and enact an appropriate response. Therefore, close communication and coordination between burn centers are essential [2].

The ABA is a multidisciplinary organization which consists of over 2000 members in the USA, Canada, Latin America, Asia, and Europe. Members include physicians, nurses, physical and occupational therapists, researchers, firefighters, social workers, and hospitals with burn centers [43]. The ABA's stated mission is to improve quality care, burn prevention, education, research, and service to its members. Its website, https://ameriburn.org, includes a plethora of resources both for members and for the public, including burn center referral criteria, a regional map of burn centers, support services for burn survivors, and disaster response resources.

It is important not to confuse *burn* capacity with *trauma* capacity; although most burn surgeons are also trained trauma surgeons, the converse is not necessarily the case, just as trauma centers are not the same as burn centers [16, 44]. So what defines a burn center?

A facility earns the title of "designated burn center" when it meets the requirements of government or other authorized entities. This burn center designation is not determined by the ABA [45]. However, the ABA provides an additional system for burn center verification.

ABA burn center verification, intended to ensure that a burn center is meeting the highest current standards of care for the burn patient, is based upon an extensive list of criteria and continuously evaluated by the ABA Verification Review Committee. This comprehensive list includes specific requirements for important burn care aspects such as patient volume, nursing and therapy staff, prehospital burn care, ambulatory care, prevention and outreach, research, emergency department care, quality improvement measures, and disaster planning [45]. Ongoing compliance with these standards by ABA-verified burn centers is reverified via periodic site visits.

There are currently 133 burn centers across the United States staffed by approximately 300 burn surgeons and comprising approximately 2000 burn specialty beds. Of these 133 burn centers, 72 are ABA verified burn centers, and represent approximately 75% of the national burn bed capacity [38].

The ABA additionally serves as a central point for unification of burn resources and coordination of burn response, especially in burn disasters on the national scale. Current data estimates that the U.S. burn care community, utilizing all burn centers across the country, could manage approximately 2000 patients within approximately 120 h of an inciting disaster event [14] if sufficient transportation resources exist to redistribute patients from initial hospital care sites to specialized burn centers [3, 46].

ABA regions do not line up with the ten designated Federal Emergency Management Agency (FEMA) regions, but rather lie along natural lines of referral and regional support [47]. There are currently five designated U.S. ABA regions: Northeast Region, Southern Region, Eastern Great Lakes Region, Midwest Region, and Western Region. While all associated with the ABA, these regions choose their own organizational structure, and the activities of each region vary to suit the individual needs of their specific geographical areas, burn providers, and patient populations [16, 47]. Additionally, each region has its own Regional Disaster Plan available for reference on the ABA website.

Federal Resources

In an MCI or BMCI response, the primary responsibility for disaster response lies with local and state agencies, as by statue the U.S. government becomes involved in a disaster only when local and state capabilities are overwhelmed. A request for federal assistance is normally initiated by a state governor and usually involves the **Department of Health and Human Services (DHHS)**, the **Department of Homeland Security (DHS)**, and may include the **Department of Justice (DOJ)** [16].

Additionally, although federal resources are available in the event of a large-scale BMCI, logistically these resources cannot be relied upon to reach the incident scene prior to 72 h after the inciting event [16]. Therefore, during the first 3 days following an event, the disaster response will be essentially limited to local and regional resources. As it is inevitable that the burn resources of a single state (and even region) will be quickly overwhelmed in a large-scale BMCI, additional coordination on the regional and national level is essential in order to maximize burn bed surge capacity [16].

Emergency Support Function # 8 (ESF-8) provides the mechanisms for coordinating federal assistance in civilian disaster response [48]. The **Secretary of Health and Human Services (HHS)** leads all such federal public health and medical response and assumes control of operational federal assets (with the exclusion of members of the Armed Forces, who remain under the authority and control of the Secretary of Defense). The Secretary of HHS (through the **Office of the Assistant Secretary for Preparedness and Response,** or **ASPR**) coordinates national ESF-8 preparedness, response, and recovery actions [48].

ASPR provides funding and technical assistance to state, local, and territorial public health departments in order to help prepare healthcare systems for disasters through the **Hospital Preparedness Program (HPP) Cooperative Agreement** [49]. ASPR also defines a set of "Healthcare Preparedness Capabilities" based on common preparedness methodologies from FEMA to assist healthcare systems with preparedness and response. These capabilities are designed to facilitate joint ESF-8 preparedness planning, ultimately assuring safer, more resilient, and better-prepared communities [49].

The **Strategic National Stockpile (SNS)**, originally called the National Pharmaceutical Stockpile, is part of the federal medical response infrastructure that can be used to supplement medical response during public health emergencies. This stockpile of medical supplies, medicines, and devices can be used as a short-term, stopgap buffer during disaster response [50]. States, territories, tribal nations, and the largest metropolitan areas may request federal assistance from the SNS in the event, their supplies are exhausted and commercial supplies are unavailable to meet disaster response needs [50]. Regional emergency coordinators assigned to each of the HHS regions throughout the country work directly with public health authorities to determine needs and assist with supply requests.

The **Biomedical Advanced Research Development Authority (BARDA)** is an HHS office responsible for the procurement and development of medical countermeasures needed in response to public health emergencies, including chemical, biological, radiological, and nuclear (CBRN) accidents, incidents, and attacks. BARDA, established in 2006 though the Pandemic and All-Hazards Preparedness Act (PAHPA), reports to ASPR and acts as an official interface between the U.S. federal government and the biomedical industry. BARDA uses grants and other assistance to promote the advancement of biomedical research, innovation, and product development. BARDA also procures and maintains supplies for the SNS [51].

Military Resources

The U.S. military involvement occurs only at the request of another federal agency, and only when the pooled assets of local, state, and federal governments are found to be insufficient. These requests are routed to the **Department of Defense (DOD),** which then assigns response tasks to the **U.S. Northern Command (NORTHCOM)**. NORTHCOM, a unified command based in Colorado, holds responsibility for the defense of North America. However, the command may also provide military support to civil authorities at the direction of the President of the United States or Secretary of Defense. When activated for civilian assistance, any asset of the military services may be requested and assigned to NORTHCOM for response to a civilian disaster, including mobile hospitals, staging facilities, and transportation resources. Military assets deployed for civilian disasters are required by federal law to be the last to be committed to a response and the first to leave a response area when no longer required [16, 51].

The **National Disaster Medical System (NDMS)**, a collaboration between HHS, DHS, DOD, and the Department of Veterans Affairs, acts to supplement local, state, tribal, territorial, and military medical resources during disaster response. It serves three major functions: onsite care, large scale patient movement, and definitive medical care. Its deployable onsite medical function consists of more than 7000 personnel organized into teams including International Medical Surgical Response Teams, Disaster Mortuary Operational Response Teams, and Disaster Medical Assistance Teams. In addition, deployed NDMS medical assets are designed to operate in dynamic/evolving environments and are able to provide their own water, food, and shelter to avoid further burdening communities impacted by disaster [16].

Guidelines for BMCI Triage and Response

The ABA's Organization and Delivery of Burn Care Committee (ODBC) develops and maintains plans to manage regional burn surge capabilities in the event of a mass casualty or other disaster [52]. This includes a list of regularly updated guidelines available to the public at https://ameriburn.org/quality-care/disaster-response/. A brief (and by no means comprehensive) overview of some highlights of the currently linked guidelines available on the ABA's website for public use is included below.

Patient Care Priorities for the First 24 h in a Burn Mass Casualty for Non-burn Physicians

Based upon *Guidelines for Burn Care Under Austere Conditions* by Jeng et al [14], this succinct outline provides a framework for establishing patient treatment priorities in the first 24 h after a BMCI. This includes guidelines for triage, initial decontamination and wound care, airway management, and burn-specific resuscitation [14].

Actionable, Revised (v.3), and Amplified American Burn Association Triage Tables for Mass Casualties: A Civilian Defense Guideline

This detailed work by Kearns et al. [38] is free to the public to download in PDF form and provides evidence-based tables that can be applied in a BMCI by those tasked with triaging and caring for large numbers of patients with burn injuries. Last revised in March of 2020, it was written by clinical burn experts and led by the ABA in order to provide clinicians evidence-based tools to maximize burn care capabilities based on realistic assumptions in the event of a BMCI [38], updating and merging findings from previous publications on the subject [53, 54]. These triage tables were examined for face validity during a functional exercise of the component of the ASPR-funded Regional Disaster Health Response System (RDHRS) pilot program in August 2019.

Additionally, this work integrates and defines newer principles and terminology that arose from the publication of *Committee on Crisis Standards of Care (CoCSoC): A Toolkit for Indicators and Triggers* by Hanfling et al. (along with previous and subsequent research by Hick et al) [36, 46]. The provided tables allow a tailored response dependent on number of burn patients, severity of burn injuries, and location/availability of resources within burn regions. These include conventional burn care (50–200 burn victims), contingency burn care (100–500 burn victims), crisis burn care (500–2000 burn victims), and catastrophic burn care (>2000 burn victims) [38]. Of course, these tables are templates only and require personalization for each disaster.

Conclusion

While the BMCI is not an everyday event, the complex needs of an adequate burn disaster response necessitate careful planning, coordination, and cooperation in order to minimize loss of life and limb. Practicing medical professionals, especially those involved in emergency response, healthcare systems, and disaster preparedness, should maintain a working knowledge of the available resources for burn disasters, including local and regional support systems, national and federal organizations, and military resources. Knowledge of these critical resources and how to activate and implement them can help reduce the significant morbidity and mortality associated with these disastrous events.

References

1. Penuel K, Statler M, Hagen R. Disasters. Encyclopedia of crisis management. 2013;2. https://doi.org/10.4135/9781452275956.
2. Kearns RD, Marcozzi DE, Barry N, Rubinson L, Hultman CS, Rich PB. Disaster preparedness and response for the burn mass casualty incident in the twenty-first century. Clin Plast Surg. 2017;44(3):441–9. https://doi.org/10.1016/j.cps.2017.02.004.
3. Kearns RD, Hubble MW, Holmes JH, Cairns BA. Disaster planning: transportation resources and considerations for managing a burn disaster. J Burn Care Res. 2014;35(1):21–32. https://doi.org/10.1097/bcr.0b013e3182853cf7.
4. DeNolf RL. EMS mass casualty management. StatPearls [Internet]. 2020. https://www.ncbi.nlm.nih.gov/books/NBK482373. Accessed 25 Sept 2021.
5. McGregor JC. Major burn disasters: lessons to be learned from previous incidents and a need for a national plan. Surgeon. 2004;2(5):249–50. https://doi.org/10.1016/s1479-666x(04)80092-1.

6. Barillo DJ, Wolf S. Planning for burn disasters: lessons learned from one hundred years of history. J Burn Care Res. 2006;27(5):622–34. https://doi.org/10.1097/01.bcr.0000236823.08124.1c.

7. Mallonee S, Shariat S, Stennies G, Waxweiler R, Hogan D, Jordan F. Physical injuries and fatalities resulting from the Oklahoma City bombing. JAMA. 1996;276(5):382–7. https://doi.org/10.1001/jama.1996.03540050042021.

8. Dellinger AM, Waxweiler RJ, Mallonee S. Injuries to rescue workers following the Oklahoma City bombing. Am J Ind Med. 1997;31(6):727–32. https://doi.org/10.1002/(sici)1097-0274(199706)31:6<727::aid-ajim9>3.0.co;2-n.

9. Turégano-Fuentes F, Caba-Doussoux P, Jover-Navalón JM, Martín-Pérez E, Fernández-Luengas D, Díez-Valladares L, et al. Injury patterns from major urban terrorist bombing in trains: the Madrid experience. World J Surg. 2008;32(6):1168–75. https://doi.org/10.1007/s00268-008-9557-1.

10. Cairns BA, Stiffler A, Price F, Peck MD, Meyer AA. Managing a combined burn trauma disaster in the post-9/11 world: lessons learned from the 2003 west pharmaceutical plant explosion. J Burn Care Rehabil. 2005;26(2):144–50. https://doi.org/10.1097/01.bcr.0000155527.76205.a2.

11. Akashi M, Maekawa K. Medical management of heavily exposed victims: an experience at the Tokaimura criticality accident. J Radiol Prot. 2021;41:S391. https://doi.org/10.1088/1361-6498/ac270d.

12. Svendsen ER, Runkle JR, Dhara VR, Lin S, Naboka M, Mousseau TA, Bennett CL. Epidemiologic methods lesson learned from environmental public health disasters: Chernobyl, the World Trade Center, Bhopal, and Graniteville, South Carolina. Int J Environ Res Public Health. 2012;9(8):2894–909. https://doi.org/10.3390/ijerph9082894.

13. Peplow M. Special report: counting the dead. Nature. 2006;440(7087):982–3. https://doi.org/10.1038/440982a.

14. Jeng J, Gibran N, Peck M. Burn care in disaster and other austere settings. Surg Clin North Am. 2014;94(4):893–907. https://doi.org/10.1016/j.suc.2014.05.011.

15. Kearns RD, Hubble MW, Holmes JH, Cairns BA. Disaster planning. J Burn Care Res. 2014;35(1):e21. https://doi.org/10.1097/bcr.0b013e3182853cf7.

16. Helminiak C, Lord G, Barillo D, Cairns BA, Goodwin C, Lamana J, Jeng J. Proceedings of the National Burn Surge Strategy

Meeting, Atlanta, Georgia, March, 2012. J Burn Care Res. 2014;35(1):e54. https://doi.org/10.1097/bcr.0000000000000033.

17. Wang T, Lin T. Responding to mass burn casualties caused by corn powder at the Formosa Water Park in 2015. J Formos Med Assoc. 2015;114(12):1151–3. https://doi.org/10.1016/j. jfma.2015.11.001.

18. Yeong E, O'Boyle CP, Huang H, Tai H, Hsu Y, Chuang S, Lai H. Response of a local hospital to a burn disaster: contributory factors leading to zero mortality outcomes. Burns. 2018;44(5):1083–90. https://doi.org/10.1016/j.burns.2018.03.019.

19. Yang C, Shih C. A coordinated emergency response: a color dust explosion at a 2015 concert in Taiwan. Am J Public Health. 2016;106(9):1582–5. https://doi.org/10.2105/ajph.2016.303261.

20. Yang C, Tsai S, Chien W, Chung C, Dai N, Tzeng Y, Chen C. The crowd-out effect of a mass casualty incident. Medicine. 2019;98(18):e15457. https://doi.org/10.1097/ md.0000000000015457.

21. Harrington DT, Biffl WL, Cioffi WG. The station nightclub fire. J Burn Care Rehabil. 2005;26(2):141–3. https://doi.org/10.1097/01. bcr.0000155537.60909.fc.

22. Mozingo D. Lessons learned from a nightclub fire: institutional disaster preparedness. Yearbook of Surgery. 2006;2006:50–51. https://doi.org/10.1016/s0090-3671(08)70337-9.

23. Seifman M, Ek EW, Menezes H, Rozen WM, Whitaker IS, Cleland HJ. Bushfire disaster burn casualty management. Ann Plast Surg. 2011;67(5):460–3. https://doi.org/10.1097/sap.0b013e3182111021.

24. Cameron PA, Mitra B, Fitzgerald M, Scheinkestel CD, Stripp A, Batey C, Cleland H. Black Saturday: the immediate impact of the February 2009 bushfires in Victoria, Australia. Med J Australia. 2009;191(1):11–6. https://doi.org/10.5694/j.1326-5377.2009.tb02666.x.

25. Mozingo DW. A regional burn center's response to a disaster: September 11, 2001, and the days beyond. Yearbook of Surgery. 2006;2006:48–49. https://doi.org/10.1016/s0090-3671(08)70335-5.

26. Mozingo DW. The pentagon attack of September 11, 2001: a burn center's experience. Yearbook of Surgery 2006;2006:49–50. doi:https://doi.org/10.1016/s0090-3671(08)70336-7.

27. Cushman JG, Pachter HL, Beaton HL. Two New York City hospitals' surgical response to the September 11, 2001, terrorist attack in New York City. J Trauma. 2003;54(1):147–55. https:// doi.org/10.1097/00005373-200301000-00018.

28. Sheridan RL, Friedstat J, Votta K. Lessons learned from burn disasters in the post-9/11 ERA. Clin Plast Surg. 2017;44(3):435–40. https://doi.org/10.1016/j.cps.2017.02.003.

29. Yurt RW, Bessey PQ, Alden NE, et al. Burn-injured patients in a disaster: September 11th revisited. J Burn Care Res. 2006;27(5):635–41. https://doi.org/10.1097/01.bcr.0000236836.46410.f2.

30. Matsunari Y, Yoshimoto N. Comparison of rescue and relief activities within 72 hours of the atomic bombings in Hiroshima and Nagasaki. Prehosp Disaster Med. 2013;28(6):536–42. https://doi.org/10.1017/s1049023x13008832.

31. Goffman TE. Nuclear terrorism and the problem of burns. Am J Emerg Med. 2011;29(2):224–8. https://doi.org/10.1016/j.ajem.2009.03.022.

32. DiCarlo AL, Maher C, Hick JL, et al. Radiation injury after a nuclear detonation: medical consequences and the need for scarce resources allocation. Disaster Med Public Health Prep. 2011;5(S1):S32–44. https://doi.org/10.1001/dmp.2011.17.

33. Phua YS, Miller JD, Wong She RB. Total care requirements of burn patients: implications for a disaster management plan. J Burn Care Res. 2010;31(6):935–41. https://doi.org/10.1097/bcr.0b013e3181f93938.

34. Sheridan R, Barillo D, Herndon D, et al. Burn specialty teams. J Burn Care Rehabil. 2005;26(2):170–3. https://doi.org/10.1097/01.bcr.0000155544.38709.6e.

35. Klein MB. Geographic access to burn center hospitals. JAMA. 2009;302(16):1774. https://doi.org/10.1001/jama.2009.1548.

36. Hick JL, Barbera JA, Kelen GD. Refining surge capacity: conventional, contingency, and crisis capacity. Disaster Med Public Health Prep. 2009;3(2 Suppl):S59–67. https://doi.org/10.1097/dmp.0b013e31819f1ae2.

37. Kearns RD, Cairns CB, Holmes JH 4th, Rich PB, Cairns BA. Thermal burn care: a review of best practices. What should prehospital providers do for these patients? EMS World. 2013;42(1):43–51.

38. Kearns RD, Bettencourt AP, Hickerson WL, et al. Actionable, revised (v.3), and amplified American Burn Association triage tables for mass casualties: a civilian defense guideline. J Burn Care Res. 2020;41(4):770–9. https://doi.org/10.1093/jbcr/iraa050.

39. Abir M, Davis MM, Sankar P, Wong AC, Wang SC. Design of a model to predict surge capacity bottlenecks for burn mass casu-

alties at a large academic medical center. Prehosp Disaster Med. 2012;28(1):23–32. https://doi.org/10.1017/s1049023x12001513.

40. Conlon KM, Bell R, Lee RA, Marano M. Determining immediate burn bed availability to support regional disaster response. J Burn Care Res. 2019;40(6):832–7. https://doi.org/10.1093/jbcr/irz094.

41. Sasser SM. In a moment's notice: surge capacity for terrorist bombings: challenges and proposed solutions. Atlanta: U.S. Dept. of Health and Human Services. Centers for Disease Control and Prevention, National Center for Injury Prevention and Control, Division of Injury Response; 2007.

42. Wachtel TL, Cowan ML, Reardon JD. Developing a regional and national burn disaster response. J Burn Care Rehabil. 1989;10(6):561–7. https://doi.org/10.1097/00004630-198911000-00021.

43. Who we are. American Burn Association. https://ameriburn.org/who-we-are/. 2017. Accessed 1 Sept 2021.

44. Kelen GD, McCarthy ML. The science of surge. Acad Emerg Med. 2006;13(11):1089–94. https://doi.org/10.1197/j.aem.2006.07.016.

45. Verification criteria effective October 1, 2019. American Burn Association. https://ameriburn.org/quality-care/verification/verification-criteria/verification-criteria-effective-october-1-2019/. 2021. Accessed 1 Sept 2021.

46. Hick JL, Einav S, Hanfling D, Kissoon N, Dichter JR, Devereaux AV, Christian MD, Task Force for Mass Critical Care; Task Force for Mass Critical Care. Surge capacity principles: care of the critically ill and injured during pandemics and disasters: CHEST consensus statement. Chest. 2014;146(4 Suppl):e1S–e16S. https://doi.org/10.1378/chest.14.

47. Harrington D, Holmes J, Conlon K, Jeng J. An update on the regional organizations of the American Burn Association. J Burn Care Res. 2014;35(3):228–32. https://doi.org/10.1097/bcr.0b013e318295789f.

48. Presidential Policy Directive 8: national preparedness. Department of Homeland Security. 2018. http://www.dhs.gov/xabout/laws/gc_1215444247124.shtm. Accessed 1 Sept 2021.

49. Office of the Assistant Secretary for preparedness and response; 2016. 2017–2022 health care preparedness and response capabilities. https://www.phe.gov/Preparedness/planning/hpp/reports/Documents/2017-2022-healthcare-pr-capabilities.pdf. Accessed 1 Sept 2021.

50. Strategic National Stockpile. phe.gov. https://www.phe.gov/about/sns/Pages/default.aspx. Accessed 1 Sept 2021.
51. Kraft M, Marks E. U.S. government counterterrorism: a guide to who does what. Boca Raton: CRC Press; 2012.
52. Hickerson WL, Ryan CM, Conlon KM, et al. What's in a name? Recent key projects of the committee on organization and delivery of burn care. J Burn Care Res. 2015;36(6):619–25. https://doi.org/10.1097/bcr.0000000000000189.
53. Saffle JR, Gibran N, Jordan M. Defining the ratio of outcomes to resources for triage of burn patients in mass casualties. J Burn Care Rehabil. 2005;26(6):478–82. https://doi.org/10.1097/01.bcr.0000185452.92833.c0.
54. Taylor SR, Jeng JG, Saffle JL, Sen S, Greenhalgh D, Palmieri T. Redefining the outcomes to resources ratio for burn patient triage in a mass casualty. J Burn Care Res. 2014;35(1):41–5. https://doi.org/10.1097/bcr.0000000000000034.

Chapter 19
Exfoliative Skin Diseases: Stevens-Johnson Syndrome and Toxic Epidermal Necrolysis

Felicia N. Williams and Jong O. Lee

Introduction

Stevens-Johnson Syndrome (SJS), Toxic Epidermal Necrolysis (TEN), and SJS/TEN overlap syndrome represent a spectrum of rare, but life-threatening type IV hypersensitive reactions to medications or infections [1–4]. The characteristic pathologic finding is complete or full-thickness necrosis or complete separation of the epidermis [1]. The reaction can present on any and every mucosal surface, as well as the skin [1]. The clinical diagnosis of SJS versus SJS/TEN overlap, versus TEN is based upon the severity or amount of skin desquamation. The loss of skin increases the risk of infection,

F. N. Williams (✉)
Department of Surgery, University of North Carolina School of Medicine, Chapel Hill, NC, USA

North Carolina Jaycee Burn Center, Chapel Hill, NC, USA
e-mail: fnwmd@med.unc.edu

J. O. Lee
Department of Surgery, University of Texas Medical Branch, Galveston, TX, USA

Shriners Children's Texas, Galveston, TX, USA

© The Author(s), under exclusive license to Springer Nature Switzerland AG 2023
J. O. Lee (ed.), *Essential Burn Care for Non-Burn Specialists*,
https://doi.org/10.1007/978-3-031-28898-2_19

sepsis, multiple organ dysfunction, and death, as skin is the patients' first line of defense against infection [5]. Mortality is related to the amount of skin desquamation, patient risk factors, and comorbidities [6, 7]. Major complications, increased morbidity and mortality related to SJS or TEN are similar in nature to those experienced by patients with major burn injuries. Upon suspicion of any of these diagnoses, patients warrant prompt transfer and treatment in a burn center [2, 4]. Burn centers have multi-disciplinary teams of specialized physicians, nurses, nutritionists, and rehabilitation personnel trained to manage patients critically ill from skin loss, and the subsequent metabolic and physiologic derangements [8]. This chapter discusses the pathophysiology of SJS and TEN, and current management guidelines.

Epidemiology

The incidence of SJS and TEN is approximately 1–10 cases per million yearly, with SJS being the most prevalent — occurring three times more commonly [9, 10]. Hypersensitive reactions to medications are responsible for up to 80% of cases [10]. Other causes are infectious (*Mycoplasma Pneumonia* or Cytomegalovirus) or vaccines [10]. There are up to 20% of cases without an identified cause [11]. It effects all ages, races, ethnicities, and gender but has been reported to be more common among older populations and more common in women [9, 10]. Significant risk factors for development of SJS and TEN include, but are not limited to having active malignancy, immune dysfunction or dysregulation, infection/sepsis, epilepsy, renal or liver dysfunction, or a genetic predisposition [4, 12]. Patients with a history of human immunodeficiency virus (HIV) have a higher incidence [4, 10]. Using the National Inpatient Sample from 2009 to 2012, which accounts for 20% of all admissions in the United States, Hsu et al. found that non-Hispanic white patients were least likely to present with SJS or TEN compared to all other races and ethnicities [4]. Like other groups, patients were more likely to be older and more likely to be women [4, 9, 10]. Patients were also more likely to have multiple comorbidities [4]. Mortality estimates are based upon degree of epidermal necrosis and detachment and have ranged from 12 to 40% in previous studies [13, 14]. Updated estimates from Hsu et al. show mortality risk for SJS at 4.8%, SJS/TEN overlap at 19.4% and TEN at 14.8% [4].

Pathophysiology (Histopathology/ Morphology)

SJS and TEN are T-cell mediated reactions [10]. For drug-induced reactions, natural killer cells and CD8+ T cells—which may be drug specific—induce apoptosis of keratinocytes and cause the activation and release of soluble cytotoxic mediators in SJS and TEN) [12]. In the cases of SJS or TEN secondary to viruses or autoimmune diseases, the factors contributing to widespread epidermal necrolysis are not completely understood [9]. Histopathological findings are subepidermal vesicles or blisters with widespread epidermal necrosis and apoptotic keratinocytes associated with mild or minimal lymphocytic infiltration [9]. Epidermal necrolysis is characterized by blister formation, partially or completely detached skin, erythematous skin, and flat, atypical target lesions. In almost all cases, mucous membranes are involved [9]. There is a temporal transition of lymphocytic infiltration in SJS and TEN. Early in the course of the syndrome, blister fluid is mainly composed of cytotoxic CD8+ T cells and natural killer cells. The composition of lymphocytes transitions to mainly monocytes later in the clinical course [9, 15]. Other noted cell types of significance are granulysin, found in cytotoxic granules, Fas-FasL, perforin, granzyme B, TNF-alpha, and nitrous oxide [10].

Clinical Presentation

SJS was first described in the 1920s. Drs. Stevens and Johnson reported on the mucocutaneous eruption in two children with concurrent ocular involvement [16]. It can result from *Mycoplasma pneumoniae* or *Herpes Simplex* virus infection or from a severe drug reaction [17]. TEN was a term used by Lyell in 1950s to describe a skin rash that appears similar to a scald [18]. The most common etiology for TEN is drug induced [17, 19]. Traditionally, patients are exposed to an inciting agent. Between days to usually up to 4 weeks, patients may then experience flu-like symptoms (fevers, chills, malaise, sore throat, myalgias, cough, rhinitis, headache, or generalized pain in the skin, eyes, or mucosal surfaces) [10, 20]. If systemic symptoms occur, they precede both mucosal and skin involvement [1]. Patients typically present secondary to the skin manifestations. They present with painful atypical targetoid lesions or bullae, or red erythematous violaceous patches or ulcers. When examined, or rubbed, the epidermal bullae will detach from the dermis—positive Nikolsky sign [1]. Up to 80% of patients have mucosal involvement—the hallmark of SJS/TEN [1]. The oral cavity is more involved than the eyes, genitals, or anus, but the entirety of the gastrointestinal and respiratory tracts may be involved [10, 11].

Acutely, patients are at risk for multi-system organ dysfunction [4, 9–11]. Over 40% of patients are at risk for pneumonia [9]. Nearly 15% of patients are at risk for renal dysfunction [9]. Gastrointestinal and cardiovascular complications are also common [9]. The loss of skin increases the risk of infection and sepsis as skin is the patients' first line of defense against infection [5]. Patients are in high risk of bacterial infections, with one single-center study reporting over 90% of patients with SJS or TEN with bacterial infections and over 60% of patients with sepsis [9, 21]. Long-term complications are often related to the extent and duration of symptoms during the acute phase. Patients may develop strictures in their gastrointestinal tract, genital adhesions, ocular impairment, or bronchiolitis obliterans [9].

Mortality is related to the amount of skin desquamation, patient risk factors, and comorbid conditions [6, 7]. Hsu et al. found that the main predictors of mortality were increasing age, number of chronic conditions, infection, malignancy, and renal failure [4]. There have been multiple scoring systems developed to help prognosticate mortality risk for SJS and TEN patients [7].

Management

Acute management of a patient suspected of having SJS or TEN is supportive and requires cessation of the causative agent, resuscitation, and evaluation or transfer to a burn center [9]. Major complications, increased morbidity and mortality related to SJS or TEN are similar in nature to those experienced by patients with major burn injuries. Upon suspicion of any of these diagnoses, patients warrant prompt transfer and treatment in a burn center [2, 4]. Burn centers have multi-disciplinary teams of specialized physicians, nurses, dietitians, and rehabilitation personnel trained to manage patients critically ill from skin loss, and the subsequent metabolic and physiologic derangements from that loss [8]. There has been an increased mortality in cases of delayed admission of 7 days or more after onset of symptoms to specialized centers [22].

One of the most critical steps in the evaluation of a patient suspected of having SJS or TEN is the history and physical examination. Identifying and stopping possible causative agents are lifesaving. The class of drug, first and last dose, half-life, and any potential previous exposures are important information in the early phases and treatment of patients with SJS and/TEN [9, 23]. Classes of drugs are important to note. If the medication was related to seizures, stopping may increase the patient's risk of seizures. If the possible causative agent is an antimicrobial, immediate cessation may increase the patient's risk of infection or sepsis which will increase their risk of mortality [4, 9]. Timing of medication may change the differential diagnosis [10]. In addition, medications with a long half-life may be associated with a higher mortality risk [23].

Clinical evaluation by dermatology is recommended. While the diagnosis is clinical, many centers prefer full-thickness skin biopsy confirmation, which may determine treatment options. In addition, determining the severity or amount of epidermal detachment is important. The clinical diagnosis of SJS versus SJS/TEN overlap, versus TEN is based upon the severity or amount of skin desquamation. Specifically, SJS involves up to 10% of (TBSA) epidermal detachment. SJS/TEN overlap involves 10–30% TBSA epidermal detachment. TEN involves over 30% TBSA epidermal detachment [9, 10, 12, 17, 23–25]. To date, there remains a lack of consensus about debridement [9, 26]. As in burns, nutrition, preferably enteral is paramount to improve outcomes [26].

Beyond supportive measures, there are a number of treatment options used to mitigate SJS and/or TEN. The ones discussed here are corticosteroids, immunoglobulins (IVIG), and cyclosporine. Corticosteroids use in SJS and TEN have not been shown to have a mortality benefit compared to supportive care alone. There have been links to higher risks of infections and sepsis [9, 26, 27].

IVIG inhibits Fas-mediated keratinocyte apoptosis [28]. Due to the suspected pathophysiology of SJS and TEN, IVIG has been used with mixed results. While there is a trend toward a mortality benefit, due to the heterogeneity of dosing and patient populations, its use remains controversial [9].

Cyclosporine is a calcineurin inhibitor, thus an inhibitor of cytotoxic T cells. It may have a potential therapy to help stop disease progression and promote healing though it is contraindicated for patients with renal failure and/or immune deficiency, or malignancy. There have been some reports with mortality benefit but these studies must be evaluated with caution due to the patient populations [9, 29, 30].

Risks and benefits of the potential therapies beyond supportive care should be weighed in a multi-disciplinary setting due to increased risks of morbidity and mortality of SJS and TEN and the potential therapies.

Conclusion

SJS and TEN, and SJS/TEN overlap syndrome represent a spectrum of rare, but life-threatening type IV hypersensitive reactions to medications or infections. The loss of skin increases the risk of infection, sepsis, multi-system organ dysfunction, and death. Major complications related to SJS or TEN are similar in nature to those experienced by patients with major burn injuries. Upon suspicion of any of these diagnoses, patients warrant prompt transfer and treatment in a burn center. Management is primarily supportive care, but steroids, IVIG, and cyclosporine are immunomodulating therapies that can be used for treatment. Most important treatment options are to stop the causative agent, resuscitate, and promptly transfer to a specialized center able to treat SJS/TEN with multi-disciplinary specialists that can effectively treat the acute syndrome and mitigate long-term consequences.

References

1. Schneider JA, Cohen PR. Stevens-Johnson syndrome and toxic epidermal necrolysis: a concise review with a comprehensive summary of therapeutic interventions emphasizing supportive measures. Adv Ther. 2017;34:1235–44.
2. Richard EB, Hamer D, Musso MW, Short T, O'Neal HR Jr. Variability in management of patients with SJS/TEN: a survey of burn unit directors. J Burn Care Res. 2018;39:585–92.
3. Pichler WJ. Delayed drug hypersensitivity reactions. Ann Intern Med. 2003;139:683–93.

4. Hsu DY, Brieva J, Silverberg NB, Silverberg JI. Morbidity and mortality of Stevens-Johnson syndrome and toxic epidermal necrolysis in United States adults. J Invest Dermatol. 2016;136:1387–97.
5. Greenhalgh DG. Management of burns. N Engl J Med. 2019;380:2349–59.
6. Bastuji-Garin S, Fouchard N, Bertocchi M, Roujeau JC, Revuz J, Wolkenstein P. SCORTEN: a severity-of-illness score for toxic epidermal necrolysis. J Invest Dermatol. 2000;115:149–53.
7. Noe MH, Rosenbach M, Hubbard RA, et al. Development and validation of a risk prediction model for in-hospital mortality among patients with Stevens-Johnson syndrome/toxic epidermal necrolysis-ABCD-10. JAMA Dermatol. 2019;155:448–54.
8. Carmichael H, Wiktor AJ, McIntyre RC, Lambert Wagner A, Velopulos CG. Regional disparities in access to verified burn center care in the United States. J Trauma Acute Care Surg. 2019;87:111–6.
9. Lerch M, Mainetti C, Terziroli Beretta-Piccoli B, Harr T. Current perspectives on Stevens-Johnson syndrome and toxic epidermal necrolysis. Clin Rev Allergy Immunol. 2018;54:147–76.
10. Oakley AM, Krishnamurthy K. Stevens Johnson syndrome. Treasure Island: StatPearls; 2020.
11. Chung WH, Wang CW, Dao RL. Severe cutaneous adverse drug reactions. J Dermatol. 2016;43:758–66.
12. Noe MH, Micheletti RG. Diagnosis and management of Stevens-Johnson syndrome/toxic epidermal necrolysis. Clin Dermatol. 2020;38:607–12.
13. Schneck J, Fagot JP, Sekula P, Sassolas B, Roujeau JC, Mockenhaupt M. Effects of treatments on the mortality of Stevens-Johnson syndrome and toxic epidermal necrolysis: a retrospective study on patients included in the prospective EuroSCAR study. J Am Acad Dermatol. 2008;58:33–40.
14. Sekula P, Dunant A, Mockenhaupt M, et al. Comprehensive survival analysis of a cohort of patients with Stevens-Johnson syndrome and toxic epidermal necrolysis. J Invest Dermatol. 2013;133:1197–204.
15. Le Cleach L, Delaire S, Boumsell L, et al. Blister fluid T lymphocytes during toxic epidermal necrolysis are functional cytotoxic cells which express human natural killer (NK) inhibitory receptors. Clin Exp Immunol. 2000;119:225–30.

16. Stevens AM, Johnson FC. A new eruptive fever associated with stomatitis and ophthalmia—report of two cases in children. Am J Dis Child. 1922;24:526–33.
17. Bastuji-Garin S, Rzany B, Stern RS, Shear NH, Naldi L, Roujeau JC. Clinical classification of cases of toxic epidermal necrolysis, Stevens-Johnson syndrome, and erythema multiforme. Arch Dermatol. 1993;129:92–6.
18. Lyell A. Toxic epidermal necrolysis—an eruption resembling scalding of the skin. Br J Dermatol. 1956;68:355–61.
19. Koh HK, Fook-Chong S, Lee HY. Assessment and comparison of performance of ABCD-10 and SCORTEN in prognostication of epidermal necrolysis. JAMA Dermatol. 2020;156(12):1294–9.
20. Schneider JA, Cohen PR. Prognosis and management of Stevens-Johnson syndrome and toxic epidermal necrolysis. J Am Acad Dermatol. 2017;77:e117.
21. Tocco-Tussardi I, Huss F, Presman B. Microbiological findings and antibacterial therapy in Stevens-Johnson syndrome/toxic epidermal necrolysis patients from a Swedish Burn Center. J Cutan Pathol. 2017;44:420–32.
22. Palmieri TL, Greenhalgh DG, Saffle JR, et al. A multicenter review of toxic epidermal necrolysis treated in U.S. burn centers at the end of the twentieth century. J Burn Care Rehabil. 2002;23:87–96.
23. Garcia-Doval I, LeCleach L, Bocquet H, Otero XL, Roujeau JC. Toxic epidermal necrolysis and Stevens-Johnson syndrome: does early withdrawal of causative drugs decrease the risk of death? Arch Dermatol. 2000;136:323–7.
24. Charlton OA, Harris V, Phan K, Mewton E, Jackson C, Cooper A. Toxic epidermal necrolysis and Steven-Johnson syndrome: a comprehensive review. Adv Wound Care (New Rochelle). 2020;9:426–39.
25. Harr T, French LE. Toxic epidermal necrolysis and Stevens-Johnson syndrome. Orphanet J Rare Dis. 2010;5:39.
26. Curtis JA, Christensen LC, Paine AR, et al. Stevens-Johnson syndrome and toxic epidermal necrolysis treatments: an internet survey. J Am Acad Dermatol. 2016;74:379–80.
27. McCullough M, Burg M, Lin E, Peng D, Garner W. Steven Johnson syndrome and toxic epidermal necrolysis in a burn unit: a 15-year experience. Burns. 2017;43:200–5.
28. Viard I, Wehrli P, Bullani R, et al. Inhibition of toxic epidermal necrolysis by blockade of CD95 with human intravenous immunoglobulin. Science. 1998;282:490–3.

29. Arevalo JM, Lorente JA, Gonzalez-Herrada C, Jimenez-Reyes J. Treatment of toxic epidermal necrolysis with cyclosporin A. J Trauma. 2000;48:473–8.
30. Zimmermann S, Sekula P, Venhoff M, et al. Systemic immunomodulating therapies for Stevens-Johnson syndrome and toxic epidermal necrolysis: a systematic review and meta-analysis. JAMA Dermatol. 2017;153:514–22.

Chapter 20
Burn Scar and Contracture Management

Jorge Leon-Villapalos ⓘ, David Zergaran ⓘ, and Tom Calderbank

Introduction

Burn scars are direct consequences of tissue repair following injury. Scars and contractures can be challenging when they become symptomatic from the physical and psychological point of view, leading to increased functional and cosmetic disability. Any strategies that accelerate healing and preserve tissue integrity will have a definitive impact in decreasing pathological burn scarring. Burn depth determines ultimate healing potential and therefore dictates initial management and the potential for scar morbidity.

Burn wounds can be broadly classified into superficial, characterised by rapid healing and epithelialisation with minimal scarring and deep, characteristically requiring surgical manage-

J. Leon-Villapalos (✉) · D. Zergaran · T. Calderbank
Department of Plastic Surgery and Burns, Chelsea and Westminster Hospital, London, UK
e-mail: Jorge.Leon-Villapalos@nhs.net; d.zargaran@ucl.ac.uk; calderbank@nhs.net

© The Author(s), under exclusive license to Springer Nature Switzerland AG 2023
J. O. Lee (ed.), *Essential Burn Care for Non-Burn Specialists*, https://doi.org/10.1007/978-3-031-28898-2_20

ment and therefore causing the most problematic and symptomatic of scars. Clinical assessment remains the most frequent technique to evaluate the depth of a burn wound although this has been shown to be accurate in up to 75% of the cases and is subject to the clinician's experience and expertise [1]

It is fair to say that burn scar management starts at the time of injury with appropriate first aid and physiology support approaches that stop the burning process, cool the burn wound, and preserve dermal perfusion and microvasculature [2, 3]. The provision of adequate cooling of the burn wound with running water has also been associated with reductions in conversion to full-thickness pattern, need for surgical debridement and ultimately, burn scarring [4]. The Jackson burn model [5] containing a classic description of concentric zones of burn injury is still relevant in highlighting the need to preserve the zone of stasis with any interventions (accurate burn assessment, fluid resuscitation) that may speed healing and therefore reduce scarring.

Delayed burn wound healing has therefore proved to greatly influence the outcome of scarring. A recent study in adult burns showed that an increase in standardised scar assessment scores, associated with worsening scar severity, is correlated with longer healing times after 21 days [6]. This study replicates the findings found in the paediatric population that concludes that there is a lower risk of hypertrophic scarring formation in scalds healed before 21 days, and that surgery is likely if healing is not achieved after that period [7].

Modern burn management comprises the attributes of being multidisciplinary and multimodal with an emphasis on dermal preservation and functional and cosmetic restoration. This approach ensures best outcomes in any circumstances of burn severity or aetiology. As burn treatment starts in the pre-hospital period with appropriate first aid, it can be stated that the first deterrent towards abnormal burn scarring is appropriate assessment and management by pre-hospital teams and emergency health professionals.

It has been reported that multidisciplinary burn team approach in the admission to specialised burn services is independently associated with significant survival benefit [8]. This is independent of the aetiology of the burn [9]. There are also definitive advantages in treating scars due to burns within a multiple team approach. The patient with a burn scar should be managed holistically focusing on functional and cosmetic improvement and rehabilitation. The non-burn specialist will need to strike the right balance and decide when referral for further management by the scar management team is necessary. This will warrant early intervention, objective scar assessment to address physical and psychological issues and will offer the patient the best choice of treatment that may include combination therapy and the use of the best technology available.

Multimodality pertains to the use of different burn wound management techniques adapted to the different initial presentation pattern (superficial vs deep) to warrant early healing and minimal scarring. This is coupled with the concept of dermal preservation. A study comparing different excisional techniques found, unsurprisingly, that "dermal preservation during acute burn excision is key to obtaining superior healing/scar outcomes, however, determining the most appropriate excision tool is an ongoing challenge" [10]. The message stated appears obvious: the better you manage the burn wound in the acute period in a multidisciplinary fashion, the better scar quality will be obtained. A superficial burn with plenty of self-regeneration potential will heal in an unproblematic fashion with minimal or no visible scarring or cosmetic mismatch. A deep burn requiring surgical excision that is performed in a too aggressive fashion will involve a much larger symptomatic scar that will impact on normal function, cosmesis, psychology, and self-image of the patient. We will assess later in the chapter the different multimodalities available in scar management.

Scar and Contracture Assessment

Continuous developments in acute burn care have reduced mortality and morbidity [11] due to improved treatment protocols, and specifically, in the assessment and management of inhalational injury, the intensive care of the critically ill burn patient, and the recognition for the need of judicious early excision and wound coverage. This has led to increased survivability and decreased hospital length of stay [12]. Despite these advances, burn scars and contractures remain a challenge. Abnormal burn scarring has been described as one of the major unmet needs in burn care [13]. Whilst ideally a burn scar should be soft, pliable, and with minimal discoloration or depigmentation, the reality is that severe deep burns may leave pathological, unsightly, symptomatic scars. These cause both functional and psychological impairment that may manifest as unsightly contractures that decrease range of motion, cause pain and itch, and exhibit cosmetically undesirable changes in pigmentation, vascularity, thickness, colour, pliability, and surface area. All these determinants affect quality of life and impact severely in the well-being of the patient [14, 15] and need to be taken into consideration when we assess the patient with a burn scar.

Burn scars can affect all ages from both the physical and psychological points of view. In children, specifically, a degree of sensitivity needs to be considered during the consultation as there can be associated long-term psychosocial and psychological difficulties and "reported lowered quality of life, particularly related to scarring and appearance" [16]. Psychological support is an important part of the management of the patients with burn scars. A recent survey highlighted that "patients with burn scars have higher levels of pre-existing psychological difficulties, carry a greater number of scars and experience more symptoms", specifically due to "appearance-related concerns, social anxiety, acceptance and coping" [17].

Scar History

A thorough history (Table 20.1) to assess and manage burn scarring should introduce first, a description that includes the mechanism of burn injury. This is an important factor in the potential outcome of burn scars. We found in the burn literature an observational study that sought to investigate the similarities and differences of wound healing and resultant scarring and stated that the mechanism of injury greatly influences wound dermal recovery [18]. The provision of first aid is also an important determinant in the development of pathological, symptomatic scarring. The description of the original assessment of the depth and extent of the burn is mandatory. It must also include the time to full healing of the burn wound. Other important determinants of burn scarring are the need for surgery to achieve healing, and any comor-

TABLE 20.1 Key points in the history taking for scar assessment

Original injury

- Mechanism of injury

- Provision of first aid at time of injury

- Depth and total body surface area of original injury

- Time to full healing / dressing free activity

- Need for acute surgery for original injury

- Comorbidities and current medications

- Skin type

- Subjective scar description or use of scar scale:

    – Functional concerns: pain, itch, decreased function, and impact on activities of daily living

    – Cosmetic concerns description: thickness, colour, relief pigmentation, pliability, vascularity, surface area

- Type of scar

- Need for referral

bidities or medications that may affect the restoration of the tissues and the ultimate quality of the scar. A number of important factors not to be missed in the scar assessment history are the skin type, colour, and ethnicity of the patient with a burn scar. Both the incidence of symptomatic pathological burn scar (atrophic vs hypertrophic vs keloid) and the response to the different modalities of scar treatment are heavily shaped by the type of skin [19].

It is widely accepted that the assessment of the scars can be broadly divided, following a thorough history as detailed above, into objective and subjective. Undoubtedly, the use of modern instrumentation for objective scar assessment provides a "more reliable evaluation of the scar, by a better reproducibility and lower inter-assessor variation" [20]. Nevertheless, the use of these objective tools may be limited for the non-burn specialist due to the need to purchase potentially expensive devices that require appropriate training, increase data collection time, and may not be used frequently enough in the management of these patients. For descriptive purposes, objective tools assess the colour and biomechanical characteristics of the scars with techniques such as laser, ultrasound, and tension measurement devices [21–23]. We will be concentrating in the subjective approach to the scar, which is the one more tailored to the non-burn specialist.

Scar Subjective Assessment and Scar Scales

We will expand on the subjective assessment. Even though a simple descriptive approach of the scar is possible by taking simple terms and applying them verbatim in the history taken from the patient (my scar is "ugly", "thick", "stiff" "dark", "red"), the potential need for referral to an expert scar centre warrants a more structured description of the pathological features of the scar. The function and cosmetic appearance can be compromised because the scar is abnormal in its colour, thickness, pliability, surface area, and causes pain and pruritus. The severity of these changes can be described using scar scales.

Even though there is no definitive consensus on the ideal scar scale, the most commonly used scar scales are the Vancouver Scar Scale (VSS) [24] and Patient and Observer Scar Assessment Scale (POSAS) [25], although there are other less frequently applied scales [26, 27]. The VSS scores pigmentation, vascularity, pliability, and scar height and thickness, but it does not take into consideration functional and psychological sequelae of scars despite several modifications [28].

The POSAS relies on two different assessment scales corresponding to the observer and to the patient. The six measures considered for the patient contain parameters similar to those measured by VSS but include functional concerns such as pain and itching in addition to colour, stiffness, thickness, and surface irregularity. The observer scale parameters include vascularisation, pigmentation, thickness, relief, pliability, and surface area. The addition of scores provides a comparison of the scar of the patient to normal, uninjured skin that defines the severity of the pathological scar.

Pathological Scar Types

The physical examination of the scar of the patient can be of immense diagnostic and therapeutic value, both to start uncomplicated lines of treatment or to provide an accurate description when making a referral to the expert scar centre. Even though a consensus scar classification has been agreed [29], this can be simplified for the scar on their way to full maturation into immature, when erythema is still present (Fig. 20.1) or mature when this feature has subsided and cannot be elicited on palpation of the scar (Fig. 20.2). On reaching maturation, characteristically the scar becomes flat and asymptomatic and can progress to atrophy with a contour defect (Fig. 20.3) in a process that may take a long time to be completed.

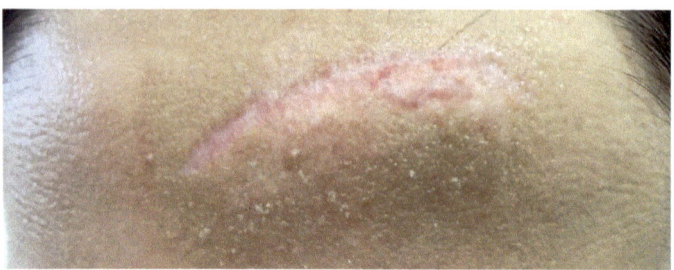

FIGURE 20.1 Atrophic immature burn scar with visible remaining hypervascularity

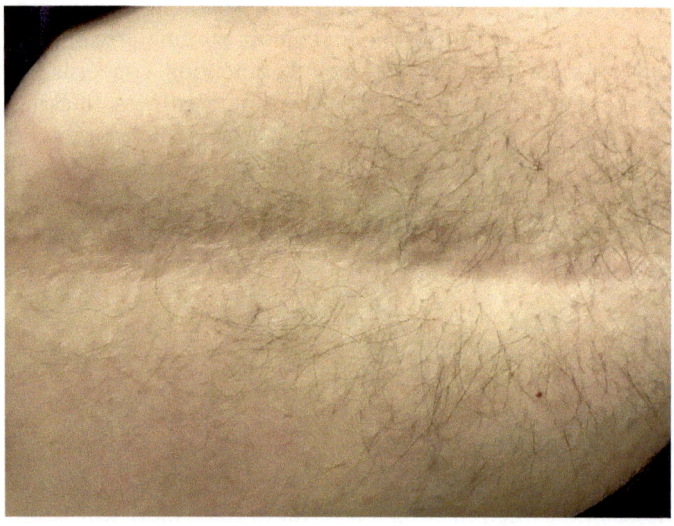

FIGURE 20.2 Atrophic mature burn scar without visible hypervascularity

Two main types of pathological scars can be identified easily based on history and physical assessment: hypertrophic and keloid scars [30]. Both types are the result of abnormal fibroblast, myofibroblast, and collagen production but express

FIGURE 20.3 Atrophic burn
scar

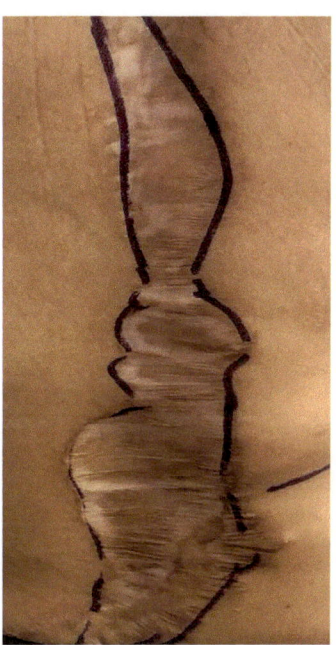

several individual peculiarities, even though both can be
symptomatic from the functional, cosmetic, and psychological
points of view.

Hypertrophic scars are common complications of burn
injuries [31] characterised by an initially raised pink or red
scar that enlarges within the first weeks of maturation and
causes symptoms such as pain and pruritus but stays within
the confinements of the original injury (Fig. 20.4).

Keloids (Fig. 20.5) are overall much more problematic
entities in their management due to their potential for recurrence. In comparison with hypertrophic scars, keloids usually
appear, with a slow growth pattern within months of the
initial burn injury and extend beyond the margin of the initial
wound.

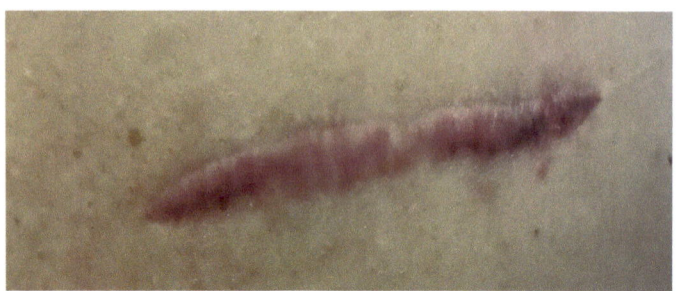

FIGURE 20.4 Hypertrophic scar

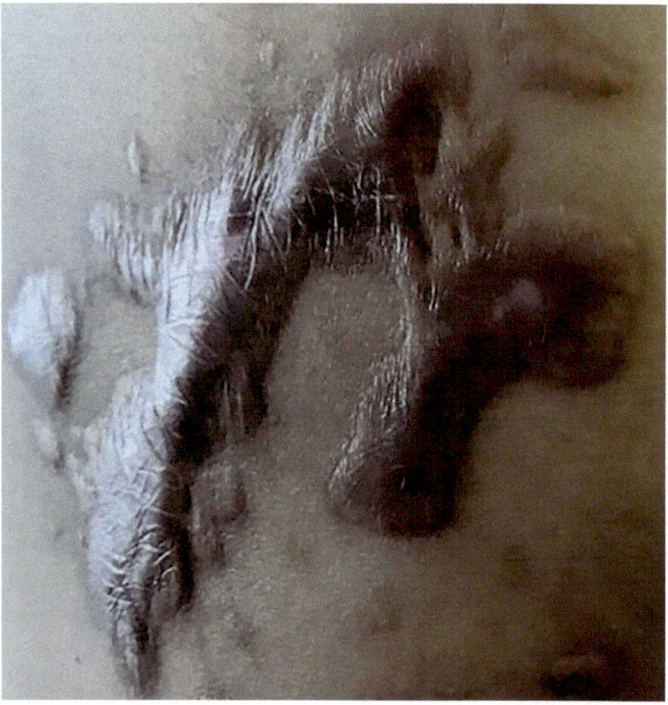

FIGURE 20.5 Keloid scar

Scar Management Options

A recent seminal paper [32] on management options for hypertrophic and keloid scars stated the following guidance:

- Conservative therapies should be administered on a case-by-case basis.
- Treatment of hypertrophic scars depends on scar severity with conservative management reserved for uncomplicated cases and surgery as first choice for the most severe presentations.
- Small and single keloids can be treated with combination of conservative therapies or radically by surgery with adjuvant therapy.
- Patients should be offered long-term follow-up.

Scar massage is one of the most basic and accessible options to provide relief to the patient's symptoms and provide changes that are most noticeable in itch and vascularity but without changes in the pliability, height, or other parameters in the scar scale. Even though patients report a noticeable and visible improvement, the lack of robust studies in the literature means that the clinician, with appropriate education, can safely choose the type of massage agent (creams vs ointments), the duration of the massage, and the technique to apply it without incurring any potential damage to the patient [33–35].

Silicone-based sheets and gels are useful therapeutic agents to prevent and treat hypertrophic and keloid scars and constitute one of the main tenets of treatment in burn scar management [36]. The mechanism of action through which scar improvement is elicited appears to be linked to scar hydration with suppression of the increased activity of the cellular components of the scar [37].

Injection of scar-modulating substances represents one of the most recognisable and minimally invasive therapeutic options in the treatment of hypertrophic and keloid scars. Even though a powerful anti-inflammatory effect can result in the scar with reduction in hypertrophic and keloid scar features with the use of injectable steroids such as triamcino-lone acetate, the variability in individual response and the potential for injection-site complications such as skin atrophy, telangiectasia, and dyspigmentation suggest caution and appropriate training in its use [38].

The use of 5-fluorouracil (5-FU) in combination with tri-amcinolone acetate preparations appears to be associated with a significant improvement in the treatment of hypertro-phic scars and keloids compared with the use of injectable steroid therapy alone [39]. Other injectable options that modulate pathological burn scarring include botulinum toxin [40], platelet-rich plasma (PRP) [41], and bleomycin [42].

The potential injection-site related complications of injected steroids have opened the possibility of using other therapeutic options that deliver steroid via transcutaneous delivery [43] using *steroid tapes*, even though their use is more limited than the injected form. Once these more conservative approaches have been exhausted as suitable options of man-agement for the scars, more complex approaches maybe nec-essary that require management within the environment of a scar service. Ultimately, surgery may be required. This chap-ter will not be dealing in detail with the multiple reconstruc-tive procedures available for reconstruction of complex scarring causing contracture, functional limitation, and cos-metic embarrassment that may include all aspects of the reconstructive ladder such as direct closure, skin grafting, tissue realignment techniques (z-plasty), flap reconstruction, and the use of dermal templates and tissue expansion. It is necessary, nevertheless, to describe the advantages that mod-ern technology has brought into scar modulation.

One of the most outstanding outcome-changing technical advancements for burn scars is the use of laser therapy, and the generalised introduction within scar services of the use of laser devices.

A review on the use of laser in the management of burn scars [44] found that laser therapy is efficacious in changing many abnormal scar scale parameters of pathological burn scarring from both functional and cosmetic points of view. Functionally, laser therapy may limit the number or complexity of the surgical reconstructive procedures required to deal with complex scars and contractures [45]. This may have improved cost-benefit advantages [46]. Cosmetically, it may improve abnormal parameters of pigmentation, vascularity, pliability, and thickness.

Fractional carbon dioxide (CO_2) laser has been found to significantly improve parameters such as thickness, pigmentation, vascularity, pliability, height of scar, and relief of burn scars [47]. It can be combined with other laser modalities such as pulsed-dye laser for hypervascularity [48] or used as a combination platform for delivery or injection of scar-modulating substances [49].

Micro needling offers an alternative to laser for atrophic, minimally raised or hyperpigmented scars [50]

Conclusion

The management of burn scars starts at the time of injury and requires a multidisciplinary and multimodal approach that preserves dermis and ultimately minimises scarring. The non-burn specialist requires a thorough approach to the scar history in order to provide conservative therapies or refer to a comprehensive scar management centre for escalation of more advanced techniques.

References

1. Monstrey S, Hoeksema H, Verbelen J, Pirayesh A, Blondeel P. Assessment of burn depth and burn wound healing potential. Burns. 2008;34(6):761–9.
2. Tan HMG, Chung L, Chong XY, Joethy J, Chong SJ. A simple mnemonic, B.U.R.N.S., for burns first aid. Burns. 2022;48(4):841–5. https://doi.org/10.1016/j.burns.2021.11.013.
3. Djärv T, Douma M, PalmierI T, et al. Duration of cooling with water for thermal burns as a first aid intervention: a systematic review. Burns. 2022;48(2):251–62. https://doi.org/10.1016/j.burns.2021.10.007.

4. Griffin BR, Frear CC, Babl F. Cool running water first aid decreases skin grafting requirements in pediatric burns: a cohort study of two thousand four hundred ninety-five children. Ann Emerg Med. 2021;75(1):75–85.

5. Jackson DM. The diagnosis of the depth of burning. Br J Surg. 1953;40:588–96.

6. Finlay V, Burrows S, Burmaz M, et al. Increased burn healing time is associated with higher Vancouver Scar Scale score. Scars Burns Healing. 2017;3:1–10.

7. Cubison TCS, Pape SA, Parkhouse N. Evidence for the link between healing time and the development of hypertrophic scars (HTS) in paediatric burns due to scald injury. Burns. 2006;32(8):992–9.

8. Win TS, Nizamoglu M, Maharaj R, et al. Relationship between multidisciplinary critical care and burn patients survival: a propensity-matched national cohort analysis. Burns. 2018;44(1):57–64.

9. Song M, Armstrong A, Murray A. Acid attacks: broadening the multidisciplinary team to improve outcomes. Burns. 2020;46(3):514–9.

10. Edmondson SJ, Ali Jumabhoy I, Murray A. Time to start putting down the knife: a systematic review of burns excision tools of randomised and non-randomised trials. Burns. 2018;44(7):1721–173.

11. Strassle PD, Williams FN, Napravnik S, van Duin D, Weber DJ, Charles A, Cairns BA, Jones SW. Improved survival of patients with extensive burns: trends in patient characteristics and mortality among burn patients in a tertiary care burn facility, 2004–2013. J Burn Care Res. 2017;38(3):187–93.

12. Latenser B. Critical care of the burn patient: the first 48 hours. Crit Care Med. 2009;37:2819–26. https://doi.org/10.1097/CCM.0b013e3181b3a08f.

13. Baumann ME, DeBruler DM, Blackstone BN, et al. Direct comparison of reproducibility and reliability in quantitative assessments of burn scar properties. Burns. 2021;47(2):466–78.

14. Finnerty C, Jeschke M, Branski L, Barret J, Dziewulski P, Herndon D. Hypertrophic scarring: the greatest unmet challenge after burn injury. Lancet. 2016;388:1427–36.

15. Greenhalgh D. Consequences of excessive scar formation: dealing with the problem and aiming for the future. Wound Repair Regen. 2007;15:52–5.

16. Maskell J, Newcombe P, Martin G, et al. Psychosocial functioning differences in pediatric burn survivors compared with healthy norms. J Burn Care Res. 2013;34(4):465–76.

17. Brewin MP, Homer SJ. The lived experience and quality of life with burn scarring—The results from a large-scale online survey. Burns. 2018;44(7):1801–10.

18. Jabeen S, Clough ECS, Thomlinson AM, Chadwick SL, et al. Partial thickness wound: does mechanism of injury influence healing? Burns. 2019;45(3):531–42.

19. Visscher MO, Bailey JK, Hom DB. Scar treatment variations by skin type. Facial Plast Surg Clin North Am. 2014;22:453–62.

20. Brusselaers N, Pirayesh A, Hoeksema H, Verbelen J, Blot S, Monstrey S. Burn scar assessment: a systematic review of objective scar assessment tools. Burns. 2010;36(8):1157–64.

21. Baumann ME, DeBruler DM, Blackstone BN, Coffey RA, Boyce ST, Supp DM, Bailey JK, Powell HM. Direct comparison of reproducibility and reliability in quantitative assessments of burn scar properties. Burns. 2021;47(2):466–78.

22. Lye I, Edgar DW, Wood FM, Carroll S. Tissue tonometry is a simple, objective measure for pliability of burn scar: is it reliable? J Burn Care Res. 2006;27(1):82–5.

23. van der Wal M, Bloemen M, Verhaegen P, Tuinebreijer W, de Vet H, van Zuijlen P, Middelkoop E. Objective color measurements: clinimetric performance of three devices on normal skin and scar tissue. J Burn Care Res. 2013;34(3):e187–94.

24. Sullivan T, Smith J, Kermode J, McIver E, Courtemanche DJ. Rating the burn scar. J Burn Care Rehabil. 1990;11(3):256–60.

25. Draaijers LJ, Tempelman FR, Botman YA, et al. The patient and observer scar assessment scale: a reliable and feasible tool for scar evaluation. Plast Reconstr Surg. 2004;113(7):1960–5; discussion 1966–1967.

26. Yeong EK, Mann R, Engrav LH, et al. Improved burn scar assessment with use of a new scar-rating scale. J Burn Care Rehabil. 1997;18(4):353–5; discussion 352.

27. Beausang E, Floyd H, Dunn KW, Orton CI, Ferguson MW. A new quantitative scale for clinical scar assessment. Plast Reconstr Surg. 1998;102(6):1954–61.

28. Tyack Z, Simons M, Spinks A, Wasiak J. A systematic review of the quality of burn scar rating scales for clinical and research use. Burns. 2012;38(1):6–18.

29. Mustoe TA, Cooter R, Gold M, et al. International clinical guidelines for scar management. Plast Reconstr Surg. 2002;110:560–72.

30. Huang C, Murphy GF, Akaishi S, et al. Keloids and hypertrophic scars: update and future directions. Plast Reconstr Surg Glob Open. 2013;1:e25.

31. Bombaro KM, Engrav LH, Carrougher GJ, Wiechman SA, Faucher L, Costa BA, et al. What is the prevalence of hypertrophic scarring following burns. Burns. 2003;29(4):299–302.

32. Ogawa R. The most current algorithms for the treatment and prevention of hypertrophic scars and keloids: a 2020 update of the algorithms published 10 years ago. Plast Reconstr Surg. 2022;149(1):79e–94e.

33. Ault P, Plaza A, Paratz J. Scar massage for hypertrophic burns scarring—a systematic review. Burns. 2018;44:24–38.

34. Shin TM, Bordeaux JS. The role of massage in scar management: a literature review. Dermatol Surg. 2012;38:414–23.

35. Valladares-Poveda S, Avendaño-Leal O, Castillo-Hidalgo H, et al. A comparison of two scar massage protocols in pediatric burn survivors. Burns. 2020;46(8):1867–74.

36. De Decker I, Hoeksema H, Verbelen J, et al. The use of fluid silicone gels in the prevention and treatment of hypertrophic scars: a systematic review and meta-analysis. Burns. 2022;48(3):491–509.

37. Bleasdale B, Finnegan S, Murray K, et al. The use of silicone adhesives for scar reduction. Adv Wound Care (New Rochelle). 2015;4:422–30.

38. Zhuang ZH, Li YT, Wei XJ. The safety and efficacy of intralesional triamcinolone acetonide for keloids and hypertrophic scars: a systematic review and meta-analysis. Burns. 2021;47(5):987–98.

39. Bao Y, Xu S, Pan Z, Deng J, Li X, Pan F, et al. Comparative efficacy and safety of common therapies in keloids and hypertrophic scars: a systematic review and meta-analysis. Aesthet Plast Surg. 2020;44(1):207–18.

40. Shaarawy E, Hegazy RA, Abdel Hay RM. Intralesional botulinum toxin type A equally effective and better tolerated than intralesional steroid in the treatment of keloids: a randomized controlled trial. J Cosmet Dermatol. 2015;14(2):161–6.

41. Hewedy ES, Sabaa BEI, Mohamed WS, Hegab DS. Combined intralesional triamcinolone acetonide and platelet rich plasma versus intralesional triamcinolone acetonide alone in treatment of keloids. J Dermatolog Treat. 2022;33(1):150–6.

42. España A, Solano T, Quintanilla E. Bleomycin in the treatment of keloids and hypertrophic scars by multiple needle punctures. Dermatol Surg. 2001;27(1):23–7.

43. Kondo A, Toyohara E, Sakae Y, Noda Y, Ogawa R. 341 effectiveness of corticosteroid tapes for hypertrophic scars and keloids. J Burn Care Res. 2019;40(Supplement_1):S147–8.
44. Willows BM, Ilyas M, Sharma A. Laser in the management of burn scars. Burns. 2017;43(7):1379–89.
45. Issler-Fisher AC, Fisher OM, Clayton NA, et al. Ablative fractional resurfacing for burn scar management affects the number and type of elective surgical reconstructive procedures, hospital admission patterns as well as length of stay. Burns. 2020;46(1):65–74.
46. Azzopardi EA, Duncan RT, Kearns M, et al. Cutaneous laser surgery for secondary burn reconstruction: cost benefit analysis. Burns. 2020;46(3):561–6.
47. Peng W, Zhang X, Kong X, Shi K. The efficacy and safety of fractional CO2 laser therapy in the treatment of burn scars: a meta-analysis. Burns. 2021;47(7):1469–77.
48. Hultman S, Edkins R. Pulsed dye laser photothermolysis versus fractional CO2 laser ablation for the treatment of hypertrophic burn scars: results from a large, rater-blinded, before-after cohort study. J Burn Care Res. 2019;40(Supplement_1):S37–8.
49. Bernabe R, Calero T, Lin J, et al. Laser-assisted drug delivery in the treatment of hypertrophic and keloid scars: a systematic review. J Burn Care Res. 2022;43(Supplement_1):S103–4.
50. Alster TS, Li MKY. Microneedling of scars: a large prospective study with long-term follow-up. Plast Reconstr Surg. 2020;145(2):358–64. https://doi.org/10.1097/PRS.0000000000006462. Erratum in: Plast Reconstr Surg. 2020 May;145(5):1341.

Chapter 21
Burn Rehabilitation

Lynne Benavides, Betsey Ferreira, Oscar E. Suman, and Jeffrey C. Schneider

Introduction

Burn care or burn rehabilitation at any level or phase of recovery can be very overwhelming to the non-burn specialist. In this chapter, we aim to provide education and practical approaches to burn rehabilitation for the non-burn specialist. With all of the significant advances in medical care for the patients that have suffered a burn injury over the past few decades, the survival rates of patients

L. Benavides (✉) · B. Ferreira
Rehabilitation Medicine, Rhode Island Hospital, Providence, RI, USA
e-mail: lbenavides@lifespan.org; BFerreira1@lifespan.org

O. E. Suman
Department of Surgery, School of Medicine, University of Texas Medical Branch, Galveston, TX, USA
e-mail: oesuman@utmb.edu

J. C. Schneider
Department of Physical Medicine and Rehabilitation, Spaulding Rehabilitation Hospital, Massachusetts General Hospital, Harvard Medical School, Boston, MA, USA
e-mail: jcschneider@mgh.harvard.edu

© The Author(s), under exclusive license to Springer Nature Switzerland AG 2023
J. O. Lee (ed.), *Essential Burn Care for Non-Burn Specialists*,
https://doi.org/10.1007/978-3-031-28898-2_21

433

with large total body surface area (TBSA) burn have greatly increased. There is evidence to support early involvement of occupational therapy (OT), physical therapy (PT), and exercise training in helping burn survivors reach their best possible outcome and continue to lead a meaningful and productive life. Implementing a rehabilitation program as soon as a patient is medically stable is imperative. This applies to a patient who has suffered a large burn and is being treated in a burn unit or to a patient who has suffered a small burn and is being treated in an outpatient setting. This chapter focuses on rehabilitation including OT and PT for the burn patients.

In rehabilitation of the burn patient, the lines between OT and PT can become blurred. The occupational therapist (OTs) and physical therapist (PTs) work as burn rehabilitation therapists. Each discipline has their specific roles and goals, however, burn therapy as a collective has many common threads. For example, goals of rehabilitation include prevention of contractures, preserving or regaining range of motion (ROM), strength, and functional abilities as well as helping patients to return to independent living. Although this is not a complete and exhaustive list, these are a few of the common threads for both OTs and PTs.

Role of OT in Care of the Burn Patient

OT theory is based on the belief that rehabilitation of dysfunction can occur through the use of occupations (daily activities and tasks) that have meaning for a patient. OTs assist the burn patient in engaging in and recovering the ability to perform Activities of Daily Living (ADLs)/ Instrumental Activities of Daily Living (IADLs), vocational and avocational activities, to help them return to their life roles as soon as possible. In burn care, OTs will screen or assess for potential for contractures, possible effects of scar, loss of skill performances, as well as evaluating for loss of motion, strength, edema, sensory injury or issues, cognition, and psychological adjustment. One of the major roles for an OT is determining the need for orthoses, positioning devices, adaptive or assistive equipment, and pressure garments. Once the screen or evaluation is complete, the OTs will establish a treatment plan. The OTs will inform and collaborate with the burn team on their plan of care. Initiation of OT should begin within 24 h of a patient being admitted after burn injury. OT will continue through the acute care phase, as well as during an acute rehabilitation stay, and in an outpatient setting. OT and /or PT should also be part of an outpatient burn clinic and care should be initiated as soon as possible to help achieve the best possible outcomes. Function, scar, and cosmesis will be the initial goals of treatment at this stage. A key point will be communication between all identified health care team.

Role of PT in Care of the Burn Patient

PTs plays a critical role in the multidisciplinary care of a patient who has sustained burns. Burns cause multisystem medical problems causing potential for prolonged hospitalizations and lengthy recovery. In the acute phase of care for hospitalized patients, PT should be initiated as early as the first 24 h. PTs primary goals are to limit loss of ROM, reduce edema, prevent predictable contractures through positioning and splinting, and prepare the patient for discharge by addressing patient function. Care for the patient will continue through rehabilitation stays and home care. The primary PT goals remain the same with the addition of assisting with initial scar management through early compression. The PTs may also assist with helping the patient adapt to any psychosocial issues related to their burn. Some key concepts to consider with acute treatment of patients with burns are maintaining effective communication with the team, scheduling therapy sessions around pain medication distribution, as well as patient and family education. As the patient progresses, outpatient services are often warranted and should be initiated as soon as possible upon the patient returning home. The outpatient PTs must continue to address any continued problem areas with ROM and edema but also progress the patient's strength and endurance through resistive exercise and cardiovascular exercise. The PTs should also address function as it pertains to return to work and any ADL. Special education should be provided on pressure garments, and scar management, and communication with the burn team should be ongoing to provide input on any skin contractures that may need reconstructive surgery.

Acute Rehabilitation of a Burn Injury

After a burn patient has been admitted to a hospital and has been stabilized medically, referrals for OT and PT should be placed. OT and PT begin in the acute care stage of burn patients and continue throughout the entire rehabilitation process. These along with familiar components of rehabilitation including evaluation, assessment of ROM, strength, sensation, edema, mobility, and ADLs are paramount to a successful initiation and plan for rehabilitation. Adaptive equipment or devices may also be used in the acute phase of treatment, and of significant importance to the progress and success in this acute stage will be positioning and orthoses. Psychological adjustment is also important to consider when treating a person who has suffered a burn injury. Even with small burns, it can have an effect psychologically and socially. These psychosocial effects should be monitored throughout the rehabilitation process, discussed, and addressed with the entire team as needed. During this acute rehabilitation stage, pain can be a limiting factor in a patient's participation in activities and exercise. Along with being aware of medication regimens, patient education regarding coping techniques should also be initiated early.

Positioning and Orthoses

Positioning

Throughout a patient's recovery, with significant emphasis in the acute phase of hospitalization, attention to positioning and prevention of contractures should be near the top of the priority after medical stability. Preventing or correcting contractures is integral in helping a burn patient return to function. Positioning a patient is all health care team's responsibility, however a rehabilitation therapist, OT, and/or PT may lead the way in determination of positioning for the best possible effect on functional performance and mitigation of possible contractures. Communication throughout the team regarding positioning will need to take place regularly. Pictures placed in the medical record or in the patient's room along with in person education for the staff and families are also a good way to ensure proper positioning. Also, if a patient is able in the acute stage, reinforcement of proper positioning verbally and with visual aids with the patient will begin to allow the patient to engage in their recovery process.

Keys to remember in a positioning program include reducing edema, reducing risk of contractures, allowing proper joint alignment, allowing facilitation of wound care, and reducing risk of possible associated iatrogenic injuries such as peripheral neuropathy and pressure sores.

There are several ways to achieve a proper antideformity positioning and neutral postures as well as protection of bony prominences. Orthoses, serial casting, foam-based troughs, wedges, pillows, straps and at times surgical intervention with pins or traction may be utilized to achieve a positioning goal.

Awareness and knowledge of contracture predisposition are important to understand for positioning and splinting purposes. Below is a table of some of the most common contracture predispositions and their splinting or orthotic recommendations (Table 21.1).

TABLE 21.1 List of recommended positioning

Affected area	Contracture predisposition	Prevention Position(s)	Device
Head		Midline, elevated 30–45°	Head of bed
Neck— anterior	Flexion	Neutral -> slight extension ~15° without rotation; no pillow use	Towel roll, anterior neck orthses, torticollis strap
Neck— posterior	Extension	Neutral ->slight flexion	Pillow behind head
Spine		Monitor for signs of scoliosis	
Shoulder/ Axilla	Adduction, protraction if anterior shoulder, chest involved	90° abduction; 15–20° horizontal adduction and 15–20° external rotation	Airplane orthoses, pillows, foam wedges, bedside tables, arm troughs
Elbow (anterior)/ Forearm	Elbow flexion	Elevation, extension	Anterior elbow orthoses, dynamic elbow flex/ext and pronation/ supination orthoses
Wrist/Hand- anterior/ palmar	Wrist and digit flexion, digit adduction, palmar cupping	Wrist extension, minimal MCP flexion, digits extended and abducted	Pan splint/orthosis

Hand-dorsal	MCP hyperextension, IP flexion, thumb adduction	Wrist extension, MP flexion, IP extension, thumb mid-palmar/radial abduction	Intrinsic + orthosis
Hip	Flexion, adduction, external rotation	Abduction 15–20°; full extension; 0° rotation	Abduction pillows; strapping
Knee	Flexion	Full extension until good quad function or mobility/ambulation	LE orthoses; knee immobilizer
Foot/Ankle	Plantar flexion	Neutral or slight dorsiflexion	Orthosis, footboard, traction, serial casting, multi podus boot
Toes (dorsal burn)	Dorsiflexion/clawing	Neutral	Foot plate, multi podus boot
Toes (plantar burn)	Curling or flexing	Neutral	Foot plate, multi podus boot
Mouth	Microstomia		Microstomia orthosis
Nostrils	Stenosis of anterior naris		Dilation device, gauges

Orthoses

The overarching goal of splinting is to assist in reaching the best functional outcome. The use of orthoses or casting can help to prevent loss of motion, preserve or improve ROM, protect vulnerable structures (skin grafts), assist in scar management and correction of contractures, support and/or assist weakened muscles as well as support, protect, and immobilize affected joints. Care should be taken so that an orthosis can allow for a reduction of edema, promotion of wound healing and maintenance of proper joint alignment. Care should also be taken that an orthosis does not cause harm in the form of pain, improper application over pressure points, and shearing of tissue or new skin grafts. An orthosis should be designed with forethought of function and ease of application and removal for dressing changes and/or exercise and function. In the acute hospital or rehabilitation stay, education for the health care team, family members and patients will be imperative to achieving the overall outcome for the use of an orthosis. In person demonstration of application/removal and proper positioning is vital, and adjunct education in the form of pictures or even videos in the patient's EMR, pictures hanging on the walls of the patient's room will assist in making sure an orthosis is utilized correctly for maximum effectiveness.

Early Mobilization

As with any critically ill patient, early mobilization is a key component of a patient's full recovery. Prolonged immobilization can lead to multiple issues such as joint immobility, weakness, deep vein thrombosis, pressure ulcers, and neuropathies. The challenge with mobilizing burn patients early in their intensive care unit stay is often limited by the need for frequent surgeries and post-operative restrictions with splints. When a patient undergoes a skin graft procedure that crosses a joint, the area is often splinted until the first dressing take down. This may limit the patient's ability to move and ambulate. However, ambulation should be started as soon as possible. The therapist will need a complete understanding of graft placement, ROM restrictions that may apply, as well as weight bearing precautions prior to initiating any mobility. A double layer of elastic compression should be applied starting from the toes and ending proximal to the grafted skin prior to ambulation. Initial ambulation should be limited in distance to avoid risk to the skin graft. Assistive devices should be utilized to aid the patient with stability and allow for adherence to weight bearing restrictions. In summary, the key points to allow early mobilization of burn patients are good communication with a multidisciplinary team, as well as the patient, good understanding of ROM and weight bearing precautions, application of a double layer of elastic compression, and sufficient assistance to allow the patient to have a successful experience.

Early Therapeutic Intervention

"Early therapeutic intervention in the burn unit has long term implications for restoration of function" [1]. Initiating therapy in the early phase of burn care in the form of stretching and exercise among other therapeutic interventions can contribute greatly to the prevention of contractures. Therapists will engage patients in either active ROM, active assisted ROM, or passive ROM depending on patients' medical condition. Ideally, active ROM is the goal as it assists in reducing edema and stretches healing tissue as well as promotes strength, endurance, and function. If a patient is having difficulty moving through their full ROM due to strength, endurance, tightness, or interference of medical equipment, active assistive ROM may be performed. For those patients who are critically ill or sedated, passive ROM is appropriate for a therapist to perform to help preserve ROM and prevent contractures. Once a patient is actively participating in their rehabilitation program, strengthening is also introduced into the program. Strengthening exercises can be in the form of isometric or isotonic exercises depending on the patient's condition. Endurance will also be a factor during therapeutic exercise. Shorter treatment sessions twice (or more) a day vs. one session per day may be beneficial if a patient is inhibited by low endurance.

Scar Management, a Rehabilitation Perspective

Scar is a natural part of the healing process and is defined as fibrous tissue replacing normal tissue that was destroyed by injury or disease [2]. Hypertrophic scar is characterized as having excess amounts of collagen which contributes to a red, raised scar but not to the extent of a keloid. It is also noted to not extend beyond the boundary of its original injury. It can promote scar contracture, but it can also regress with time. A keloid scar can appear as rounded protuberances that can be anywhere from pink to purple in color and extend beyond the boundaries of the original wound. Scar contracture is not common with keloids, but they do not regress over time and can recur after surgical intervention. The concerns for scarring in a burn injury are functional deficits as well as the psychosocial impact of scarring and its effect on cosmesis. It is important to provide education to patients and families regarding scar formation—the what, why, and how of development and treatment as well as to provide resources for psychological support for a patient and their family.

Burn patients are at risk for hypertrophic scarring. The time it takes for healing of a burn wound or skin graft (>2–3 weeks) contributes to hypertrophic scarring. Burn scars can take up to 2 years for full maturation.

Assessment

Assessment of scars falls into the realm of rehabilitation. Their impact on functional, cosmetic, and psychosocial outcomes makes them an important part of the rehabilitation process.

There are several outcome measures, scar scales, and tools that have been developed to assist in the process of scar assessment and evaluation of the efficacy of treatment. However, "no ideal scale that is suitable for all assessment purposes has emerged" [3]. The qualities of scar that are looked at can include, pigmentations, texture, thickness, pliability, size, as well as pain and pruritus [3].

The following table lists simple, easy to use, noninvasive, and inexpensive scar assessment scales as well as a list of more technical, expensive, and sometimes invasive tools (Table 21.2).

TABLE 21.2 Scar assessment and outcome tools

Simple, non-invasive, inexpensive
Vancouver Scar Scale
Modified Vancouver Scar Scale
Patient and Observer Scar Assessment Scale
Manchester Scar Scale
Matching Assessment of Scars and Photographs Scale
Technical, expensive, invasive
Photography
Ultrasound
Elastometer
Extensometer
Tonometer
Pneumatonometer

(continued)

Table 21.2 (continued)

Durameter/Durometer
Cutometer
Laser Doppler
Biopsy
Three-dimensional mould
Dermaspectrometer
Chromameter
Spectrocolorimeter
Infrared camera
Three-dimensional imaging
Oximetry
Planimetry

The simpler scales/tools are rated as more subjective and the more complex scales/tools are more objective. According to a study from 2009 by Forbes et al., they found that burn therapists believe that using a Burn Scar Outcome Measure is important and that they should be reliable, valid, quick, easy, and noninvasive [4].

Treatment

Compression or pressure therapy is one of the oldest and most utilized methods for prevention and treatment of hypertrophic scars. This can begin early when wounds are healed and skin can tolerate the shearing forces that can occur from a prefabricated or custom fabricated garment, wraps such as Coban, silicone or foam inserts, or conforming orthoses such as a transparent facial orthosis. Pressure garments can include elastic wrap bandages, tubular pressure bandages, an interim prefabricated garment, and a custom fabricated garment. Benefits of compression therapy include improvement in scar pliability and thickness, reduction of itching and pain, and prevention of contractures. It has been found that a compression pressure of 20–30 mmHg is an effective pressure to achieve the desired results [1, 5, 6]. One of the biggest threats to the successful outcome of use of compression is patient compliance. Non-adherence to use of compression can be attributed to discomfort, skin irritation/pain, and length of treatment time with garment. It is recommended that compression garments be used for 23 h per day for about 1 year or until the scar has matured.

The use of silicone gel sheets has also been widely used for burn scars. It can be used in conjunction with pressure garments. Elastomer putties and prosthetic foam are also other types of inserts available for use under pressure garments to enhance pressure over anatomical locations that are difficult to achieve adequate compression.

Other Scar Therapies

Scar massage has also been widely used in the treatment of post-burn scars. This should only be initiated once a scar has matured enough to tolerate a shearing force. Scar massage effects include assisting in softening or remodeling of scar tissue by affecting adherent fibrous bands which can assist in mobility of tissue as well. Scar massage techniques begin with pressure to blanch skin and mobilize skin surface without friction. Once the skin and scar can tolerate greater friction, the scar massage can include manipulation of tissue in circular, parallel, and perpendicular motions. Patients and families should be educated regarding scar massage techniques for optimal outcomes. Therapeutic heat may also be used in conjunction with scar massage as it assists in the extensibility of connective tissue [7]. Heat modalities can include moist hot packs, paraffin wax, fluidotherapy, and ultrasound and are completed prior to initiation of scar massage. Care should be taken when using a heat modality for patient tolerance and sensitivity (hypersensitivity or loss of sensation) after a burn injury. Low load prolonged stretching after use of a heat modality is also a utilized method for obtaining positive effects on ROM when scar is involved.

Outpatient Rehabilitation of Burn Injury

Burn rehabilitation does not end with discharge from the hospital after an acute injury. Burn rehabilitation starts on the day of admission and continue for several months to years after burn injury. Burn scar tissue is most active 3–4 months after an injury. Scar maturation can take up to a year or more. After suffering burn, patients can struggle with psychological or emotional issues, scars, contractures, and functional limitations as well as issues with re-entering community, school, or work. All of these issues can contribute to a decreased quality of life. Ensuring patients are part of a multidisciplinary outpatient burn clinic is paramount in helping them receive the services that they need to assist in improving quality of life. If the availability of a multidisciplinary clinic is not possible, ongoing communication between all caregivers is essential.

Wound care, splinting or casting, scar assessment and management, including compression garment, range of motion, stretching, strengthening, endurance, and exercise, as well as psychological/emotional adjustment, return to work needs and peer support are all part of an outpatient burn rehabilitation program. OTs and PTs continue to evaluate evolving problems during outpatient treatments, and communication with the burn team or current caregivers regarding ongoing issues with wounds or contractures can assist the surgeon in formulating reconstructive plans.

Conclusion

Rehabilitation is an important piece of treatment in helping patients put their lives back together. This is never truer than in the care of a burn survivor. Burn rehabilitation has unique challenges and requires persistence, patience, ingenuity, and compassion. It also requires a multidisciplinary team with effective communication skills. Taking on the challenges of burn care and rehabilitation can be overwhelming, however, knowing that your burn survivors have returned to all of their pre-burn functions and activities is proof that the challenge of burn rehabilitation is worth it.

References

1. Cheng JC, Evans JH, Leung KS, et al. Pressure therapy in the treatment of post-burn hypertrophic scar—a critical look into its usefulness and fallacies by pressure monitoring. Burns Incl Therm Inj. 1984;10:154–63.
2. "Scar" Def 1. www.lexico.com. Oxford English and Spanish Dictionary, Thesaurus, and Spanish to English Translator. 2020 Lexico.com.
3. Tredget E, Shupp JW, Schneider JC. Scar management following burn injury. J Burn Care Res. 2017;38(3):146–7.
4. Forbes-Duchart L, Cooper J, Nedelec B, Ross L, Quanbury A. Burn therapists' opinion on the application and essential characteristics of a burn scar outcome measure. J Burn Care Res. 2009;30(5):792–800.
5. Sharp P, Pan B, Yakuboff K, Rothchild D. Development of a best evidence statement for the use of pressure therapy for management of hypertrophic scarring. J Burn Care Res. 2016;37(4):255–64.
6. Herndon D. Total burn care e-book. Philadelphia: Elsevier; 2017.
7. Ward RS, Richard RL, Staley MJ. The use of physical agents in burn care. Burn care and rehabilitation principles and practice. Philadelphia: FA Davis; 1994. p. 419–46.

Chapter 22
Anesthesia for Burn Patients

Jamie L. Sparling ⓘ **and J. A. Jeevendra Martyn**

Introduction

Burn patients frequently present to the operating room (OR) during both the acute and chronic phases of their burn injury. Anesthesia clinicians are frequently called to undertake specific challenges with respect to airway management and vascular access, but they must also thoroughly understand and be prepared to address the pathophysiologic changes in each organ system affected by burn. Clinicians also must accommodate the pharmacologic changes induced by the body's response to the injury and adapt their anesthetic plan accordingly. In the chronic phase, anesthesia clinicians may utilize techniques to mitigate the effect of recurrent general anesthetics in vulnerable populations while accommodating the psychological impact of burn trauma and the associated pain and anxiety during repeated returns to the OR. Finally, knowledge of and experience in burn injury will enable clinicians to plan anesthetics during the chronic phase that facilitate ambulatory reconstructive procedures, when possible.

J. L. Sparling · J. A. J. Martyn (✉)
Department of Anesthesiology, Critical Care and Pain Medicine, Massachusetts General Hospital, Shriners Hospitals for Children—Boston, Harvard Medical School, Boston, MA, USA
e-mail: jlsparling@mgh.harvard.edu; jmartyn@mgh.harvard.edu

© The Author(s), under exclusive license to Springer Nature Switzerland AG 2023
J. O. Lee (ed.), *Essential Burn Care for Non-Burn Specialists*, https://doi.org/10.1007/978-3-031-28898-2_22

Anesthesia Considerations

Airway Management

Airway management may prove difficult in both the acute and chronic phases of burn injury. In the acute phase, direct thermal skin and inhalation injury may cause macroglossia or edema of the subglottic airway and the glottis. In the subacute and chronic phases, contractures may limit mouth opening (microstomia), jaw thrust, and neck extension. Even nasal passages can be blocked by contractures. Inhalation injury is more frequent in patients with burns sustained in a closed space, and clinical signs that predict inhalation injury include soot in mouth and pharynx, singed nasal hairs, vocal changes, stridor, and hoarseness. For patients with predicted difficult intubation, fiberoptic intubation—whether awake, anesthetized, or under sedation—is advantageous to navigate edematous airways and narrow mouth openings. Ketamine or dexmedetomidine may be utilized with minimal respiratory depression and may be especially useful in children for whom awake intubation is not possible. Manual distraction of the tongue utilizing gauze or a suction catheter, as well as jaw thrust by an assistant, may improve fiberoptic visualization. Video laryngoscopy with any of a large number of commercially available products (e.g., GlideScope, C-MAC, McGRATH MAC video laryngoscope) also offers improved visualization of laryngeal structures; however, their use may be limited in cases of microstomia [1].

Placement of a supraglottic or laryngeal mask airway (LMA) may be used as a rescue technique during difficult intubation, or as a planned conduit through which to intubate the trachea. Alternative airway techniques include retrograde wires following tracheotomy, fiberoptic stylets, or lightwand intubation. In patients for whom intubation is expected to be difficult due to contractures of the neck or face, the patient may be induced with anesthesia while maintaining spontaneous ventilation (e.g., ketamine, inhalation induction) until the surgeon releases the contracture to facilitate airway instrumentation. Finally, as in all difficult intubations, surgical airway equipment and a qualified surgeon should be available as a back-up plan, per the American Society of Anesthesiologists (ASA) Difficult Airway Algorithm [2].

Vascular Access

Adequate venous access is crucial to support the initial resuscitation and ongoing care of acutely burned patients. Several factors may hinder venous access including large total body surface area (TBSA) affected, peripheral edema from fluid resuscitation, and multiple graft donor sites. Ultrasound guidance is the current standard for internal jugular central venous and femoral vein cannulation and is a useful adjunct for other types of central lines, peripheral venous catheters, and arterial lines. Cannulation through burn wounds is occasionally necessary, and in such cases, it is important to meticulously disinfect the area. Ultrasound examination prior to cannulation attempts can evaluate for in situ clot of either peripheral or central veins, for which burn patients are at risk due to repeated cannulations, prolonged immobility, and hypercoagulability. Intraosseous (IO) catheters may be a useful alternative for up to 48 h, if venous access is difficult or impossible [3]. When transferring from a peripheral, nontertiary care hospital, where personnel experienced in placing central lines may not be available, intraosseous route is a good temporary alternative.

Volume Status/Fluid Resuscitation

Critically ill burn patients should receive prompt intravascular fluid resuscitation to reverse hypovolemic shock and prevent organ failure. Overly aggressive fluid resuscitation, on the other hand, contributes to pulmonary, gut, and peripheral edema—and if continued, may result in intra-abdominal hypertension or abdominal compartment syndrome.

Traditionally, initial fluid resuscitation has been guided by estimates based on the TBSA affected by burn. The "Rule of Nines" is used in adults, while the Lund-Browder chart may be useful in children who have variable body proportions depending on age. Patients with burns affecting less than 15% TBSA may receive oral hydration or intravenous fluids at 100–150% of the calculated maintenance rate. The Parkland and modified Brooke formulas have historically been used to guide initial fluid resuscitation for larger burns based on TBSA estimate, but more recent literature suggests that less aggressive resuscitation may be associated with improved survival and less edema. More important than following calculated volume targets, clinicians must incorporate clinical and laboratory parameters to guide resuscitation. Conventionally used parameters include urine output (target 0.5–1.0 mL/kg/h in adults), heart rate, blood pressure, lactate, base deficit, central venous pressure (CVP), BUN/Cr ratio, and fractional excretion of sodium (FE_{Na}). Several caveats are notable, however—for instance, urine output may be deceptively low due to the release of arginine vasopressin with acute burn, or it may be elevated despite hypovolemia due to the increased glomerular filtration rate during hyperdynamic state (48–72 h after injury), osmotic effects of breakdown products, and tubular dysfunction. FE_{Na} may be unreliable after administration of sodium-containing fluids or after diuresis.

Because of the limitations of these measures, novel methods have been studied to assess fluid status, and specifically to predict fluid responsiveness. Such examples include the use of a "mini" fluid bolus, a straight leg raise, or the end-expiratory occlusion (EEO) test [4]. The EEO test consists of pausing the ventilator for 15–30 s at the end of expiration, and cardiac output is assessed to determine whether the increase in right ventricular preload transmitted to the left ventricle improves stroke volume and thus cardiac output [5]. Pulse pressure variation (a surrogate for stroke volume variation) and inferior vena cava (IVC) size and collapsibility have been studied extensively, but both are reliable only under strict conditions [6]. Non-invasive cardiac output monitors (NICOM) utilize these and other principles.

Crystalloid is typically administered for initial resuscitation, with balanced crystalloid solutions preferred over normal saline to avoid its propensity for causing hyperchloremic metabolic acidosis. Colloid solutions, however, may reduce the degree of peripheral edema, at least transiently, and many burn centers have begun to incorporate colloid into earlier resuscitation [7]. Recent meta-analysis concluded that albumin infusion in the first 24 h was associated with reduced mortality and decreased occurrence of compartment syndrome [8]. Non-glucose containing fluids are typically utilized due to the insulin resistance and resultant hyperglycemia seen in major burns; however, glucose should be added for infants and others at risk for hypoglycemia.

Capillary wall permeability returns to normal in non-burned tissue around 36–48 h after burn, and consequently, peripheral edema begins to resolve over the subsequent 1–2 weeks. Fluids are restricted during this time, and diuretics may be administered to augment mobilization of the edema.

Blood product administration is frequently required in patients with major burns. As no standard hemoglobin threshold for transfusion in burn patients is established, clinicians must make individualized decisions based on levels required to restore circulation and maintain metabolic homeostasis. A survey of United States burn center directors revealed that the hemoglobin level below which respondents would transfuse increased with increasing TBSA, history of cardiac disease, acute respiratory distress syndrome (ARDS), and age [9]. Considerable bleeding may occur during excision and grafting procedures, and blood loss may be underrecognized due to losses into the surgical drapes, soaked wet sponges, and onto the floor. Thus, blood products may be transfused preoperatively in anticipation of blood loss or preemptively in the OR at the beginning of these procedures. Massive transfusion, when required, should occur in a balanced fashion with one fresh frozen plasma (FFP) for every one or two packed red blood cells (RBC), 1:1 or 1:2 transfusion ratio.

Temperature Regulation

Maintenance of normal body temperature in the severely burned patient requires the communication and collaboration of the perioperative team in both the OR and the ICU. Burn patients are particularly vulnerable to heat loss due to the lost thermal regulatory function of intact skin. Initial resuscitation is a susceptible period, and consideration should be given to utilizing warmed fluids or an in-line fluid warmer. Subsequently, dressing changes and dressing removal are an additional vulnerability. During the hypermetabolic phase, the inflammatory response causes an increase in the hypothalamic temperature set point, and hypermetabolism occurs to maintain this set point. Shivering increases oxygen consumption, which exacerbates catabolism in burn injury. Hypothermia below 35 °C contributes to coagulopathy through platelet inhibition [10], and hypothermia during surgery despite aggressive intraoperative warming is correlated with the development of postoperative acute lung injury (ALI). [11] Interventions to improve intraoperative body temperature maintenance include increased ambient temperature (80–100 °F), use of underbody fluid warmers, forced air warming blankets, radiant warmers, intravenous fluid warmers, minimization of exposed skin, and wrapping exposed skin in plastic insulation, especially the head. Patient temperature should be communicated with the surgical and nursing teams intraoperatively, so that, if necessary, surgery may be paused to allow the patient to warm to acceptable levels.

Analgesia

Burns necessitate aggressive pain management, as many aspects of burn treatment are inherently painful, including dressing changes, excision and grafting procedures, and physical and occupational therapy. Pain severity depends not only on the extent and depth of burns, but also on psychosocial factors that influence a patient's experience of pain. Inadequate analgesia may provoke anxiety with subsequent procedures, leading to a vicious cycle of pain and anxiety. Burn patients may also develop hyperalgesia and allodynia in the affected areas of burned skin and/or skin graft donor sites, in addition to the tolerance and opioid-induced hyperalgesia that follows from prolonged opioid therapy.

Opioids are the cornerstone of pain treatment in burn patients. While long-term opioid dependence has been a concern, addiction after therapeutic use of opioids for burn pain is rare. Opioids may be delivered via continuous infusion in ventilated patients, with intermittent IV boluses, enterally, or via patient-controlled analgesia (PCA) pumps with or without a continuous background rate. Opioid requirements generally decrease significantly after successful wound closure, which should be targeted as early as possible.

Myriad analgesic adjuncts have been reported in the literature. Ketamine has been shown to counteract the hyperalgesic effects of upregulated N-methyl-D-aspartate (NMDA) receptors after burn, and it may also possess anti-inflammatory effects [12]. Ketamine may be administered as a continuous background infusion during anesthesia or in the awake patient, or it may be administered via IV bolus for painful bedside procedures. Ketamine has a superb margin of safety in terms of dosing. Methadone offers the advantage of concomitant opioid agonism and NMDA antagonism, limiting opioid tolerance and opioid-induced hyperalgesia. Methadone's utility is limited, however, by its variable half-life due to cytochrome p450-dependent elimination and potential for drug–drug interactions [13].

Dexmedetomidine is an intravenous α_2-agonist with sedative, anxiolytic, and analgesic properties; preoperative administration reduced postoperative opioid requirements in adults [14]. Dexmedetomidine use with ketamine can produce adequate sedation and analgesia for pediatric patients undergoing burn wound procedures, though its use is consistently associated with hypotension and bradycardia [15, 16].

Perioperative use of gabapentinoids (i.e., gabapentin, pregabalin) has an uncertain effect on pain and opioid requirements, with a higher rate of dizziness and visual disturbances [17]. Further, gabapentinoids have been associated with potentiation of the respiratory depressant effects of opioids [18, 19].

Acetaminophen has opioid-sparing effects demonstrated for burn and other types of surgery, but generally must be used in conjunction with other analgesics for all but the smallest burns. Nonsteroidal anti-inflammatory drugs (NSAIDs) are generally avoided in the acute phase due to the increased risk of peptic ulcers, gastrointestinal bleeds, and renal impairment.

Regional anesthesia should be considered in all burn patients to improve both intraoperative and postoperative analgesia and facilitate early participation in physical and occupational therapy. Frequently, split-thickness skin graft donor sites are more painful than the actual burn wound, which may be addressed with either tumescent local anesthesia or regional nerve blocks. The surface area covered by tumescent anesthesia is limited by maximally allowable local anesthetic dose (e.g., lidocaine with epinephrine 7 mg/kg), but has been shown to be safe and effective with this constraint [20]. Regional nerve block may be delivered as a single injection or via a continuous catheter. Lateral femoral cutaneous block may be particularly useful as the lateral thigh is a frequent donor site, and this block affects only sensory innervation permitting early ambulation. This block may be combined with a fascia iliaca block if coverage of the anterior and medial thigh is also desired. Epidural analgesia or truncal blocks—such as transversus abdominal plane (TAP), rectus sheath, paravertebral, pectoralis I or II, or erector spinae plane—may be utilized for wounds affecting the chest, abdomen, or back. Meticulous care must be taken during regional anesthesia with respect to sterility and management of prophylactic and therapeutic anti-coagulation, according to nationally recognized guidelines [21].

Echocardiography and Point of Care Ultrasonography (POCUS)

Point of care ultrasonography (POCUS) and echocardiography have many uses in the perioperative care of severely burned patients. To date, small studies have examined the use of transesophageal echocardiography (TEE) on burn patients. These studies have reported reduced left ventricular (LV) systolic function, impaired diastolic function, valvular vegetation (i.e., with bacteremia), pulmonary hypertension, pericardial effusion, fluid overload, and right heart failure [22, 23]. TEE overcomes the challenges of access to the chest in patients with anterior chest and abdominal burns, yet placement of the TEE probe is invasive and may be difficult in patients with acute facial burns. Transthoracic echocardiography (TTE) is more readily available at the bedside in the Intensive Care Unit (ICU) and in many ORs.

Increasing attention has been given to perioperative use of POCUS, with recent recommendations published by the American Society of Regional Anesthesia and Pain Medicine (ASRA) for use of POCUS by anesthesiologists [24]. The ASRA recommendations include acquiring competency in airway evaluation (for confirmation of endotracheal, orogastric, and nasogastric tube placement), lung evaluation (for diagnosis of pneumothorax, complicated and uncomplicated effusions, interstitial fluid, diaphragmatic paresis), cardiac evaluation (as above), gastric ultrasound (for unknown fasting status, characterization of stomach contents, and aspiration risk), and FAST examination (Focused Assessment with Sonography for Trauma, for presence of abdominal fluid). Gastric ultrasound, in particular, may be an important tool to assess patients' gastric volume and stratify risk of aspiration. This evaluation may safely allow enteral nutrition to be continued with shorter required fasting times preoperatively for nutritionally vulnerable burn patients.

Perioperative Communication and Teamwork

The critical nature of extensive burn injury makes interprofessional communication and collaboration between surgery, anesthesiology, and nursing clinicians essential. Structured handoff procedures should be utilized for critically ill patients preoperatively and postoperatively to ensure that all essential information is conveyed and that the receiver is adequately prepared to assume clinical responsibility for the patient. During prolonged procedures, regular communication as to the progress of the surgical procedure, the patient's hemodynamic, fluid, and temperature status, and any recent laboratory analysis should occur. This dialogue allows for shared decision-making, for example—as to whether ongoing debridement will be tolerated or should be terminated, or whether a brief pause to allow for further fluid resuscitation

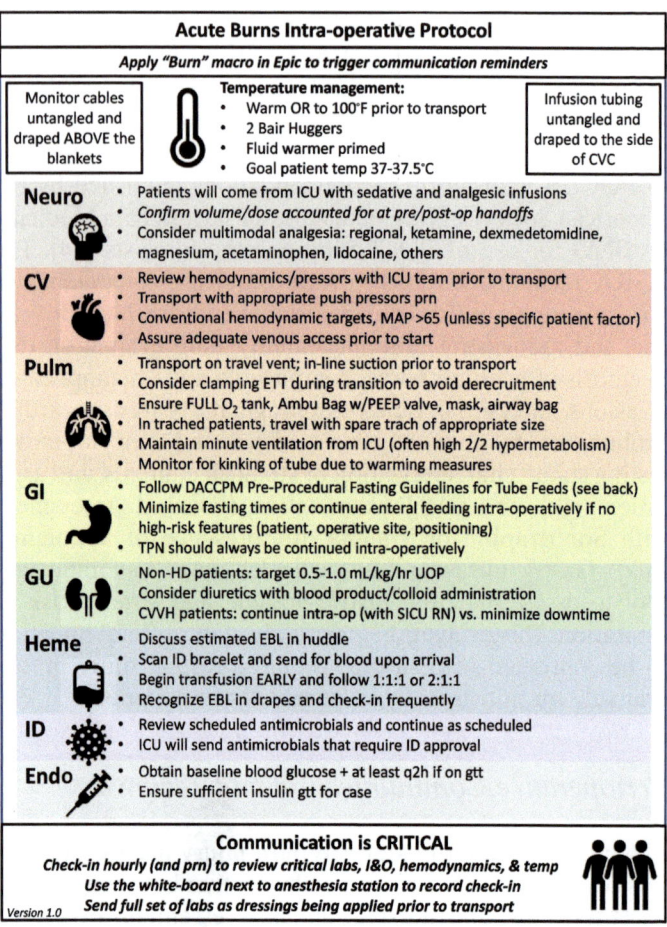

Acute Burns Intra-operative Protocol

Apply "Burn" macro in Epic to trigger communication reminders

| Monitor cables untangled and draped ABOVE the blankets | **Temperature management:**
• Warm OR to 100°F prior to transport
• 2 Bair Huggers
• Fluid warmer primed
• Goal patient temp 37-37.5°C | Infusion tubing untangled and draped to the side of CVC |

Neuro
• Patients will come from ICU with sedative and analgesic infusions
• *Confirm volume/dose accounted for at pre/post-op handoffs*
• Consider multimodal analgesia: regional, ketamine, dexmedetomidine, magnesium, acetaminophen, lidocaine, others

CV
• Review hemodynamics/pressors with ICU team prior to transport
• Transport with appropriate push pressors prn
• Conventional hemodynamic targets, MAP >65 (unless specific patient factor)
• Assure adequate venous access prior to start

Pulm
• Transport on travel vent; in-line suction prior to transport
• Consider clamping ETT during transition to avoid derecruitment
• Ensure FULL O_2 tank, Ambu Bag w/PEEP valve, mask, airway bag
• In trached patients, travel with spare trach of appropriate size
• Maintain minute ventilation from ICU (often high 2/2 hypermetabolism)
• Monitor for kinking of tube due to warming measures

GI
• Follow DACCPM Pre-Procedural Fasting Guidelines for Tube Feeds (see back)
• Minimize fasting times or continue enteral feeding intra-operatively if no high-risk features (patient, operative site, positioning)
• TPN should always be continued intra-operatively

GU
• Non-HD patients: target 0.5-1.0 mL/kg/hr UOP
• Consider diuretics with blood product/colloid administration
• CVVH patients: continue intra-op (with SICU RN) vs. minimize downtime

Heme
• Discuss estimated EBL in huddle
• Scan ID bracelet and send for blood upon arrival
• Begin transfusion EARLY and follow 1:1:1 or 2:1:1
• Recognize EBL in drapes and check-in frequently

ID
• Review scheduled antimicrobials and continue as scheduled
• ICU will send antimicrobials that require ID approval

Endo
• Obtain baseline blood glucose + at least q2h if on gtt
• Ensure sufficient insulin gtt for case

Communication is CRITICAL
Check-in hourly (and prn) to review critical labs, I&O, hemodynamics, & temp
Use the white-board next to anesthesia station to record check-in
Send full set of labs as dressings being applied prior to transport
Version 1.0

FIGURE 22.1 Intraoperative cognitive aid for burn anesthesia. Cognitive aids standardize intraoperative approaches to management of the critically ill burn patient and facilitate regular intraoperative communications between surgical, anesthesia, and nursing teams to align on patient status and inform shared clinical decision-making

and active warming may occur. Cognitive aids posted in the OR or embedded in the medical record may help facilitate these communications. (See Fig. 22.1.)

Anesthesia Implications, by System

Cardiovascular

Cardiac output is reduced immediately following a major burn due to (1) a decline in effective blood volume secondary to insensible and intravascular fluid loss from the burn in the first 24–36 h after major burn, (2) a decrease in venous return due to circumferential burns of the chest and abdomen, (3) impaired cardiac contractility, and (4) increased systemic vascular resistance (SVR) [25, 26]. TEE may be a useful adjunct to guide fluid resuscitation and administration of vasopressors or inotropes in the acute setting [23]. In scenarios where adequate fluid resuscitation fails to normalize the cardiac output, the impairment is likely due to a combination of inflammation-mediated myocardial depression and elevated SVR due to release of endogenous vasopressin, pain- or anxiety-induced catecholamines, and elevated viscosity due to hemoconcentration [25]. Early burn wound excision may help to attenuate these inflammatory-mediated changes and development of hypermetabolism [27].

Cardiac output in patients with substantial burns (e.g., involving more than 40% TBSA) evolves into a hypermetabolic phase within 3–5 days following an acute burn [28]. A deviance from these expected trends should prompt investigation into other causes of decreased cardiac output such as persistent hypovolemia or a stress-induced cardiomyopathy. Hypertension may occur during this phase due to increased catecholamines (pain- or anxiety-induced), angiotensin II, neuropeptide Y, vasopressin, and activation of the renin–angiotensin–aldosterone system (RAAS) [25, 29, 30]. Adrenergic antagonists, such as propranolol, have been found to modulate the hypermetabolic response in burn injury and may be initiated early in the acute phase [31]. Elevated oxygen consumption associated with hypermetabolism is reduced following complete excision and closure [32], but cardiac output may continue to be elevated for up to 24 months following injury [28].

Pulmonary

The American Burn Association's National Burn Repository reports a 10.3% incidence of inhalation injury among burn patients, although this figure is likely higher in those who present for anesthetic care in the acute phase [33, 34]. Mortality increases more than ten-fold in those patients with some degree of inhalation injury, and this fact has not changed despite advances in diagnosis and treatment [35]. Thermal damage is generally confined to the upper (supraglottic) airways as heat is effectively dissipated in the oropharynx and nasopharynx, and the vocal cords tend to close preventing heat from reaching the lower airways [34, 36]. However, supraglottic edema occurs within hours following injury, leading to airway obstruction and difficult intubation. "Thermal epiglottitis" may develop after intraoral scalds or ingestion of a toxic agent [37, 38].

Conversely, subglottic inhalation injury typically arises from the inhalation of noxious chemicals such as halogen acids, unsaturated aldehydes, and formaldehydes, depending on the type of product burnt. Inhaled nitrogen dioxide and sulfur dioxide form nitric and sulfuric acid, respectively, causing damage to the distal bronchi and alveoli. Hydrochloric acid, sulfuric acid, and phosgene exist as aerosols and can themselves reach the distal tracheobronchial tree and cause disruption of surfactant and produce direct injury to the alveolar membrane. These substances inflict direct irritation and trigger inflammation via neuropeptide production leading to hyperemia, mucosal sloughing, loss of surfactant, impaired mucociliary function, bronchospasm, and inducible nitric oxide synthase (iNOS) activation impairing hypoxic pulmonary vasoconstriction [39]. Cast formation can occur due to the sloughing of damaged mucosal epithelium, together with impaired mucociliary clearance; inhaled heparin and acetylcysteine have been studied to reduce airway cast formation and mucous plugging, with mixed reports of their efficacy [40].

Physical examination findings such as presence of facial burns, singed nasal hairs, or carbonaceous sputum have traditionally been associated with inhalation injury, however, these signs have poor discriminative value in predicting patients with inhalation injury and poor agreement with bronchoscopic diagnosis [41]. Clinical interventions for inhalation injury should rather be considered given a comprehensive assessment including estimated length of exposure, degree of enclosure, type of material burned, and any accompanying mental status changes. Flexible fiberoptic bronchoscopy is a useful adjunct to evaluate for inhalation injury, and more limited indirect (fiberoptic) laryngoscopy may help to evaluate for laryngeal edema. Xenon-133 scan is also a validated tool for diagnosis of inhalation injury, which measures the delayed clearance of Xenon-133 via damaged terminal airways, but its clinical utility is limited [42, 43].

Difficulty ventilating patients may arise due to reduced chest wall compliance from circumferential chest or abdominal burns and rarely pleural effusion [26]. Optimization of the functional residual capacity (FRC) through best positive end-expiratory pressure (PEEP) titration and recruitment maneuvers may improve ventilation-perfusion mismatching, but escharotomy may ultimately be necessary to relieve elevated thoracic or abdominal compartment pressures precluding adequate ventilation. Hypoxemia may also develop in the absence of direct inhalation injury, through the development of cardiogenic or noncardiogenic pulmonary edema due to fluid resuscitation or blood product transfusion (i.e., transfusion-associated circulatory overload (TACO)), or transfusion-related acute lung injury (TRALI). Acute respiratory distress syndrome (ARDS) may also occur independent of inhalation injury. The P_aO_2/F_iO_2 ratio at presentation predicts burn-related mortality [44].

Systemic poisoning from carbon monoxide (CO) or cyanide may drive tissue hypoxia. Diagnosis may be challenged by non-specific symptoms causing a delay in diagnosis, and thus CO poisoning should be suspected in enclosed (e.g., house) fires.

Renal

A variety of mechanisms may lead to acute kidney injury (AKI) following substantial burns. Myoglobinuria is more common following electrical burns and is associated with high-voltage exposure, prehospital cardiac arrest, full-thickness burns, and compartment syndrome [45]. Patients may present with some degree of prerenal AKI due to volume depletion and peripheral vasoconstriction caused by catecholamine surge, activation of the RAAS, upregulation of vasopressin receptors, and release of endothelin-1 and vasopressin [46]. Persistence of hypovolemia, hypotension, and hypoxemia may lead to acute tubular necrosis (ATN) manifesting as intrinsic renal injury.

Initial fluid resuscitation and the release of these mediators result in fluid retention commonly being seen in the first 2–5 days following a burn, which is followed by diuresis and an increase in glomerular filtration rate (GFR) concomitant with the increase in cardiac output and basal metabolic rate. However, this increase in GFR occurs even in the presence of hypovolemia, as the tubular dysfunction may limit the ability to concentrate urine. Thus, urine output may be a poor indicator of intravascular volume status. This may be reflected by a blood urea nitrogen (BUN) to creatinine ratio greater than 20.

Hepatic

Early liver injury may represent ischemic hepatopathy or "shock liver" because of hypoperfusion, direct injury from inhaled toxins, or reperfusion injury once intravascular volume has been adequately restored. Later liver injury may occur as a sequelae of the proinflammatory cytokine cascade. Functional assays such as the plasma disappearance rate of indocyanine green (PDR_{ICG}) may offer an advantage over static laboratory tests in predicting mortality [47].

The hypermetabolic response to burns is characterized by increased hepatic blood flow, hepatic oxygen uptake, synthesis of acute phase reactants, and gluconeogenesis [48, 49]. Other etiologies of later hepatic impairment include iatrogenic drug toxicity, blood transfusions, or sepsis. Fatty liver may also develop due to peripheral lipolysis induced by the hypermetabolic response, including in the absence of total parental nutrition [50].

Alterations to the hepatic clearance of common anesthetic medications are important to consider. Increased hepatic blood flow and enzyme induction in the hypermetabolic phase may decrease the half-life of perfusion-dependent (e.g., lidocaine, fentanyl) and enzyme-dependent (methadone, diazepam) drugs [51]. Variation among many factors, including magnitude of burn, timeframe following burn injury, co-administration, degree of protein-binding, and volume of distribution, make clinical studies of these drugs challenging to interpret.

Central Nervous System

Central nervous system (CNS) injury may occur in burn patients due to neurotoxin inhalation, hypoxic encephalopathy, sepsis, electrolyte abnormalities (particularly in the setting of volume resuscitation), or cytokine-related neuroinflammation [52].

Coma, delirium, seizure, or focal neurologic deficits may develop because of these injuries. Brain imaging upon presentation may be useful to diagnose the presence of cerebral edema and signs of elevated intracranial pressure, due to either concomitant injuries or hypoxic damage during the initial phase. Imaging can prompt neurologic or neurosurgical consultation as indicated. It is further helpful to establish a preanesthetic baseline neurologic status, when able, but this is proven difficult for patients who present from the ICU already receiving several sedative or analgesic infusions.

Hematologic

Following initial burn injury, prior to adequate fluid resuscitation, patients may experience hemoconcentration, which together with elevated plasma proteins as a component of acute phase reactants, increase blood viscosity. The anemia of thermal injury begins to develop approximately 2 days following injury and is multifactorial due to a combination of hemorrhage, hemolysis, and a decline in erythropoiesis [53]. Serial phlebotomy may also contribute. Some studies of recombinant erythropoietin in severely burned patients have shown a mortality benefit, while others have shown to have impact on mortality, blood transfusion requirements, or rate of thromboembolic complications [54]. Erythropoietin is also posited to mitigate burn-induced muscle wasting and secondary burn progression in animal models [55, 56].

Following major burn, platelets exhibit a biphasic response. Initially, thrombocytopenia occurs due to platelet aggregation and trapping in the lungs. Lower platelet nadirs and a longer duration of thrombocytopenia correlate with increased mortality. Additionally, patients are at higher risk of disseminated intravascular coagulopathy (DIC) in the first 3–5 days. Approximately 10–14 days following injury, thrombocytosis occurs due to inflammation. Later fluctuations in platelet count may be attributed to medication effect, sepsis, and dilutional effects [57].

Gastrointestinal

Acutely following burn injury, patients develop delayed gastric emptying and ileus. Because of this, all acute burns should be considered to have a full stomach prompting rapid sequence intubation (RSI). Additionally, prompt decompression of the stomach should occur, and appropriate gastric ulcer prophylaxis should be initiated. Bowel edema begins to resolve 2–3 days following injury, and early enteral feeding should be established to improve caloric intake, prevent stress ulcer formation, limit the requirement for gluconeogenesis, diminish muscle catabolism, and reduce bacterial translocation from the gut. Early enteral feeding is associated with reduced mortality and shorter hospitalizations [58]. Post-pyloric (e.g., naso-duodenal or nasojejunal) feeding tubes may be helpful in patients who do not tolerate gastric feeds due to impaired gastric emptying from edema or opioids [59].

Endocrine

Several endocrinologic alterations occur in patients with severe burn. Vasopressin is highest at the time of ICU admission and correlates with the percentage TBSA affected. Atrial natriuretic peptide (ANP) peaks around the fifth to sixth postburn day and plays an important role in restoring intravascular fluid homeostasis. Catecholamines remain elevated through at least the first week following injury [60]. Testosterone levels decline in the acute phase of burn, but replacement with the testosterone analogue oxandrolone has been demonstrated to shorten hospital length of stay, maintain lean body mass, improve body composition, and increase hepatic protein synthesis [61].

Alterations in the insulin signaling pathway occur following severe burn, resulting in insulin resistance, altered glucose metabolism, and hyperglycemia. These changes occur due to increased cortisol, proinflammatory cytokines, and free radical formation [62]. Patients with larger burns, older age, and increased body fat percentage are at higher risk for the development of insulin resistance [63].

Hypocalcemia develops in many patients with large burns due to altered calcium and magnesium metabolism, reduced secretion of PTH, and citrate toxicity due to blood product administration [64]. Aggressive calcium repletion is necessary to avoid the impaired cardiovascular function associated with ionized hypocalcemia.

Skin

Large TBSA burns impair temperature regulation, fluid and electrolyte maintenance and create a breakdown in the ability to physically block bacterial entry, with increased depth of burns correlating with the degree of permeability. Body heat may be preserved by elevating ambient temperature and utilizing radiant and forced air warmers, plastic coverings around the extremities, reflective insulated barriers, heat-and-moisture exchangers (HMEs) in ventilator circuits, and fluid warmers. In the chronic phase of burn injury, contractures may occur and limit respiratory excursion, reduce mouth opening, and make vascular access difficult. Wound infection rates may be reduced by topical antimicrobial therapies [65].

Metabolic

Interleukin-1 (IL-1), tumor necrosis factor (TNF), catecholamines, and stress hormones mediate the development of hypermetabolism in burn injury. Increased glucose, fat, and protein metabolism lead to increased oxygen demand and carbon dioxide production, which can be further exacerbated by fever or neurogenic hyperthermia. Nutritional demands are increased in burn patients, but carbohydrate-rich parenteral or enteral nutrition will further increase carbon dioxide production and require a higher minute ventilation to maintain normal carbon dioxide balance [66]. Energy expenditure is further increased by postoperative shivering, which may be mitigated by meperidine or dexmedetomidine [67].

Psychiatric

Anesthesia clinicians should be cognizant of the psychological trauma faced by many burn patients from both their initial injuries and sequelae. Burn patients and their caregivers commonly face depression, anxiety, acute stress disorder, and post-traumatic stress disorder (PTSD) [68, 69]. These issues should be anticipated and planned for by the anesthesia team caring for a patient through measures such as attention to such issues during informed consent, pharmacologic preoperative anxiolysis, and parental presence for pediatric patients where appropriate.

Special Populations

Pediatric

Children under 16 years represent 26% of admission to the United States burn centers. They are at increased risk for burns due to their immature motor and cognitive abilities, inability to self-rescue, and dependence on others for supervision. Young children also have thinner dermal layers leading to deeper injury at the same temperature and exposure duration, and the same quantity of hot liquid will affect a larger TBSA in children due to their smaller size [70]. Children are more susceptible to hypothermia due to the heat loss from altered skin integrity, as they have a greater ratio of surface area to mass. Further, the effects of hypermetabolism are accentuated due to children's baseline higher oxygen consumption on a weight basis. Children have even less respiratory reserve during airway management for this reason. Difficult intravenous access in small children is compounded in burn injury. Children may also require general anesthesia for procedures which may be done in the awake or less sedated adult, including dressing changes and line changes.

Children with burn may require multiple general anesthetics in both their acute injuries and the chronic phase of injury, raising concern for the neurocognitive effects of anesthetics on the developing brain [71]. Further prospective research is needed for children with repeat exposures, prolonged exposures, and in vulnerable populations.

Geriatric

Physical and cognitive limitations place elderly patients at increased risk for burn and make more difficult to manage due to the presence of medical comorbidities. In these patients, the hypermetabolic phase of burn injury may be delayed or absent. The increase in cardiac output may be poorly tolerated in patients with ischemic heart disease due to increased myocardial oxygen demand. Likewise, patients with diastolic dysfunction may develop pulmonary edema due to fluid resuscitation and peri-capillary leak. Medication clearance of anesthetics, analgesics, and sedatives may also be altered by impaired renal or hepatic function, and elderly patients are at increased risk of delirium perioperatively. The American Geriatrics Society recommends electroencephalographic (EEG) use during general anesthesia, regional analgesia when feasible, and optimization of non-opioid pain medications to prevent delirium in high risk elders [72].

Pharmacologic Considerations

Pharmacodynamics and pharmacokinetics are both affected following major burn, i.e., those exceeding 40% TBSA. In the initial resuscitative phase of burn injury, hypovolemia, myocardial impairment, reduced SVR, and increased blood viscosity compromise cardiac output and therefore organ perfusion, resulting in reduced clearance [51]. However, once the patient enters the hypermetabolic phase, usually around 48 hours after injury, provided resuscitation has been adequate, clearance may be enhanced by hepatic enzyme induction and increases in hepatic and renal blood flow depending on the drug [51]. Edema may result in increased volume of distribution, necessitating increased bolus doses and higher maintenance rates of infusions. Additionally, plasma protein concentrations are altered during both the acute and hypermetabolic phases, with a reduction in serum albumin and an increase in α_1-acid glycoprotein (AAG, an acute phase reactant). The activity of plasma protein bound drugs depends on the unbound portion, so small changes in plasma protein concentrations may result in large changes in the clinical effect of a given dose. The effective (unbound) concentration of drugs that bind albumin, such as benzodiazepines, is increased. On the contrary, the effective (unbound) concentration of drugs that bind AAG (e.g., tricyclic antidepressants, beta blockers, and local anesthetics) is reduced [73].

Tolerance

Receptor-mediated drug effects are altered in acute burn injury due to the up- or down-regulation of the corresponding receptors. For instance, extrajunctional acetylcholine receptors, specifically the α-7 acetylcholine receptors, emerge throughout the muscle membrane following large burn. Thus, 48–72 h following burn, patients demonstrate an increased sensitivity to depolarizing neuromuscular relaxants and a propensity for the development of succinylcholine-induced hyperkalemia. Risk factors for development of this hyperkalemic response include the dose of succinylcholine, time since burn injury, and severity of burn [51]. Conversely, the presence of extrajunctional acetylcholine receptors results in tolerance to the non-depolarizing neuromuscular relaxants.

Tolerance in burn patients may also develop to β-adrenergic antagonists, such as propranolol. This tolerance is hypothesized to be related to both high levels of circulating catecholamines and increased binding to plasma AAG, as above [74]. Antibiotic clearance is often augmented in burn patients, due to the enhanced glomerular filtration rate; this results in subtherapeutic serum levels unless larger and more frequent doses are administered. Similarly, renal clearance of H2-receptor antagonists is increased in the hypermetabolic phase, requiring increased doses for prophylaxis against gastric and duodenal ulcers [51]. Both tolerance and the potential for opioid-induced hyperalgesia occur in burn patients receiving narcotics for analgesia, yet these agents remain the cornerstone of pain control [75]. Finally, increased doses of intravenous anesthetics such as propofol are necessary due to both the increased volume of distribution and increased hepatic clearance. Caution should be exercised due to the potential for hypotension associated with large doses, particularly in hypovolemic patients.

Multimodal Analgesia

A multimodal approach to analgesia is necessary to address pain and anxiety in critically ill burned patients and to mitigate the risk for developing opioid-induced hyperalgesia. This approach will require modulation over time due to changes in sensitivity and the development of tolerance. Opioid-induced hyperalgesia and tolerance both occur with continuous opioid infusions and potentiate the need for further opioids. Opioid rotation, that is substitution of one opioid agent for alternative, can reduce opioid tolerance and is usually achievable with a ~25–50% decrease in equivalent dose [76].

As discussed above, adjunctive acetaminophen, NMDA-antagonists (e.g., ketamine), α2-antagonists (i.e., dexmedetomidine, clonidine), gabapentinoids (i.e., gabapentin, pregabalin), and/or local anesthetics reduce overall opioid requirements and improve pain control. Additionally, selection of methadone as an agent with both opioid and NMDA-antagonism activity offers theoretical advantages, but its pharmacokinetics is highly variable and has not yet been studied in burn patients. Observational studies have shown that early methadone initiation may reduce duration of mechanical ventilation [77]. A meta-analysis of four studies in burn patients concluded that dexmedetomidine, a selective α_2-antagonist, may provide deeper sedation and prevent hypertension in burn patients [78]. With each of these agents, pharmacokinetics depend on the phase of burn injury and individual heterogeneity, and thus they should be titrated based on clinical criteria and laboratory analysis of serum concentrations, when available.

Conclusion

Anesthesia care of severely burned patients must address the complex pathophysiologic changes affecting every organ system in burn injury. Careful attention to the pharmacologic changes in burn is necessary to choose and dose medications optimally for burn patients, depending on their phase of injury. Preparation and planning for the challenges of airway management, vascular access, and analgesia will afford the best opportunity for successful closure and subsequent care of severely burned patients. Through these efforts, anesthesia clinicians play an essential role in the multidisciplinary burn care team.

References

1. Woo CH, Kim SH, Park JY, Bae JY, Kwak IS, Mun SH, et al. Macintosh laryngoscope vs. Pentax-AWS video laryngoscope: comparison of efficacy and cardiovascular responses to tracheal intubation in major burn patients. Korean J Anesthesiol. 2012;62(2):119–24.
2. Apfelbaum JL, Hagberg CA, Connis RT, Abdelmalak BB, Agarkar M, Dutton RP, et al. 2022 American Society of Anesthesiologists practice guidelines for management of the difficult airway*. Anesthesiology. 2022;136(1):31–81.
3. Davlantes C, Puga T, Montez D, Philbeck T, Miller L, DeNoia E. 253: 48 hours dwell time for intraosseous access: a longer-term infusion using a temporary solution. Crit Care Med. 2016;44(12):140.
4. Guerin L, Monnet X, Teboul JL. Monitoring volume and fluid responsiveness: from static to dynamic indicators. Best Pract Res Clin Anaesthesiol. 2013;27(2):177–85.
5. Gavelli F, Teboul J-L, Monnet X. The end-expiratory occlusion test: please, let me hold your breath! Crit Care. 2019;23(1):274.

6. Monnet X, Marik PE, Teboul JL. Prediction of fluid responsiveness: an update. Ann Intensive Care. 2016;6(1):111.

7. Lawrence A, Faraklas I, Watkins H, Allen A, Cochran A, Morris S, et al. Colloid administration normalizes resuscitation ratio and ameliorates "fluid creep". J Burn Care Res. 2010;31(1):40–7.

8. Navickis RJ, Greenhalgh DG, Wilkes MM. Albumin in burn shock resuscitation: a meta-analysis of controlled clinical studies. J Burn Care Res. 2016;37(3):e268–78.

9. Palmieri TL, Greenhalgh DG. Blood transfusion in burns: what do we do? J Burn Care Rehabil. 2004;25(1):71–5.

10. Polderman KH. Hypothermia and coagulation. Crit Care. 2012;16(Suppl 2):A20–A.

11. Oda J, Kasai K, Noborio M, Ueyama M, Yukioka T. Hypothermia during burn surgery and postoperative acute lung injury in extensively burned patients. J Trauma. 2009;66(6):1525–9; discussion 9–30.

12. Hofbauer R, Moser D, Hammerschmidt V, Kapiotis S, Frass M. Ketamine significantly reduces the migration of leukocytes through endothelial cell monolayers. Crit Care Med. 1998;26(9):1545–9.

13. Kharasch ED. Current concepts in methadone metabolism and transport. Clin Pharmacol Drug Dev. 2017;6(2):125–34.

14. Unlugenc H, Gunduz M, Guler T, Yagmur O, Isik G. The effect of pre-anaesthetic administration of intravenous dexmedetomidine on postoperative pain in patients receiving patient-controlled morphine. Eur J Anaesthesiol. 2005;22(5):386–91.

15. Frestadius A, Grehn F, Kildal M, Huss F, Fredén F. Intranasal dexmedetomidine and rectal ketamine for young children undergoing burn wound procedures. Burns. 2022;48(6):1445–51.

16. Shank ES, Sheridan RL, Ryan CM, Keaney TJ, Martyn JA. Hemodynamic responses to dexmedetomidine in critically injured intubated pediatric burned patients: a preliminary study. J Burn Care Res. 2013;34(3):311–7.

17. Verret M, Lauzier F, Zarychanski R, Perron C, Savard X, Pinard A-M, et al. Perioperative use of gabapentinoids for the management of postoperative acute pain: a systematic review and meta-analysis. Anesthesiology. 2020;133(2):265–79.

18. Cavalcante AN, Sprung J, Schroeder DR, Weingarten TN. Multimodal analgesic therapy with gabapentin and its association with postoperative respiratory depression. Anesth Analg. 2017;125(1):141–6.

19. Myhre M, Diep LM, Stubhaug A. Pregabalin has analgesic, ventilatory, and cognitive effects in combination with remifentanil. Anesthesiology. 2016;124(1):141–9.
20. Bussolin L, Busoni P, Giorgi L, Crescioli M, Messeri A. Tumescent local anesthesia for the surgical treatment of burns and postburn sequelae in pediatric patients. Anesthesiology. 2003;99(6):1371–5.
21. Horlocker TT, Vandermeuelen E, Kopp SL, Gogarten W, Leffert LR, Benzon HT. Regional anesthesia in the patient receiving antithrombotic or thrombolytic therapy: American Society of Regional Anesthesia and Pain Medicine evidence-based guidelines (Fourth Edition). Reg Anesth Pain Med. 2018;43(3):263–309.
22. Maybauer MO, Asmussen S, Platts DG, Fraser JF, Sanfilippo F, Maybauer DM. Transesophageal echocardiography in the management of burn patients. Burns. 2014;40(4):630–5.
23. Etherington L, Saffle J, Cochran A. Use of transesophageal echocardiography in burns: a retrospective review. J Burn Care Res. 2010;31(1):36–9.
24. Haskins SC, Bronshteyn Y, Perlas A, El-Boghdadly K, Zimmerman J, Silva M, et al. American Society of Regional Anesthesia and Pain Medicine expert panel recommendations on point-of-care ultrasound education and training for regional anesthesiologists and pain physicians-part II: recommendations. Reg Anesth Pain Med. 2021;46(12):1048–60.
25. Crum RL, Dominic W, Hansbrough JF, Shackford SR, Brown MR. Cardiovascular and neurohumoral responses following burn injury. Arch Surg. 1990;125(8):1065–9.
26. Turbow ME. Abdominal compression following circumferential burn: cardiovascular responses. J Trauma. 1973;13(6):535–41.
27. Barret JP, Herndon DN. Modulation of inflammatory and catabolic responses in severely burned children by early burn wound excision in the first 24 hours. Arch Surg. 2003;138(2):127–32.
28. Williams FN, Herndon DN, Suman OE, Lee JO, Norbury WB, Branski LK, et al. Changes in cardiac physiology after severe burn injury. J Burn Care Res. 2011;32(2):269–74.
29. Murton SA, Tan ST, Prickett TC, Frampton C, Donald RA. Hormone responses to stress in patients with major burns. Br J Plast Surg. 1998;51(5):388–92.
30. Kulp GA, Herndon DN, Lee JO, Suman OE, Jeschke MG. Extent and magnitude of catecholamine surge in pediatric burned patients. Shock. 2010;33(4):369–74.

31. Williams FN, Herndon DN, Kulp GA, Jeschke MG. Propranolol decreases cardiac work in a dose-dependent manner in severely burned children. Surgery. 2011;149(2):231–9.
32. Lalonde C, Demling RH. The effect of complete burn wound excision and closure on postburn oxygen consumption. Surgery. 1987;102(5):862–8.
33. Mosier M, Bernal N, Faraklas I, Kahn S, Karanas Y, Lee J, et al. National burn repository. Chicago: American Burn Association; 2017.
34. Foncerrada G, Culnan DM, Capek KD, González-Trejo S, Cambiaso-Daniel J, Woodson LC, et al. Inhalation injury in the burned patient. Ann Plast Surg. 2018;80(3 Suppl 2):S98–S105.
35. Dyamenahalli K, Garg G, Shupp JW, Kuprys PV, Choudhry MA, Kovacs EJ. Inhalation injury: unmet clinical needs and future research. J Burn Care Res. 2019;40(5):570–84.
36. Moritz AR, Henriques FC, McLean R. The effects of inhaled heat on the air passages and lungs: an experimental investigation. Am J Pathol. 1945;21(2):311–31.
37. Verhees V, Ketharanathan N, Oen IMMH, Baartmans MGA, Koopman JSHA. Beware of thermal epiglottis! A case report describing 'teapot syndrome'. BMC Anesthesiol. 2018;18(1):203.
38. Dye DJ, Milling MA, Emmanuel ER, Craddock KV. Toddlers, teapots, and kettles: beware intraoral scalds. BMJ. 1990;300(6724):597–8.
39. Westphal M, Cox RA, Traber LD, Morita N, Enkhbaatar P, Schmalstieg FC, et al. Combined burn and smoke inhalation injury impairs ovine hypoxic pulmonary vasoconstriction. Crit Care Med. 2006;34(5):1428–36.
40. Deutsch CJ, Tan A, Smailes S, Dziewulski P. The diagnosis and management of inhalation injury: an evidence based approach. Burns. 2018;44(5):1040–51.
41. Ching JA, Shah JL, Doran CJ, Chen H, Payne WG, Smith DJ Jr. The evaluation of physical exam findings in patients assessed for suspected burn inhalation injury. J Burn Care Res. 2015;36(1):197–202.
42. Peters WJ. Inhalation injury caused by the products of combustion. Can Med Assoc J. 1981;125(3):249–52.
43. Agee RN, Long JM 3rd, Hunt JL, Petroff PA, Lull RJ, Mason AD Jr, et al. Use of 133xenon in early diagnosis of inhalation injury. J Trauma. 1976;16(3):218–24.
44. Hassan Z, Wong JK, Bush J, Bayat A, Dunn KW. Assessing the severity of inhalation injuries in adults. Burns. 2010;36(2):212–6.

45. Rosen CL, Adler JN, Rabban JT, Sethi RK, Arkoff L, Blair JA, et al. Early predictors of myoglobinuria and acute renal failure following electrical injury. J Emerg Med. 1999;17(5):783–9.

46. Aikawa N, Wakabayashi G, Ueda M, Shinozawa Y. Regulation of renal function in thermal injury. J Trauma. 1990;30(12 Suppl):S174–8.

47. Steinvall I, Fredrikson M, Bak Z, Sjoberg F. Incidence of early burn-induced effects on liver function as reflected by the plasma disappearance rate of indocyanine green: a prospective descriptive cohort study. Burns. 2012;38(2):214–24.

48. Jeschke MG, Barrow RE, Herndon DN. Extended hypermetabolic response of the liver in severely burned pediatric patients. Arch Surg. 2004;139(6):641–7.

49. Wilmore DW, Goodwin CW, Aulick LH, Powanda MC, Mason AD Jr, Pruitt BA Jr. Effect of injury and infection on visceral metabolism and circulation. Ann Surg. 1980;192(4):491–504.

50. Barret JP, Jeschke MG, Herndon DN. Fatty infiltration of the liver in severely burned pediatric patients: autopsy findings and clinical implications. J Trauma. 2001;51(4):736–9.

51. Martyn J. Clinical pharmacology and drug therapy in the burned patient. Anesthesiology. 1986;65(1):67–75.

52. Flierl MA, Stahel PF, Touban BM, Beauchamp KM, Morgan SJ, Smith WR, et al. Bench-to-bedside review: burn-induced cerebral inflammation—a neglected entity? Crit Care. 2009;13(3):215.

53. Wallner SF, Vautrin R. The anemia of thermal injury: mechanism of inhibition of erythropoiesis. Proc Soc Exp Biol Med. 1986;181(1):144–50.

54. Lundy JB, Hetz K, Chung KK, Renz EM, White CE, King BT, et al. Outcomes with the use of recombinant human erythropoietin in critically ill burn patients. Am Surg. 2010;76(9):951–6.

55. Wu SH, Lu IC, Tai MH, Chai CY, Kwan AL, Huang SH. Erythropoietin alleviates burn-induced muscle wasting. Int J Med Sci. 2020;17(1):33–44.

56. Tobalem M, Harder Y, Rezaeian F, Wettstein R. Secondary burn progression decreased by erythropoietin. Crit Care Med. 2013;41(4):963–71.

57. Warner P, Fields AL, Braun LC, James LE, Bailey JK, Yakuboff KP, et al. Thrombocytopenia in the pediatric burn patient. J Burn Care Res. 2011;32(3):410–4.

58. Khorasani EN, Mansouri F. Effect of early enteral nutrition on morbidity and mortality in children with burns. Burns. 2010;36(7):1067–71.

59. Sefton EJ, Boulton-Jones JR, Anderton D, Teahon K, Knights DT. Enteral feeding in patients with major burn injury: the use of nasojejunal feeding after the failure of nasogastric feeding. Burns. 2002;28(4):386–90.

60. Matsui M, Kudo T, Kudo M, Ishihara H, Matsuki A. The endocrine response after burns. Agressologie: revue internationale de physio-biologie et de pharmacologie appliquees aux effets de l'agression. 1991;32(4):233–235.

61. Jeschke MG, Finnerty CC, Suman OE, Kulp G, Mlcak RP, Herndon DN. The effect of oxandrolone on the endocrinologic, inflammatory, and hypermetabolic responses during the acute phase postburn. Ann Surg. 2007;246(3):351–60; discussion 60–2.

62. Berlanga-Acosta J, Iglesias-Marichal I, Rodríguez-Rodríguez N, Mendoza-Marí Y, García-Ojalvo A, Fernández-Mayola M, et al. Review: insulin resistance and mitochondrial dysfunction following severe burn injury. Peptides. 2020;126:170269.

63. Chondronikola M, Meyer WJ, Sidossis LS, Ojeda S, Huddleston J, Stevens P, et al. Predictors of insulin resistance in pediatric burn injury survivors 24 to 36 months postburn. J Burn Care Res. 2014;35(5):409–15.

64. Szyfelbein SK, Drop LJ, Martyn JA. Persistent ionized hypocalcemia in patients during resuscitation and recovery phases of body burns. Crit Care Med. 1981;9(6):454–8.

65. Cancio LC. Topical antimicrobial agents for burn wound care: history and current status. Surg Infect. 2021;22(1):3–11.

66. Masch JL, Bhutiani N, Bozeman MC. Feeding during resuscitation after burn injury. Nutr Clin Pract. 2019;34(5):666–71.

67. Liu ZX, Xu FY, Liang X, Zhou M, Wu L, Wu JR, et al. Efficacy of dexmedetomidine on postoperative shivering: a meta-analysis of clinical trials. Can J Anaesth. 2015;62(7):816–29.

68. Lodha P, Shah B, Karia S, De Sousa A. Post-traumatic stress disorder (Ptsd) following burn injuries: a comprehensive clinical review. Ann Burns Fire Disasters. 2020;33(4):276–87.

69. Boersma-van Dam E, van de Schoot R, Geenen R, Engelhard IM, Van Loey NE. Prevalence and course of posttraumatic stress disorder symptoms in partners of burn survivors. Eur J Psychotraumatol. 2021;12(1):1909282.

70. American Burn Association. Burn incident and treatment in the United States. Chicago: American Burn Association; 2016.

71. SmartTots. Consensus statement on the use of anesthetic and sedative drugs in infants and toddlers. San Francisco. p. 1.

72. American Geriatrics Society abstracted clinical practice guideline for postoperative delirium in older adults. J Am Geriatr Soc. 2015;63(1):142–50.
73. Martyn JA, Abernethy DR, Greenblatt DJ. Plasma protein binding of drugs after severe burn injury. Clin Pharmacol Ther. 1984;35(4):535–9.
74. Piafsky KM, Borgá O, Odar-Cederlöf I, Johansson C, Sjöqvist F. Increased plasma protein binding of propranolol and chlorpromazine mediated by disease-induced elevations of plasma alpha1 acid glycoprotein. N Engl J Med. 1978;299(26):1435–9.
75. Holtman JR Jr, Jellish WS. Opioid-induced hyperalgesia and burn pain. J Burn Care Res. 2012;33(6):692–701.
76. Nalamachu SR. Opioid rotation in clinical practice. Adv Ther. 2012;29(10):849–63.
77. Jones GM, Porter K, Coffey R, Miller SF, Cook CH, Whitmill ML, et al. Impact of early methadone initiation in critically injured burn patients: a pilot study. J Burn Care Res. 2013;34(3):342–8.
78. Asmussen S, Maybauer DM, Fraser JF, Jennings K, George S, Maybauer MO. A meta-analysis of analgesic and sedative effects of dexmedetomidine in burn patients. Burns. 2013;39(4):625–31.

Index

A

Abbreviated Injury Score (AIS), 149
Abdominal escharotomy, 128
Ablative fractional resurfacing (AFR) laser, 190
Acetaminophen, 317, 319
Acetic acid, 291
Acids, 288
ActiveFX™, 190
Acute lung injury (ALI), 454
Acute respiratory distress syndrome (ARDS), 159, 305, 308, 453
Adaptic™, 203
Adaptive immune system, 214
Adipose tissue (AT), 42
Advanced Burn Life Support (ABLS), 147, 256
Advanced Trauma Life Support (ATLS), 147, 152, 272
Airspace injury, 305
Airway compromise, 146
Airway injury, 304
Airway management, 151, 450
Airway security, 88
Alkalis, 295–296
Alkyl mercuric compounds, 297
AlloDerm®, 176
Allograft skin, 176, 215
Alpha-2 receptor agonists, 320

American Burn Association (ABA), 114, 152, 171, 216, 366, 391, 393, 394
Analgesia, 454
Anesthesia considerations
  airway management, 450
  analgesia, 455–457
  fluid resuscitation, 451, 452
  perioperative communication, 457
  temperature regulation, 454
  vascular access, 451
Anesthesia implications
  cardiovascular, 459
  central nervous system, 463
  endocrine, 465
  gastrointestinal, 465
  hematologic, 464
  hepatic, 462, 463
  metabolic, 466
  psychiatric, 466
  pulmonary, 460, 461
  renal, 462
  skin, 466
Anesthetics, 318, 323
Anticoagulants, 259
Antimicrobial agents, 187
Antiplatelets, 259
Antisialagogue/anticholinergic agent, 149
Anxiolytics, 318, 323

© The Editor(s) (if applicable) and The Author(s), under exclusive license to Springer Nature Switzerland AG 2023
J. O. Lee (ed.), *Essential Burn Care for Non-Burn Specialists*,
https://doi.org/10.1007/978-3-031-28898-2

Apocrine glands, 183
Arc injury, 268
Arm escharotomies, 203
Arterial blood gas analysis, 185
Aspergillus infections, 223
Aspergillus species, 219
Assessment, 443
Autograft skin, 175

B
Bases, 288
Benefits Improvement and
        Protection Act, 2000,
        376
Benzodiazepines, 149
Beta-2 agonists, 158
Biodegradable Temporizing
        Matrix (BTM),
        177, 189
Biodegradable Temporizing
        Matrix (BTM) plus
        STSG, 191
Biomedical Advanced Research
        Development
        Authority (BARDA),
        396
Blisters, 202
Bronchoscopy, 151, 158
Burn depth determination, 201
Burn disaster, 384, 385
Burn excision, 174, 175
Burn extent, 200
Burn injuries, 183, 389–390
    global and local inequities,
        7–8
    hypermetabolism, 31–34
    incidence, 3–4
    initial assessment of, 101
        airway security, 88
        burn-specific history,
            90–91
        checklist of, 87
        chemical burn injuries, 103
        chest and abdomen, 94
        clinical characteristics, 98
        cold induced injuries, 104
        electrical injuries, 106, 107
        extremity, 95–96
        first aid, 86–87
        genitourinary, 94
        neurological evaluation, 92
        non-accidental injuries,
            107–109
        ocular examination, 92, 93
        otolaryngology
            assessment, 93
        prehospital considerations,
            86–87
        primary survey, 88–90
        "Rule of Nines", 99
        secondary survey, 91
        tertiary survey, 102, 103
        treatment of minor burns,
            101
    metabolic consequences,
        34–39
    mortality, 6–7
    nutritional therapy, 46, 49–52
    pharmacological intervention,
        52–59
    prevention and control, 18–19
    pyramid of, 4
    risk factors for
        age, 8–11
        climate and seasonality,
            14–15
        comorbidities, 15, 16
        gender, 11–13
        interpersonal and
            collective violence,
            16–18
        occupational exposure, 13
    targeting organ systems,
        39–46
Burn injuries non-specialist
        providers, 367
Burn injury pain, 324
Burn mass casualty incidents
        (BMCIs), 384
Burn mobile phone app, 373
Burn model system (BMS), 358

Burn rehabilitation, 446
  acute rehabilitation, 436
  assessment, 443
  early mobilization, 440, 441
  early therapeutic
      intervention, 441
  orthoses, 440
  OT theory, 434, 435
  positioning, 437
  scar management, 442
  treatment, 444, 445
Burn resuscitation, 302
  checklist, 136
  complication, 126–128
  decision support system, 128
  deep burns, 117
  fluid resuscitation, 118–121
  management of, 129–131
  monitoring, 121–126
  pain management, 132
  positioning programs, 134
  rehabilitation, 133
  Rule of Nines, 114
  supportive care, 132–133
  symptomatic inhalation
      injury, 115
  teamwork, 135–136
  wound care, 132
Burn scar, 415–417
  continuous developments, 418
  contractures, 182
  history, 419, 420
  management options, 425–427
  pathological scar types, 421,
      423
  subjective assessment, 420
Burn surgeons, 342
Burn surgery services, 342
Burn therapy services, 344
Burn wound
  evaluation, 96–101
  infection, 306, 308
      diagnosis, 215–218
      microbiology, 218, 219
      prevention, 224
      treatment, 220, 222, 223

management
  burn surgery, 174, 177
  care algorithm, 169
  major burns treatment,
      172, 173
  minor burns treatment,
      170, 171
  skin anatomy, 168, 169

C
CAGE Alcohol Questionnaire,
      348
Capability, 390, 391
Carbolic acid, 291
Cardiovascular system, 302–304,
      459
  burn resuscitation, 302
  fluid creep, 304
  invasive monitoring, 303
Casting, 352
Cement, 296
Central nervous system (CNS),
      463
Central venous pressure (CVP),
      452
Chemical assault, 16
Chemical burns, 103, 368, 341,
      341
  acetic acid, 291
  alkalis, 295, 296
  alkyl mercuric compounds,
      297
  carbolic acid, 291
  cement, 296
  chromic acid, 292
  clinical background, 285, 286
  epichlorohydrin acid, 292
  formic acid, 292
  general management, 289, 290
  hydrocarbons, 297
  hydrofluoric acid, 293, 294
  hypochlorite solutions, 297
  mechanisms of action, 287
  muriatic acid, 293
  nitric acid, 294

Chemical burns (*cont.*)
  oxalic acid, 295
  pathophysiology, 286
  phosphorus, 295
  sulfuric acid, 293
  tar, 297
  vesicant chemical warfare
      agents, 298
Chest x-ray, 185
Child life and scholastic support
      services, 346
Chromic acid, 291
Chronic obstructive pulmonary
      disease (COPD), 258,
      259
Circulatory system, 257
Clinical Practice Guidelines, 223
Clinical Pulmonary Infection
      Score (CPIS), 308
Cognitive behavioral therapy
      (CBT), 327, 328, 345
Cognitive techniques, 327, 328
Cold induced injuries, 104
Collective violence, 17
Colloidal oatmeal baths, 208
Committee on Crisis Standards
      of Care (CoCSoC), 398
Compression, 441
Consensus-based burn nursing
      competencies, 343
Conservative approach, 189, 190
Continuous development, 418
Continuous renal replacement
      therapy (CRRT), 311
Cool water, 86
Coronavirus (COVID-19), 377
Corrosion, 287
Corticotrophin-releasing
      hormone (CRH), 45
Critical-care pain observation
      tool (CPOT), 316
Crystalloid resuscitation, 302
Cyclosporine, 410
Cytokines, 33

D
Dakin's solution, 222
Debridement, 200
DeepFX™, 190
Delayed debridement, 214
Denver criteria, 152
Dermis, 183
Desiccation, 287
Distraction techniques, 327
Doppler flowmetry, 130
Dry dressings, 202
Dyspnea, 155

E
Early mobilization, 441
Early therapeutic intervention,
      441
Eastern Association for the
      Surgery of Trauma, 152
Echocardiography, 123
Ectropion, 184
Elderly burns
  initial assessment and
      resuscitation, 256–258
  medications, 259
  non-accidental injury, 261
  nutritional supplementation,
      260
  outcomes, 262
  pain control, 260
  pre-existing conditions, 258
  surgical treatment, 261
Electrical injuries, 106, 107, 341
  acute management, 272
  aggressive resuscitation, 275
  compartment syndrome, 268,
      272, 275, 276
  complications, 271, 277, 278
  electrocardiographic
      monitoring, 273
  high voltage injuries, 270
  lightning strikes, 271, 272
  low voltage injuries, 270

pathophysiology, 268
rhabdomyolysis, 274
wound care, 268, 276
Endocrine system, 257
Endotoxin, 33
Endotracheal tube, 116
Epichlorohydrin acid, 292
Epidermis, 183
Escharotomy, 117, 130, 172, 174
Extracorporeal membrane
    oxygenation (ECMO),
    305
Extubation guidelines, 154

F
Facial burns, 148, 182
    anatomy and pathophysiology
        of, 182–184
    deep facial burns, 187–189
    inhalation injury, 184–186
    management of, 182, 186, 187
        burn reconstruction of
            anatomical regions,
            191, 192
        conservative approach,
            189, 190
        laser therapy, 190, 191
        surgical approach, 190
Facial landmarks, 182
Facial subunits, 182
Federal resources, 395
Fiberoptic endoscopic evaluation
    of swallowing (FEES),
    310
First aid, 86–87
Flame injury, 268
Flexible bronchoscopy, 148
Flexor sparing, 109
Fluid creep, 303–304
Fluid resuscitation, 118–121
5-Fluorouracil (5-FU), 426
Foley catheters, 107
Formic acid, 292
Fractional excretion of sodium
    (FENa), 452

French/McCauley technique, 191
Functional residual capacity
    (FRC), 461
Fungal burn, 217
Fungal infections, 223
Fungal pathogens, 219

G
Gabapentin, 317, 319, 320
Gastrointestinal (GI) changes, 40
Gender-based (GBV)/intimate
    partner violence (IPV),
    17
General anesthesia, 116
Geriatric, 468
Global Burden of Disease Study
    (GBD), 6
Glomerular filtration rate
    (GFR), 462
Glucose homeostasis, 34
Glucose metabolism, 34–36
Gram-negative organisms, 218
Gram-positive organisms, 225
Growth hormone-releasing
    hormone (GHRH), 45

H
Haddon Matrix, 19–21
Hair follicles, 183
Hand burn treatment
    aim of, 199
    anatomy of hand skin, 198
    etiology of, 198
    initial hand burn evaluation,
        199
    long-term issues in, 207, 208
    maintain circulation, 203
    range of motion, 206, 207
    wound closure, 204–206
    wound healing environment,
        202
Hand splints, 206
Health and Human Services
    (HHS), 395

Health Insurance Portability and
  Accountability Act
  (HIPAA), 375
Hemoglobin binds carbon
  monoxide (CO), 154
High voltage injuries, 97, 268, 270,
  276, 368
Home oxygen, 259
Hormone sensitive lipase (HSL),
  44
Hospital Preparedness Program
  (HPP), 395
Human GH, 54
Hydrocarbons, 297
Hydrochloric acid, 287, 292–293
Hydrofluoric acid, 288, 293, 294
Hydroxocobalamin, 155
Hyperglycemia, 308, 310
Hypermetabolism, 31–34, 51
Hypertrophic scarring, 187
Hypnosis, 327, 328
Hypochlorite solutions, 297
Hypotension, 155
Hypovolemia, 118
Hypoxemia, 147

I
Immersion hydrotherapy, 214
Immunosuppression, 214
Inducible nitric oxide synthase
  (iNOS), 460
Industrial accidents, 387
Infectious Diseases Society of
  America, 219
Inflammatory agents, 156
Inflammatory response, 146
Inhalation injury, 184–186, 304,
  305, 309, 339, 340, 368
  airway management, 151–154
  assessment and grading, 147,
    149, 150
  carbon monoxide and
    hydrogen cyanide, 154

complications, 158, 160
  mechanical ventilation, 155,
    156
  medical therapy, 156, 158
  pathophysiology, 146, 147
Inhaled hydrogen cyanide
  (HCN), 155
Inhaled nitrous oxide, 323
Innate immune system, 214
Inorganic solutions, 288
Insulin, 56–57
Integra®, 176
Integra Dermal Regeneration
  Template, 191
Interleukin 6 (IL-6), 33
Invasive fungal infections, 223

J
Joint fixation, 206

K
Ketamine, 116, 318, 322
Kirschner wires, 206

L
Lactic acidosis, 155
Laser Doppler imaging, 100
Laser therapy, 190
Lidocaine, 322, 323
Lipid metabolism, 36
Lipolysis, 50
Lipopolysaccharide (LPS), 32
Local tissue rearrangement
  techniques, 192
Local V-Y advancement flaps,
  192
Lower airway inhalation injury,
  305
Low voltage injuries, 268, 270,
  276, 278
Lund-Browder method, 99

M
Mafenide acetate, 220, 276–277
Mass casualty incident, 383
Mass gatherings, 385, 386
Material Safety Data Sheets
    (MSDS), 289
Matriderm®, 177
Mean arterial pressure (MAP),
    303
Mechanical ventilation, 155, 156
Medical therapy, 156, 158
Metformin, 57
Methicillin-resistant
    Staphylococcus aureus,
    218
Meticulous hemostasis, 188
Microbiology, 218, 219
Military resources, 397
Mobile phone app, 374
Model Systems Knowledge
    Translation Center
    (MSKTC), 353
Modern burn management, 214
Modified barium swallow (MBS),
    310
Mucolytic agents, 158
Multimodal analgesia, 350, 470
Multiple modalities, 148
Mupirocin, 222
Muriatic acid, 293
Muscle relaxants, 321
Music alternate engagement
    (MAE), 327
Music-based imagery (MBI), 327
Mycoplasma Pneumonia, 406

N
N-acetylcysteine (NAC), 158
Nail bed burns, 198
Narcotics, 149
Nasal intubation, 186
Nasopharyngoscopy, 149, 151
Nasotracheal intubation, 153
National Disaster Medical
    System (NDMS), 397

National Institute of Disability,
    Independent Living
    and Rehabilitation
    Research (NIDILRR),
    358
National Trauma Data Bank, 340
Natural disasters, 387
Negative pressure wound
    therapy (NPWT), 276,
    277
Neuraxial blocks, 325
Nexobrid, 131
Nitric acid, 294
Non-accidental injuries, 107–109
Nonsteroidal anti-inflammatory
    drugs (NSAIDs), 319,
    455
Non-surgical scar management
    services, 345
Novel skin grafting techniques,
    146
Nursing services, 343
Nutrition, 309
Nutritional supplementation, 260
Nutritional therapy, 46, 49–52

O
Opioid, 318–322, 324, 326–328
Optimal management, 160
Organic solutions, 288
Organization and Delivery of
    Burn Care Committee
    (ODBC), 397
Orthoses, 440
Outpatient burn care
    electrical and chemical
        injuries, 341
    functions
        burn surgery services, 342
        burn therapy services, 344
        child life and scholastic
            support services, 346
        non-surgical scar
            management services,
            345

Outpatient burn care (*cont.*)
   psychology and social
     services, 344, 345
   vocational rehabilitation
     services, 345
   wound care and nursing
     services, 343
  inhalation injury, 340
  inpatient to outpatient
    transitions, 341
  interdisciplinary
    management, 336–338
  outcome measures, quality
    improvement for, 358
  pathways, 355, 356
  patient selection, 338
  principles
    dressing plan, 349
    long-term follow-up, 354
    pain, anxiety and acute
     stress symptoms, 349,
     350
    patient and wound
     assessment, 348
    patient education and
     support system, 353
    range of motion, 351
    return conditions and
     schedule, 353
    signs, symptoms and
     impairments, 347, 348
    stretching and exercise
     plans, 352
    wound cleansing, 349
  psychosocial comorbidities
    and social support, 340
  quality improvement, 356
  training programs, 357
Oxalic acid, 295
Oxandrolone, 58
Oxidation, 287

P
Pain control, 260
Pain management
  acetaminophen, 319
  alpha-2 receptor agonists, 320
  anesthetics, 323
  anxiolytics, 323
  gabapentinoids, 319
  initial treatment approach,
    328–329
  ketamine, 322
  lidocaine, 322
  muscle relaxants, 321
  neuraxial anesthesia, 325
  non-pharmacological therapy,
    327
  NSAIDs, 319
  opioids, 321
  peripheral nerve blocks, 325
  pharmacological therapy, 326
  regional anesthesia, 323
  serotonin-norepinephrine
    reuptake inhibitors,
    320–321
  tricyclic antidepressants, 320
Palliative care, burn patients, 311
Palm blisters, 202
Paravertebral blocks, 325
Partial-thickness burns, 168
Patient and Observer Scar
    Assessment Scale
    (POSAS), 421
Patient Health Questionnaire-2
    (PHQ-2), 348
Patient-Reported Outcomes
    Measurement
    Information System®
    (PROMIS) Global-10,
    348
Pediatric, 467
Peripheral nerve blocks, 325
Pharmacodynamics, 468
Pharmacologic considerations,
    469
Phosphoric acid, 295
Phosphorus, 295
Plane blocks, 326
Plasma-Lyte A, 119
Platelet-rich plasma (PRP), 426

Point of care ultrasonography (POCUS), 456
Positioning, 437
Postburn management, 182
Post-extubation stridor, 157
Pre-existing conditions (PECs), 258
Pregabalin, 319
Pressure garments, 207
Pressure therapy, 190
Prolonged mechanical ventilation, 159
Propranolol, 53–54
Protein, 50
Protein metabolism, 37–39
Protoplasmic poisons, 288
Pruritus, 344, 347, 350, 351
Psychology and social services, 344, 345
PTSD Checklist 5-Civilian (PCL-C), 348
Pulmonary artery (PA) catheter, 123
Pulmonary compliance/ bronchospasm, 147
Pulmonary system, 304
    airspace injury, 305
    inhalation injury, 304, 305
    toxins, 306
    ventilation, 305
Pulmonary vasodilators, 160
Pulse oximetry, 185
Purposeful hostilities, 388

Q
Quadratus lumborum (QL) blocks, 326
Quality improvement (QI) programs, 356
Quantitative cultures, 215

R
Reduction, 287
Regional anesthesia, 323, 324

Rehabilitation, 133
Relaxation exercises, 345
Relaxation therapy, 327
Renal replacement therapy, 311
Renal tubular acidosis, 122
Respiratory management, 156
Rhabdomyolysis, 274, 275

S
Scalp alopecia, 191
Scar assessment, 420
Scar contractures, 193
Scar management, 442, 445
Sebaceous glands, 183
Sedation adjuncts, 149
Seizures, 155
Sepsis, 301, 305, 307, 308, 310
Sepsis-induced acute kidney injury (AKI), 129
Serotonin-norepinephrine reuptake inhibitors, 320–321
Silicone gel, 190
Silver-based therapies, 220
Silver sulfadiazine, 204
Skin anatomy, 198
Skin grafts, 175, 188, 208
Skin substitutes, 176
Smoke inhalation, 145, 185
Spinal and epidural techniques, 325
Splinting, 352
Split thickness skin graft (STSG), 191
Steroids, 156
Stevens-Johnson syndrome (SJS), 405
    clinical presentation, 408, 409
    epidemiology, 406
    management, 409, 410
    morphology, 407
Strategic National Stockpile (SNS), 396
Stratum basale, 168
Stratum corneum, 168

Stratum granulosum, 168
Stratum lucidum, 168
Stratum spinosum, 168
Sulfuric acid, 293
Superficial burns, 192
Superficial partial-thickness
    burns, 186
Surgical burn scar contracture
    release, 207
Sympathetic nervous system
    (SNS), 122
Systemic antibiotics, 222, 223

T
Tar, 297
Targeting organ systems, 39–46
Telemedicine, 336–338, 342, 345,
    346, 354, 359
    adoption and usage of, 376
    advantages, 366
    associated technologies, 366
    definition, 365
    long-term scar management,
        377
    medical community, 366
    quality improvement effort,
        373
    rapid and widespread
        adoption, 377
    reduction of unnecessary
        transfers, 373
    reimbursement, 376
    widespread adoption, 367
Testosterone, 59
Therapeutic nebulized agents,
    156
Thermal injury, 146, 304
Tissue hypoxia, 155
Toddler-aged children, 9
Topical antibiotic ointments, 187
Topical antimicrobials, 220
Total body surface area (TBSA),
    213, 367, 368, 374, 451

Tourniquets, 204
Toxic Epidermal Necrolysis
    (TEN), 405, 406, 408,
    410
Toxins, 306
Tracheal rupture, 160
Tracheal stenosis, 160
Tracheoesophageal fistula, 160
Tracheostomy, 154
Transesophageal
    echocardiography
    (TEE), 456
Transverse abdominus plane
    (TAP) blocks, 326
Tricyclic antidepressants (TCA),
    317, 320
True electrical injury, 268
Tumor necrosis factor (TNF), 33

U
Ultraviolet radiation, 183
Upper extremity blocks, 326
Upper lip eversion, 192
U.S. Department of Health and
    Human Services
    (HHS), 392

V
Vancouver Scar Scale (VSS), 421
Vascular access, 451
Ventilation, 305–306
Ventilator-associated pneumonia
    (VAP), 308
Vesicant chemical warfare
    agents, 298
Vesication, 287
Virtual reality (VR), 327–329
Visual analog scale
    (VAS), 316
Vocational rehabilitation
    services, 345
Volume status, 451, 452

W
World Health Organization
(WHO), 169
Wound care, 172, 174, 276, 343
Wound healing, 183

Wrist and ankle injuries, 269

X
Xeroform™, 203